# Pathology, Diagnosis and Treatment of Kidney Diseases

# Pathology, Diagnosis and Treatment of Kidney Diseases

Editor: Kevin Lewis

AMERICAN
MEDICAL PUBLISHERS
www.americanmedicalpublishers.com

AMERICAN
MEDICAL PUBLISHERS
www.americanmedicalpublishers.com

**Cataloging-in-Publication Data**

Pathology, diagnosis and treatment of kidney diseases / edited by Kevin Lewis.
p. cm.
Includes bibliographical references and index.
ISBN 978-1-63927-711-7
1. Kidneys--Disease. 2. Kidneys--Disease--Diagnosis. 3. Kidneys--Diseases--Treatment.
4. Kidneys--Diseases--Etiology. 5. Nephrology. I. Lewis, Kevin.
RC902 .P38 2023
616.61--dc23



American Medical Publishers,
41 Flatbush Avenue,
1st Floor, New York,
NY 11217, USA

ISBN 978-1-63927-711-7 (Hardback)

# Contents

# Preface

The main aim of this book is to educate learners and enhance their research focus by presenting diverse topics covering this vast field. This is an advanced book which compiles significant studies by distinguished experts in the area of analysis. This book addresses successive solutions to the challenges arising in the area of application, along with it; the book provides scope for future developments.

Kidney disease is a condition or disease that affects or damages the kidneys and their functions. Kidneys play an essential role in the normal functioning of the body. The functions of kidneys involve expelling waste products and impurities from the blood. There are several types of kidney diseases, such as chronic kidney disease, kidney stones, glomerulonephritis, polycystic kidney disease and urinary tract infections. Chronic kidney disease is the most common form of nephropathy caused by increased blood pressure and diabetes. Various tests like glomerular filtration rate (GFR), ultrasound or computed tomography (CT) scan, kidney biopsy and blood creatinine test are used to examine the stage of kidney disease. Treatment varies, depending on the stage of the disease. Preventive measures such as sufficient water intake, less salt and sugar consumption, and reduced smoking can be adopted to help reduce the risk of developing a kidney disease. The topics included in this book on kidney diseases are of utmost significance and bound to provide incredible insights to readers. It outlines the pathology, diagnosis and treatment of these diseases. Those with an interest in the study and treatment of kidney diseases will find this book helpful.

It was a great honour to edit this book, though there were challenges, as it involved a lot of communication and networking between me and the editorial team. However, the end result was this all-inclusive book covering diverse themes in the field.

Finally, it is important to acknowledge the efforts of the contributors for their excellent chapters, through which a wide variety of issues have been addressed. I would also like to thank my colleagues for their valuable feedback during the making of this book.

**Editor**

1

# Acute Kidney Injury and In-Hospital Mortality: A Retrospective Analysis of a Nationwide Administrative Database of Elderly Subjects in Italy

**Fabio Fabbian [1,2,*], Caterina Savriè [1], Alfredo De Giorgi [2], Rosaria Cappadona [1,2], Emanuele Di Simone [2], Benedetta Boari [2], Alda Storari [2], Massimo Gallerani [2] and Roberto Manfredini [1,2]**

1 Faculty of Medicine, Surgery and Prevention, University of Ferrara, via Ludovico Ariosto 35, 44121 Ferrara, Italy
2 Azienda Ospedaliero-Universitaria 'S. Anna', Via Aldo Moro 8, 44123 Cona, Ferrara, Italy
* Correspondence: f.fabbian@ospfe.it

**Abstract:** Background: The aim of this study was to investigate the association between acute kidney injury (AKI) and in-hospital mortality (IHM) in a large nationwide cohort of elderly subjects in Italy. Methods: We analyzed the hospitalization data of all patients aged ≥65 years, who were discharged with a diagnosis of AKI, which was identified by the presence of the International Classification of Diseases, 9th Revision, Clinical Modification (ICD-9-CM), and extracted from the Italian Health Ministry database (January 2000 to December 2015). Data regarding age, gender, dialysis treatment, and comorbidity, including the development of sepsis, were also collected. Results: We evaluated 760,664 hospitalizations, the mean age was 80.5 ± 7.8 years, males represented 52.2% of the population, and 9% underwent dialysis treatment. IHM was 27.7% (210,661 admissions): Deceased patients were more likely to be older, undergoing dialysis treatment, and to be sicker than the survivors. The population was classified on the basis of tertiles of comorbidity score (the first group 7.48 ± 1.99, the second 13.67 ± 2,04, and third 22.12 ± 4.13). IHM was higher in the third tertile, whilst dialysis-dependent AKI was highest in the first. Dialysis-dependent AKI was associated with an odds ratios (OR) of 2.721; 95% confidence interval (CI) 2.676–2.766; $p < 0.001$, development of sepsis was associated with an OR of 1.990; 95% CI 1.948–2.033; $p < 0.001$, the second tertile of comorbidity was associated with an OR of 1.750; 95% CI 1.726–1.774; $p < 0.001$, and the third tertile of comorbidity was associated with an OR of 2.522; 95% CI 2.486–2.559; $p < 0.001$. Conclusions: In elderly subjects with AKI discharge codes, IHM is a frequent complication affecting more than a quarter of the investigated population. The increasing burden of comorbidity, dialysis-dependent AKI, and sepsis are the major risk factors.

**Keywords:** acute kidney injury; in-hospital mortality; comorbidity; International Classification of Diseases; 9th Revision; Clinical Modification (ICD-9-CM)

---

## 1. Introduction

Comorbidity is a risk factor for in-hospital mortality (IHM) and appears to be high in admitted elderly patients [1]. In elderly subjects, admissions due to acute medical complications, determinants of health status decline, and prediction of negative outcomes could be based on comorbidities [2]. Mortality has been associated with the development of acute kidney injury (AKI) [3]. In western society, multi-morbidity is frequently and increasingly reported, causing increased complexity in elderly subjects with different burdens of organ dysfunction [4–6]. The presence of comorbidities could increase the risk of AKI, and in previous studies, our group, utilizing administrative databases, evaluated the relationship between renal dysfunction, comorbidities, and IHM in individuals hospitalized with myocardial infarction, pulmonary embolism, stroke, and severe chronic obstructive pulmonary disease [7–10]. Even a small increase in serum creatinine during admission has been significantly associated with mortality, hospital length-of-stay (LOS), and costs, after adjustment for age, gender, severity of illness, and chronic kidney disease in a sample of 19,982 adults [11]. It has been recently reported that in a large USA database, AKI increased hospitalization costs and LOS, especially if dialysis was required [12]. More than 50% of elderly adults have three or more chronic diseases and poor general conditions are associated with many adverse consequences. A comorbidity index is able to summarize all the coexistent illnesses in a single numeric score, allowing comparisons between different groups—the index suggests the severity of the patient's conditions [13]. In clinical practice, the Elixhauser Index is a well-known score able to summarize comorbidity into an index providing a single parameter [14]; however, because it was conceived in 1998, our group decided to modify and adapt it for our hospitalized patients [1]. Management of a specific disease in the presence of comorbidity is complex [15], and recognition of the high risk related to AKI in an aging population may help to avoid further morbidity and mortality. Elderly subjects are often treated similarly to the general population regardless of the comorbidity; this practice is unrealistic due to the fact that survival in sexagenarians is significantly different to survival in nonagenarians [16,17]. The risk factors for AKI in older adults are multiple comorbidities and polypharmacy [18,19], and AKI is a common complication in hospitalized older individuals [20]. The aim of this retrospective study was to evaluate the relationship between AKI, comorbidities, dialysis treatment, and IHM in a large sample of Italian elderly subjects.

## 2. Experimental Section

### *2.1. Patient Selection and Eligibility*

The total number of hospitalizations due to AKI between 1 January 2000, and 31 December 2015, recorded in the Italian National Hospital database, provided by the Ministry of Health (SDO Database, Ministry of Health, General Directorate for Health Planning) were considered in this analysis. All hospitalizations of patients in public and private Italian hospitals are recorded in the National database of Hospital Discharge Records (HDR). Gender, age, date of hospital admission and discharge, department of admission and discharge, vital status at discharge (in-hospital death vs. discharged alive), main diagnosis, up to five co-morbidities, and up to six procedures/interventions, based on the International Classification of Diseases, 9th Revision, Clinical Modification (ICD-9-CM), are recorded in the HDR file. Because of the national disposition-by-law in terms of privacy, patients' names and all other potential identifiers were removed by the Ministry of Health from the database for this analysis. The only identifier, allowing us to search the database for possible recurrence of hospital admissions of the same patient, was a consecutive number for each patient. Administrative database codes usually make reference to acute renal failure, but in clinical settings, the term AKI has largely replaced that term. AKI was identified using as first or second discharge diagnosis ICD-9-CM code 584.xx. Finally, diagnosis of sepsis and diabetes were taken into consideration, and LOS was calculated.

### *2.2. Data Analysis*

The outcome of this analysis was IHM being a hard clinical outcome indicator; therefore, fatal cases (death during hospitalization) were compared with non-fatal ones (patient discharged alive). The comorbidity score was evaluated using ICD-9-CM, and a novel score recently proposed by our group was calculated for considering the comorbidity burden [1]. The conditions of age, gender, presence of chronic kidney disease, neurological disorders, lymphoma, solid tumor with metastasis, ischemic heart disease, congestive heart disease, coagulopathy, fluid and electrolyte disorders, liver disease, weight loss, and metastatic cancer were taken into account for score calculation. The original score was corrected, removing the diagnosis of previous AKI, therefore points assigned to renal diseases were considered only if chronic kidney disease was recorded during admission. The points for each condition ranged from 0 to 16, and the total score calculated could vary between 0 and 89. When the score was >40, the risk of IHM was >60%. The score, developed using administrative data, was calculated automatically. The points assigned to different conditions in order to calculate the risk score of IHM are reported in Table 1 [1]. Finally, data of IHM related to these patients were extracted from the general database.

**Table 1.** Points assigned to different conditions in order to calculate the score for risk of in-hospital mortality (IHM).

| Items | Score |
|---|---|
| Age 0–60 (years) | 0 |
| Age 61–70 (years) | 3 |
| Age 71–80 (years) | 7 |
| Age 81–90 (years) | 11 |
| Age 91+ (years) | 16 |
| Chronic kidney disease | 1 |
| Male gender | 2 |
| Neurological disorders | 3 |
| Lymphoma | 4 |
| Solid tumor without metastasis | 4 |
| Ischemic heart disease | 5 |
| Congestive heart failure | 5 |
| Coagulopathy | 8 |
| Fluid and electrolyte disorders | 8 |
| Liver disease | 10 |
| Cachexia | 11 |
| Metastatic cancer | 12 |

### 2.3. Statistical Analysis

Absolute numbers, percentages, and means ± SD were used to present data. A descriptive analysis of the whole population was performed, followed by a comparison of survivors and deceased during admission. The population was divided in tertiles based on the comorbidity score, and the three groups were compared according to all the parameters investigated. The analysis of the variables was done by using the Chi-Squared test, Student *t*-tests, Mann–Whitney *U* test, and ANOVA as appropriate. Moreover, in order to assess the independent parameters associated with IHM, the latter was considered as a dependent variable in a logistic regression analysis and demography; tertiles of the comorbidity score, dialysis treatment, and sepsis were considered as independent ones. Odds ratios (ORs) and their 95% confidence intervals (95% CI) were reported. All $p$-values were 2-tailed, and $p$-value $< 0.5$ was considered significant. SPSS 13.0 for Windows (SPSS IN., Chicago, IL, USA, 2004) was used for statistical analysis.

### 2.4. Ethical Issues

This retrospective study was conducted in agreement with the declaration of Helsinki of 1975, revised in 2013. Subject identifiers were deleted before the analysis of the database in order to maintain data anonymity and confidentiality. None of the patients could be identified, either in this paper or in the database. The study was conducted in agreement with the existent Italian disposition-by-law (G.U. n.76, 31/03/2008), and due to the study design ethics committee approval was not necessary.

## 3. Results

We analyzed 760,664 records, of which 52.2% were males. The mean age of the population was 80.5 ± 7.8 years, and mean LOS was 13.72 ± 15.49 days. The mean comorbidity score was 14.57 ± 6.21. The distribution of the score in the population is shown in Figure 1.

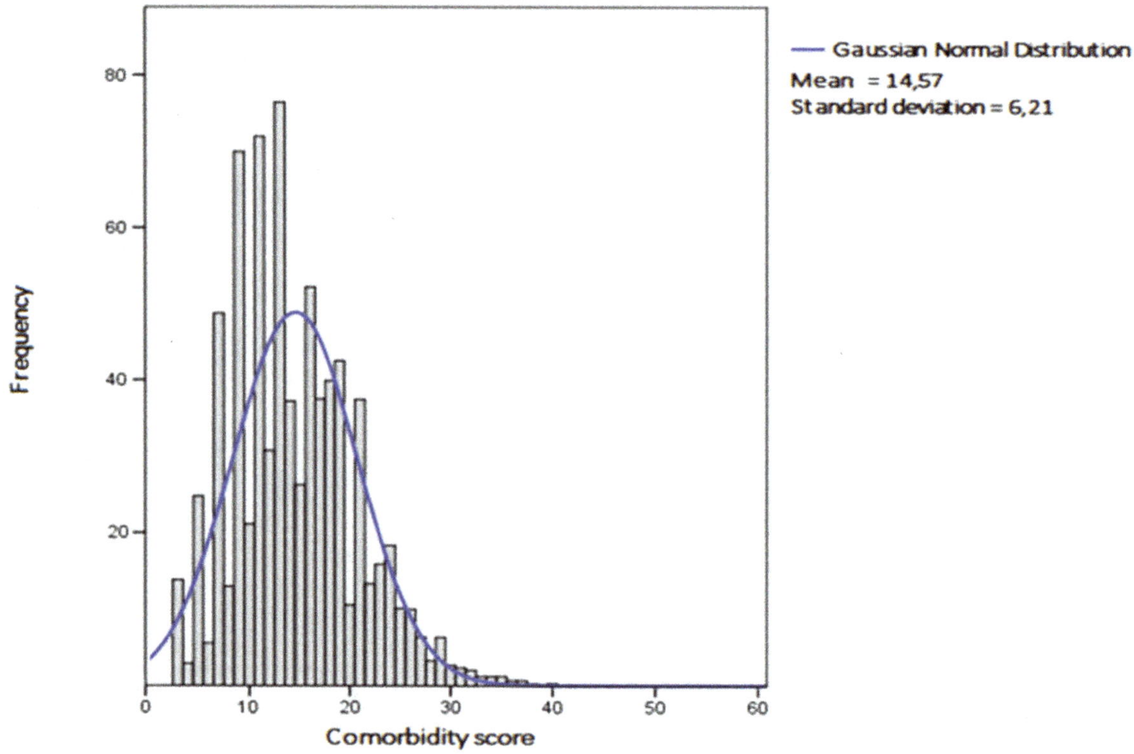


**Figure 1.** Distribution of the comorbidity score values in the population investigated.

The main characteristics of the investigated population are reported in Table 2.

**Table 2.** Characteristics of the considered population with acute kidney injury.

| Total Number of Records | 760,664 |
|---|---|
| Men, (n (%)) | 397,174 (52.2) |
| Women, (n (%)) | 363,490 (47.8) |
| Age (years) | 80.5 ± 7.8 |
| Comorbidity score | 14.57 ± 6.21 |
| Dialysis-dependent acute kidney injury (AKI), (n (%)) | 68,653 (9) |
| Diabetes, (n (%)) | 115,238 (15.6) |
| Sepsis, (n (%)) | 39,144 (5.1) |
| Length-of-stay (LOS) (days) | 13.72 ± 15.49 |
| Deceased subjects, (n (%)) | 210,661 (27.7) |

Heart failure was diagnosed in 146,359 (19.2%), fluid and electrolyte disorders in 126,702 (16.7%), chronic kidney disease in 115,238 (15.1%), cancer in 71,624 (9.4%,), ischemic heart diseases in 34,943 (4.6%), liver diseases in 34,015 (4.5%), metastatic cancer in 30,425 (4%), neurological disorders in 17,912

(2.4%), lymphoma in 16,443 (2.2%), cachexia in 15,363 (2%), and coagulopathy in 8266 (1.1%). Diabetics were 15.6% (n = 118,299) and patients with diagnosis of sepsis 5.1% (n = 39,144). Nine percent of the population underwent dialysis treatment, and overall IHM was 27.7% (210,661 hospitalizations). The frequency of survivors and deceased patients during the study period is reported in Figure 2.

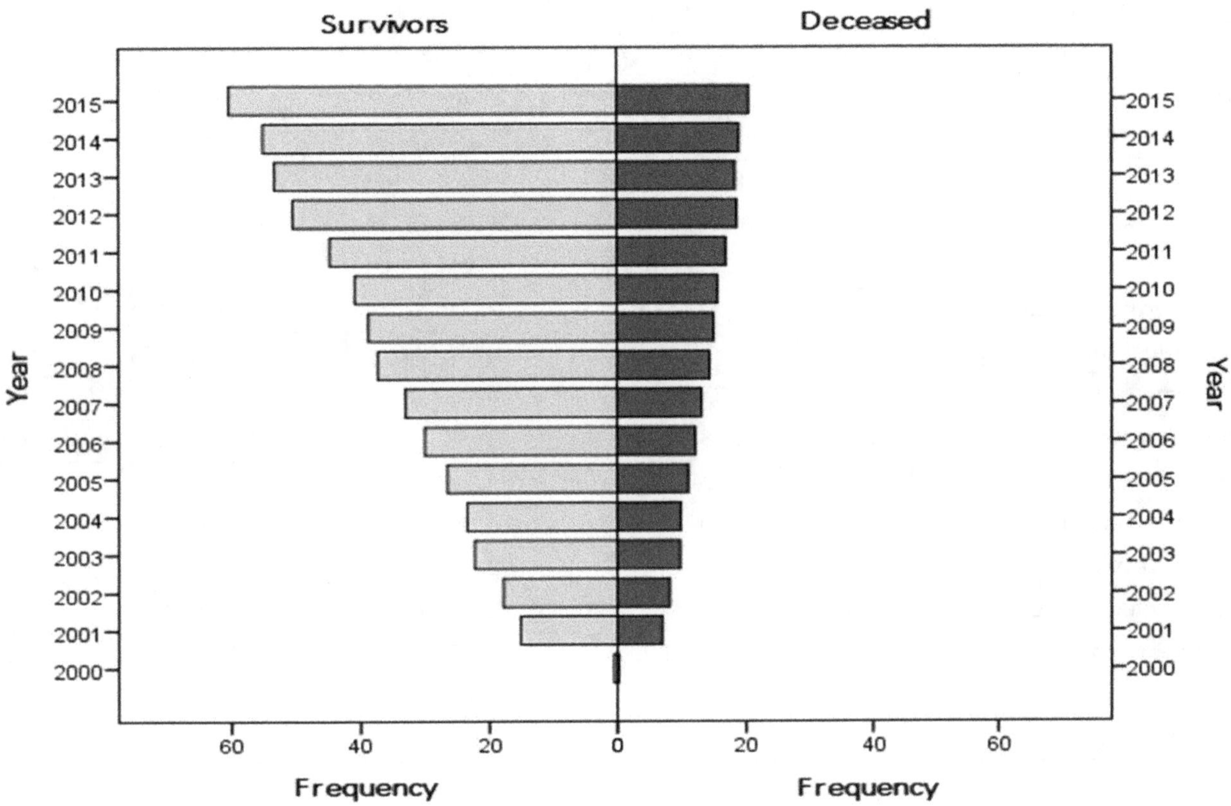


**Figure 2.** Prevalence of survivors and in-hospital mortality during the study period.

Deceased patients were older and the prevalence of women was higher. Moreover, deceased subjects had higher rates of sepsis diagnosis, were more likely to be on dialysis treatment, and were sicker than survivors; however, diabetes was more frequent in survivors (Table 3).

**Table 3.** Comparison of survivors and deceased individuals with acute kidney injury.

| Parameters | Survivors | Deceased | *p* |
|---|---|---|---|
| | n = 550,003 | n = 210,661 | |
| Men, (n (%)) | 288,120 (52.4) | 109,054 (51.8) | <0.001 |
| Women, (n (%)) | 261,883 (47.6) | 101,607 (48.2) | |
| Age (years) | 80 ± 7.72 | 81.9 ± 7.9 | <0.001 |
| Comorbidity score | 14.04 ± 6.02 | 15.96 ± 6.48 | <0.001 |
| Dialysis-dependent AKI, (n (%)) | 37,598 (6.8) | 31,055 (14.7) | <0.001 |
| Diabetes, (n (%)) | 95,433 (17.4) | 22,866 (10.9) | <0.001 |
| Sepsis, (n (%)) | 23,230 (4.2) | 15,914 (7.6) | <0.001 |

The comorbidity score of the population was classified on the basis of tertiles: in the first tertile, the score was lower than 11; in the second, it was between 11 and 17; and in the third, it was higher than 17. Comparison between the three groups is reported in Table 4.

**Table 4.** Comparison of subjects divided into tertiles.

| **Parameters** | **First Tertile (Score < 11)** | **Second Tertile (11 ≤ Score ≤ 17)** | **Third Tertile (Score > 17)** | *p* |
|---|---|---|---|---|
| Number of subjects | 200,131 (26.3%) | 332,533 (43.7%) | 228,000 (30%) | |
| Length-of-stay (days) | 15.6 ± 19 | 13.59 ± 14.5 | 12.28 ± 13.1 | <0.001 |
| Comorbidity score | 7.48 ± 1.99 | 13.67 ± 2,04 | 22.12 ± 4.13 | <0.001 |
| Males, (n (%)) | 119,798 (59.9%) | 144,464 (43.4%) | 132,912 (58.3%) | <0.001 |
| Females, (n (%)) | 80,333 (40.1%) | 188,069 (56.6%) | 95,088 (41.7%) | |
| Deceased, (n (%)) | 38,740 (19.4%) | 92,987 (28%) | 78,934 (34.6%) | <0.001 |
| Dialysis-dependent AKI, (n (%)) | 26,901 (13.4%) | 29,054 (8.7%) | 12,698 (5.6%) | <0.001 |
| Sepsis, (n (%)) | 12,652 (6.3%) | 17,944 (5.4%) | 8,548 (3.7%) | <0.001 |
| Chronic kidney disease (n (%)) | 32,217 (16.1%) | 49,308 (14.8%) | 33,713 (14.8%) | <0.001 |
| Neurological disorders (n (%)) | 2609 (1.3%) | 8661 (2.6%) | 6642 (2.9%) | <0.001 |
| Lymphoma (n (%)) | 2856 (1.4%) | 9145 (2.8%) | 4442 (1.9%) | <0.001 |
| Solid tumor without metastasis (n (%)) | 5888 (2.9%) | 29,907 (9%) | 35,829 (15.7%) | <0.001 |
| Ischemic heart disease (n (%)) | 2042 (1%) | 14,001 (4.2%) | 18,900 (8.3%) | <0.001 |
| Congestive heart failure (n (%)) | 7109 (3.6%) | 67,211 (20.2%) | 72,039 (31.6%) | <0.001 |
| Coagulopathy (n (%)) | 0 | 2780 (0.8%) | 5486 (2.4%) | <0.001 |
| Fluid and electrolyte disorders (n (%)) | 0 | 33,322 (10%) | 93,380 (41%) | <0.001 |
| Liver disease (n (%)) | 0 | 8578 (2.6%) | 25,437 (11.2%) | <0.001 |
| Cachexia (n (%)) | 0 | 441 (0.1%) | 14,922 (6.5%) | <0.001 |
| Metastatic cancer (n (%)) | 0 | 2009 (0.6%) | 28,416 (12.5%) | <0.001 |

IHM was independently associated with dialysis-dependent AKI (OR 2.721; 95% CI 2.676–2.766; $p < 0.001$), development of sepsis (OR 1.990; 95% CI 1.948–2.033; $p < 0.001$), the second tertile of comorbidity (OR 1.750; 95% CI 1.726–1.774; $p < 0.001$), and the third tertile of comorbidity (OR 2.522; 95% CI 2.486–2.559; $p < 0.001$) (Figure 3, the first tertile was used as the reference).

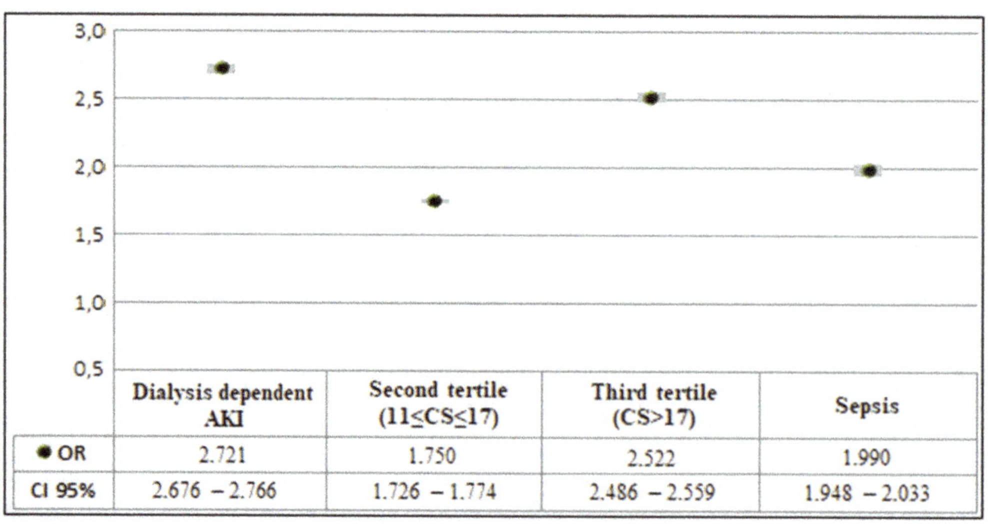


**Figure 3.** Multivariate analysis results relating the association between in-hospital mortality, comorbidity, and dialysis treatment in individuals with acute kidney injury. CS: Comorbidity Score (in all cases $p < 0.001$; Hosmer and Lemeshow test $p < 0.001$).

## 4. Discussion

To the best of our knowledge, this is the first national Italian study testing the impact of comorbidity on IHM in elderly subjects admitted with AKI. The score tested had an approximately normal distribution, and the population showed a gradual increase in the number of admissions and IHM during the study period. The mean score in the whole population was 14.57, and the mean score in deceased subjects was 15.96. However, when the tertiles were analyzed, in the highest tertile, we detected a mean score value of 22.12, and more than one-third of subjects belonging to this group died during hospitalization. Univariate analysis showed that the group of patients in the third tertile had a higher comorbidity burden due to a higher prevalence of cancer and cardiovascular morbidity, the two major causes of death in western societies. Such a burden of comorbidity was not related to sepsis or to dialysis-dependent AKI. Our data suggest that physicians did not think that dialyzing AKI patients with a high comorbidity burden could be beneficial. Probably, as a result of this finding, LOS in patients with a high comorbidity score was lower. Previously, we reported that the score used in this study and sepsis diagnosis were able to predict IHM in patients hospitalized for infectious diseases [21]. In this study, sepsis had a lower prevalence in the third tertile of the comorbidity burden; however, as well as increasing comorbidity, it was independently associated with IHM. In this study, a diagnosis of sepsis was made more frequently in the group of patients with a lower comorbidity burden, and in the same group, dialysis-dependent AKI had a higher prevalence, suggesting that there was a relationship between the two findings, i.e., subjects with sepsis developed dialysis-dependent AKI. Diabetes, a well-known risk factor for mortality, was recorded in 15.6% of cases, and appeared to be more frequent in survivors. However, this finding could be ascribed to a bias associated with our study design. Conditions pre-existing at the time of admission, such as diabetes, are poorly coded if the hospitalization procedure is complicated and if the patient dies [22]. In studies analyzing administrative databases, diabetes usually appears to be protective. The comparison of survivors and deceased patients could not show the real difference in the comorbidity burden, but the analysis of tertiles of the comorbidity burden and logistic regression analysis suggested that the three factors related to IHM were increasing comorbidity score due to cardiovascular and liver disease, cachexia and cancer, diagnosis of sepsis, and advanced renal damage requiring dialysis treatment. Increasing the tertiles of comorbidity score had an impact on mortality similar to dialysis-dependent AKI and sepsis.

We run the Hosmer–Lemeshow test in order to evaluate the goodness of fit of our logistic regression, and we could detect that our data were not fitting well into the model. The Hosmer–Lemeshow test calculates if the observed event rates match the expected event rates in population subgroups. By this analysis, data are grouped by ordering the predicted probabilities and forming the number of groups. The small *p*-value indicates mean that the fit of the model is poor, however, large *p*-values don't necessarily mean that the model is a good fit. Changing the number of subgroups by very small amounts may result in wild changes in *p*-values. Therefore, we do not think that Hosmer–Lemeshow calculated by our data could be of any significance, due to the fact that, we analyzed a very large population at a national level.

The real-world epidemiology of AKI in western societies is still a matter of debate. The different figures reported in the medical literature are due to the different clinical settings in which studies have been carried out. Several comorbidities have been reported in the list of risk factors for AKI, including diabetes mellitus, cardiovascular disease, chronic liver disease, cancer, and complex surgery [23]; moreover, in individuals with AKI, mortality appears to be related to the stage of the syndrome [24,25]. AKI is a complex condition related to different etiologies and pathophysiological mechanisms; it is commonly diagnosed in hospitalized patients, and leads to increased morbidity, mortality, and health care costs [26]. Different biomarkers have been investigated in order to predict AKI outcomes [27,28], however, we think that consideration of the clinical history of patients developing AKI could improve risk stratification.

Similar to our study, Hsu et al. [29] evaluated dialysis-requiring AKI cases using ICD-9-CM codes. Over a decade (2000–2009), incidence of dialysis-requiring AKI increased, and the risk factors for its development were older age, male sex, black race, and sepsis, as well as acute heart failure, and invasive procedures; mortality was associated with dialysis-requiring AKI and showed an increased frequency [29].

We detected an increasing number of hospitalizations with AKI during the study period. Similar findings were reported by a study analyzing administrative databases between 1988 and 2002. During this period, the incidence of AKI increased from 61 to 288 per 100,000; the incidence of AKI requiring dialysis rose from 4 to 27 per 100,000. On the contrary, IHM decreased from 40.4% to 20.3% in patients with AKI and from 41.3% to 28.1% in those with AKI that required dialysis [30]. The increasing number of admissions and deaths during the study period would be ascribed to two different factors, the first one could be related to a better way of coding by physicians, the second one, could be related to the aging of the population and the change in the organization of Italian health system.

Similar to our study, Liangos et al. [31] defined the epidemiology of AKI using the United States national administrative ICD-9-CM database. AKI was frequent in older, male, black individuals and was associated with chronic kidney disease, congestive heart failure, chronic lung disease, sepsis, and cardiac surgery. In our study, diagnosis of chronic kidney disease was higher in the lowest tertile of the comorbidity score, the same group with a higher prevalence of dialysis-dependent AKI. We cannot exclude the possibility that this group included elderly patients with a low comorbidity burden with decreasing renal function who needed dialysis treatment. Moreover, AKI can be a post-surgical complication, but even in these cases, comorbidity appears to be crucial in determining patients' prognosis, as shown by Thakar et al. [32] in their study on open-heart surgery. Female gender, congestive heart failure with low ejection fraction, preoperative use of an intra-aortic balloon pump, chronic obstructive pulmonary disease, diabetes, previous surgery, and serum creatinine were associated with mortality and AKI. As in our study, the authors classified subjects in different risk categories of increasing severity [32].

Several studies stratified populations with AKI using different scores, but these indexes were mainly developed in intensive care settings. On the contrary, we tried to stratify our population using a simple score based on administrative data and derived from internal medicine admitted patients. The use of the APACHE II score, especially when modified by the presence or absence of oliguria, should help in predicting the outcome when evaluating interventions for patients with AKI [33]. In 2000, Fiaccadori et al. [34] tested the predictive ability of three general prognostic models: version II of the Acute Physiology and Chronic Health Evaluation (APACHE II), version II of the Simplified Acute Physiology Score, and version II of the Mortality Probability Model at 24 h in a prospective, single-center cohort of patients with AKI in a nephrology setting. They concluded that the APACHE II score was slightly better in predicting mortality. Again, the score used in this study was simple, taking into consideration a small amount of demographic data; in fact, the score included only age and gender; we did not consider race. In Italy, the great majority of hospitalized patients were Caucasian. In 2006, Xue et al. [35] determined the incidence and mortality of AKI in Medicare beneficiaries. They found that older age, male sex, and black race were associated with development of AKI. IHM was 15.2% if AKI was the principal diagnosis at the time of discharge, and 32.6% in discharges with AKI as a secondary diagnosis [35].

Even small acute changes in serum creatinine levels in hospitalized patients increased short-term mortality [36]. In our study, we included elderly patients with AKI without considering different hospital settings. AKI is encountered in 5%–10% of hospitalized patients and up to 60% in individuals admitted to the intensive care unit [37]. In 1996, the epidemiology of AKI was evaluated in 13 tertiary-care Spanish hospitals, covering a population of 4.2 million persons. During a nine-month period, the incidence of AKI was 209 cases per million. Mortality was calculated to be 45%; however, negative outcome in many cases was attributed to underlying diseases, reducing the mortality caused by AKI to 26.7%. Dialysis-dependent AKI was recorded in 36% of individuals [37]. Our mortality was similar, but the percentage of dialysis-dependent AKI was much lower, suggesting that a different selection of the population was investigated. Our data are in agreement with results reported by

Chertow et al. [38] who showed that dialysis-dependent AKI and sepsis were independently associated with IHM.

*Limitations*

We are aware of several limitations of our study: (i) The design was retrospective, based on administrative data, and we could not assess complications due to AKI such as fluid overload, electrolyte abnormalities, and coagulopathy. It has been reported that complications related to AKI such as fluid overload could be associated with a risk of death [39]. However, our results suggest that conditions diagnosed well before the detection of AKI could be associated with IHM; (ii) we did not provide reasons for admission, specific cause of death, intensive care level, including aggressive therapy and/or device use, neither did we identify AKI on the basis of international Kidney Disease Improving Global Outcomes (KDIGO) guidelines [40]; (iii) we could not evaluate the impact of clinical or biochemical parameters due to the fact that they were not available. There are evident disadvantages in studies based on administrative databases, such as a lack of specific clinical information, the effects of administrative use (i.e., reimbursement), possible misclassification of outcomes, and difficulties in controlling confounding factors [41]. Moreover, as previously stated, race and clinical settings (i.e., surgical and intensive care settings) were not considered; (iv) patients could be wrongly coded, and subjects that are nowadays coded with AKI may have suffered a less severe renal insult than previously. This could be because awareness of AKI has improved; (v) we did not differentiate patients on the basis of the cause of AKI and the treatment setting, we only considered dialysis treatment. On the other hand, only advanced stages of AKI undergo renal replacement therapy. Furthermore, we could not distinguish if AKI happened before or during admission. In 2006, Waikar et al. [42] calculated the performance of ICD-9-CM for acute renal failure and found that the sensitivity was 35.4%, specificity 97.7%, positive predictive value 47.9%, and negative predictive value 96.1% [42]. The validity of AKI codes in administrative databases was analyzed in 2011 in Canada: sensitivity was poor, the median value was 29% (in the range 1%–81%), and median of the positive predictive value was 67% (in the range 15%–96%) [43]. In 2013, Tomlinson et al. [44] calculated a positive predictive value for patients with AKI of 95%. In 2014, Grams et al. [45] validated administrative codes for AKI against the KDIGO AKI definition. They calculated a sensitivity of 17.2% if the comparison was the evaluation of serum creatinine criteria, and 11.7% if the comparison was serum creatinine and urine output-based criteria, whilst specificity was >98% in both cases. Sensitivity was significantly higher when they considered a more recent time period and individuals aged ≥65 years. AKI diagnosed by administrative data was related to more severe disease and higher in-hospital mortality [45]. All these data seem to reinforce our results.

Our study also has some strengths: (i) The high number of records derived from a national administrative database, recording all real diagnoses of AKI; (ii) the long period considered; (iii) the choice of IHM as hard outcome indicator.

## 5. Conclusions

Nowadays, multi-morbidity is receiving greater attention [15], and our findings confirm that comorbidity stratification is crucial to understanding the reasons for IHM of hospitalized elderly patients with AKI. The results of this study emphasize that in elderly subjects, IHM is associated with a degree of renal impairment (especially if the damage needs dialysis treatment), sepsis development, and an increasing burden of comorbidity. Increasing comorbidity score, ascribed to cardiovascular and liver disease, cachexia and cancer, diagnosis of sepsis and advanced renal damage requiring dialysis treatment should be taken into account when evaluating the risk of IHM in hospitalized elderly subjects with AKI.

**Author Contributions:** Conceptualization, F.F., M.G., A.S., and R.M.; methodology, C.S., A.D.G.; software, A.D.G.; validation, C.S., R.C., E.D.S., and B.B.; formal analysis, C.S., A.D.G., E.D.S., R.C., and B.B.; investigation, F.F., E.D.S., R.C., and B.B.; resources, M.G., A.S., and R.M.; data curation, F.F. and M.G.; writing—original draft preparation,

F.F. and C.S.; writing—review and editing, R.M.; supervision, A.S. and M.G.; project administration, M.G.; funding acquisition, R.M.

**Acknowledgments:** We would thank Franco Guerzoni and Nicola Napoli, Center for Health Statistics, Azienda Ospedaliero-Universitaria "S.Anna", Ferrara, Italy, for precious and valuable collaboration.

## References

1. Fabbian, F.; De Giorgi, A.; Maietti, E.; Gallerani, M.; Pala, M.; Cappadona, R.; Manfredini, R.; Fedeli, U. A modified Elixhauser score for predicting in-hospital mortality in internal medicine admissions. *Eur. J. Intern. Med.* **2017**, *40*, 37–42. [CrossRef] [PubMed]
2. Clegg, A.; Young, J.; Iliffe, S.; Rikkert, M.O.; Rockwood, K. Frailty in elderly people. *Lancet* **2013**, *381*, 752–762. [CrossRef]
3. Hounkpatin, H.O.; Fraser, S.D.S.; Glidewell, L.; Blakeman, T.; Lewington, A.; Roderick, P.J. Predicting risk of recurrent acute kidney injury: A systematic review. *Nephron* **2019**, *142*, 83–90. [CrossRef] [PubMed]
4. Xu, X.; Mishra, G.D.; Jones, M. Evidence on multimorbidity from definition to intervention: An overview of systematic reviews. *Ageing Res. Rev.* **2017**, *37*, 53–68. [CrossRef] [PubMed]
5. Klompstra, L.; Ekdahl, A.W.; Krevers, B.; Milberg, A.; Eckerblad, J. Factors related to health-related quality of life in older people with multimorbidity and high health care consumption over a two-year period. *BMC Geriatr.* **2019**, *19*, 187. [CrossRef] [PubMed]
6. Millá-Perseguer, M.; Guadalajara-Olmeda, N.; Vivas-Consuelo, D.; Usó-Talamantes, R. Measurement of health-related quality by multimorbidity groups in primary health care. *Health Qual. Life Outcomes* **2019**, *17*, 8. [CrossRef] [PubMed]
7. Fabbian, F.; Pala, M.; De Giorgi, A.; Manfredini, F.; Mallozzi Menegatti, A.; Salmi, R.; Portaluppi, F.; Gallerani, M.; Manfredini, R. In-hospital mortality in patients with renal dysfunction admitted for myocardial infarction: The Emilia-Romagna region of Italy database of hospital admissions. *Int. Urol. Nephrol.* **2013**, *45*, 769–775. [CrossRef] [PubMed]
8. Fabbian, F.; Gallerani, M.; Pala, M.; De Giorgi, A.; Salmi, R.; Manfredini, F.; Portaluppi, F.; Dentali, F.; Ageno, W.; Mikhailidis, D.P.; et al. In-hospital mortality for pulmonary embolism: Relationship with chronic kidney disease and end-stage renal disease. The hospital admission and discharge database of the Emilia Romagna region of Italy. *Intern. Emerg. Med.* **2013**, *8*, 735–740.
9. Fabbian, F.; Gallerani, M.; Pala, M.; De Giorgi, A.; Salmi, R.; Dentali, F.; Ageno, W.; Manfredini, R. Association between in-hospital mortality and renal dysfunction in 186 219 patients hospitalized for acute stroke in the Emilia-Romagna region of Italy. *Angiology* **2014**, *65*, 906–910. [CrossRef]
10. Fabbian, F.; De Giorgi, A.; Manfredini, F.; Lamberti, N.; Forcellini, S.; Storari, A.; Gallerani, M.; Caramori, G.; Manfredini, R. Impact of renal dysfunction on in-hospital mortality of patients with severe chronic obstructive pulmonary disease: A single-center Italian study. *Int. Urol. Nephrol.* **2016**, *48*, 1121–1127. [CrossRef]
11. Chertow, G.M.; Burdick, E.; Honour, M.; Bonventre, J.V.; Bates, D.W. Acute kidney injury, mortality, length of stay, and costs in hospitalized patients. *J. Am. Soc. Nephrol.* **2005**, *16*, 3365–7330. [CrossRef] [PubMed]
12. Silver, S.A.; Long, J.; Zheng, Y.; Chertow, G.M. Cost of Acute Kidney Injury in Hospitalized Patients. *J. Hosp. Med.* **2017**, *12*, 70–76. [CrossRef] [PubMed]
13. Gijsen, R.; Hoeymans, N.; Schellevis, F.G.; Ruwaard, D.; Satariano, W.A.; van den Bos, G.A. Causes and consequences of comorbidity: A review. *J. Clin. Epidemiol.* **2001**, *54*, 661–674. [CrossRef]
14. Elixhauser, A.; Steiner, C.; Harris, D.R.; Coffey, R.M. Comorbidity measures for use with administrative data. *Med. Care* **1998**, *36*, 8–27. [CrossRef] [PubMed]
15. Barnett, K.; Mercer, S.W.; Norbury, M.; Watt, G.; Wyke, S.; Guthrie, B. Epidemiology of multimorbidity and implications for health care, research, and medical education: A cross-sectional study. *Lancet* **2012**, *380*, 37–43. [CrossRef]
16. Randall, G.K.; Martin, P.; Bishop, A.J.; Poon, L.W.; Johnson, M.A. Age differences and changes in resources essential to aging well: A comparison of sexagenarians, octogenarians, and centenarians. *Curr. Gerontol. Geriatr. Res.* **2011**, *2011*, 357896. [CrossRef] [PubMed]
17. Santoni, G.; Angleman, S.; Welmer, A.K.; Mangialasche, F.; Marengoni, A.; Fratiglioni, L. Age-related variation in health status after age 60. *PLoS ONE* **2015**, *10*, e0120077.
18. Ge, S.; Nie, S.; Liu, Z.; Chen, C.; Zha, Y.; Qian, J.; Liu, B.; Teng, S.; Xu, A.; Bin, W.; et al. Epidemiology and outcomes of acute kidney injury in elderly Chinese patients: A subgroup analysis from the EACH study.

*BMC Nephrol.* **2016**, *17*, 136. [CrossRef]

19. Chao, C.T.; Tsai, H.B.; Wu, C.Y.; Lin, Y.F.; Hsu, N.C.; Chen, J.S.; Hung, K.Y. Cumulative cardiovascular polypharmacy is associated with the risk of acute kidney injury in elderly patients. *Medicine* **2015**, *94*, e1251. [CrossRef]
20. Gong, Y.; Zhang, F.; Ding, F.; Gu, Y. Elderly patients with acute kidney injury (AKI): Clinical features and risk factors for mortality. *Arch. Gerontol. Geriatr.* **2012**, *54*, e47–e51. [CrossRef]
21. Fabbian, F.; De Giorgi, A.; Boari, B.; Misurati, E.; Gallerani, M.; Cappadona, R.; Cultrera, R.; Manfredini, R.; Rodrìguez Borrego, M.A.; Lopez-Soto, P.J. Infections and internal medicine patients: Could a comorbidity score predict in-hospital mortality? *Medicine* **2018**, *97*, e12818. [CrossRef] [PubMed]
22. Grimes, D.A. Epidemiologic research using administrative databases—Garbage in, garbage out. *Obstet. Gynecol.* **2010**, *116*, 1018–1019. [CrossRef] [PubMed]
23. Lameire, N.H.; Bagga, A.; Cruz, D.; De Maeseneer, J.; Endre, Z.; Kellum, J.A.; Liu, K.D.; Mehta, R.L.; Pannu, N.; Van Biesen, W.; et al. Acute kidney injury: An increasing global concern. *Lancet* **2013**, *382*, 170–179. [CrossRef]
24. Moore, P.K.; Hsu, R.K.; Liu, K.D. Management of acute kidney injury: Core curriculum 2018. *Am. J. Kidney Dis.* **2018**, *72*, 136–148. [CrossRef] [PubMed]
25. Joannidis, M.; Metnitz, B.; Bauer, P.; Schusterschitz, N.; Moreno, R.; Druml, W.; Metnitz, P.G. Acute kidney injury in critically ill patients classified by AKIN versus RIFLE using the SAPS 3 database. *Intensive Care Med.* **2009**, *35*, 1692–1702. [CrossRef] [PubMed]
26. Gameiro, J.; Fonseca, J.A.; Jorge, S.; Lopes, J.A. Acute Kidney Injury Definition and Diagnosis: A Narrative Review. *J. Clin. Med.* **2018**, *7*, 307. [CrossRef] [PubMed]
27. Wu, V.-C.; Shiao, C.-C.; Chi, N.-H.; Wang, C.-H.; Chueh, S.-C.J.; Liou, H.-H.; Spapen, H.D.; Honore, P.M.; Chu, T.-S. Outcome Prediction of Acute Kidney Injury Biomarkers at Initiation of Dialysis in Critical Units. *J. Clin. Med.* **2018**, *7*, 202. [CrossRef]
28. Douvris, A.; Zeid, K.; Hiremath, S.; Brown, P.A.; Sood, M.M.; Abou Arkoub, R.; Malhi, G.; Clark, E.G. Safety Lapses Prior to Initiation of Hemodialysis for Acute Kidney Injury in Hospitalized Patients: A Patient Safety Initiative. *J. Clin. Med.* **2018**, *7*, 317. [CrossRef]
29. Hsu, R.K.; McCulloch, C.E.; Dudley, R.A.; Lo, L.J.; Hsu, C.Y. Temporal changes in incidence of dialysis-requiring AKI. *J. Am. Soc. Nephrol.* **2013**, *24*, 37–42. [CrossRef]
30. Waikar, S.S.; Curhan, G.C.; Wald, R.; McCarthy, E.P.; Chertow, G.M. Declining mortality in patients with acute renal failure, 1988 to 2002. *J. Am. Soc. Nephrol.* **2006**, *17*, 1143–1150. [CrossRef]
31. Liangos, O.; Wald, R.; O'Bell, J.W.; Price, L.; Pereira, B.J.; Jaber, B.L. Epidemiology and outcomes of acute renal failure in hospitalized patients: A national survey. *Clin. J. Am. Soc. Nephrol.* **2006**, *1*, 43–51. [CrossRef] [PubMed]
32. Thakar, C.V.; Arrigain, S.; Worley, S.; Yared, J.P.; Paganini, E.P. A clinical score to predict acute renal failure after cardiac surgery. *J. Am. Soc. Nephrol.* **2005**, *16*, 162–168. [CrossRef] [PubMed]
33. Parker, R.A.; Himmelfarb, J.; Tolkoff-Rubin, N.; Chandran, P.; Wingard, R.L.; Hakim, R.M. Prognosis of patients with acute renal failure requiring dialysis: Results of a multicenter study. *Am. J. Kidney Dis.* **1998**, *32*, 432–443. [CrossRef]
34. Fiaccadori, E.; Maggiore, U.; Lombardi, M.; Leonardi, S.; Rotelli, C.; Borghetti, A. Predicting patient outcome from acute renal failure comparing three general severity of illness scoring systems. *Kidney Int.* **2000**, *58*, 283–292. [CrossRef] [PubMed]
35. Xue, J.L.; Daniels, F.; Star, R.A.; Kimmel, P.L.; Eggers, P.W.; Molitoris, B.A.; Himmelfarb, J.; Collins, A.J. Incidence and mortality of acute renal failure in Medicare beneficiaries, 1992 to 2001. *J. Am. Soc. Nephrol.* **2006**, *17*, 1135–1142. [CrossRef]
36. Coca, S.G.; Peixoto, A.J.; Garg, A.X.; Krumholz, H.M.; Parikh, C.R. The prognostic importance of a small acute decrement in kidney function in hospitalized patients: A systematic review and meta-analysis. *Am. J. Kidney Dis.* **2007**, *50*, 712–720. [CrossRef]
37. Liaño, F.; Pascual, J. Epidemiology of acute renal failure: A prospective, multicenter, community-based study. Madrid Acute Renal Failure Study Group. *Kidney Int.* **1996**, *50*, 811–818. [CrossRef]
38. Chertow, G.M.; Soroko, S.H.; Paganini, E.P.; Cho, K.C.; Himmelfarb, J.; Ikizler, T.A.; Mehta, R.L. Mortality after acute renal failure: Models for prognostic stratification and risk adjustment. *Kidney Int.* **2006**, *70*, 1120–1126. [CrossRef]

39. Bouchard, J.; Soroko, S.B.; Chertow, G.M.; Himmelfarb, J.; Ikizler, T.A.; Paganini, E.P.; Mehta, R.L. Fluid accumulation, survival and recovery of kidney function in critically ill patients with acute kidney injury. *Kidney Int.* **2009**, *76*, 422–427. [CrossRef]
40. Kidney Disease: Improving Global Outcomes (KDIGO) Acute Kidney Injury Work Group. KDIGO. clinical practice guideline for acute kidney injury. *Kidney Int. Suppl.* **2012**, *2*, 1–138.
41. Mazzali, C.; Duca, P. Use of administrative data in healthcare research. *Intern. Emerg. Med.* **2015**, *10*, 517–524. [CrossRef] [PubMed]
42. Waikar, S.S.; Wald, R.; Chertow, G.M.; Curhan, G.C.; Winkelmayer, W.C.; Liangos, O.; Sosa, M.A.; Jaber, B.L. Validity of International Classification of Diseases, Ninth Revision, Clinical Modification Codes for Acute Renal Failure. *J. Am. Soc. Nephrol.* **2006**, *17*, 1688–1694. [CrossRef] [PubMed]
43. Vlasschaert, M.E.; Bejaimal, S.A.; Hackam, D.G.; Quinn, R.; Cuerden, M.S.; Oliver, M.J.; Iansavichus, A.; Sultan, N.; Mills, A.; Garg, A.X. Validity of administrative database coding for kidney disease: A systematic review. *Am. J. Kidney Dis.* **2011**, *57*, 29–43. [CrossRef] [PubMed]
44. Tomlinson, L.A.; Riding, A.M.; Payne, R.A.; Abel, G.A.; Tomson, C.R.; Wilkinson, I.B.; Roland, M.O.; Chaudhry, A.N. The accuracy of diagnostic coding for acute kidney injury in England—A single centre study. *BMC Nephrol.* **2013**, *14*, 58. [CrossRef] [PubMed]
45. Grams, M.E.; Waikar, S.S.; MacMahon, B.; Whelton, S.; Ballew, S.H.; Coresh, J. Performance and limitations of administrative data in the identification of AKI. *Clin. J. Am. Soc. Nephrol.* **2014**, *9*, 682–689. [CrossRef]

2

# Effect of Anesthetic Technique on the Occurrence of Acute Kidney Injury after Total Knee Arthroplasty

**Ha-Jung Kim, Hee-Sun Park, Yon-Ji Go, Won Uk Koh *, Hyungtae Kim, Jun-Gol Song and Young-Jin Ro**

Department of Anesthesiology and Pain Medicine, Asan Medical Center, University of Ulsan, College of Medicine, Seoul 05505, Korea; alexakim06@gmail.com (H.-J.K.); lenadiar@naver.com (H.-S.P.); goyunji426@gmail.com (Y.-J.G.); ingwei2475@gmail.com (H.K.); jungol.song@amc.seoul.kr (J.-G.S.); yjro@amc.seoul.kr (Y.-J.R.)

* Correspondence: koh9726@naver.com

**Abstract:** Recent studies have reported the advantages of spinal anesthesia over general anesthesia in orthopedic patients. However, little is known about the relationship between acute kidney injury (AKI) after total knee arthroplasty (TKA) and anesthetic technique. This study aimed to identify the influence of anesthetic technique on AKI in TKA patients. We also evaluated whether the choice of anesthetic technique affected other clinical outcomes. We retrospectively reviewed medical records of patients who underwent TKA between January 2008 and August 2016. Perioperative data were obtained and analyzed. To reduce the influence of potential confounding factors, propensity score (PS) analysis was performed. A total of 2809 patients and 2987 cases of TKA were included in this study. A crude analysis of the total set demonstrated a significantly lower risk of AKI in the spinal anesthesia group. After PS matching, the spinal anesthesia group showed a tendency for reduced AKI, without statistical significance. Furthermore, the spinal anesthesia group showed a lower risk of pulmonary and vascular complications, and shortened hospital stay after PS matching. In TKA patients, spinal anesthesia had a tendency to reduce AKI. Moreover, spinal anesthesia not only reduced vascular and pulmonary complications, but also shortened hospital stay.

**Keywords:** acute kidney injury; anesthetic technique; total knee arthroplasty

---

## 1. Introduction

Total knee arthroplasty (TKA) is the primary treatment option for advanced inflammatory and degenerative knee osteoarthritis. With an increase in the elderly population, the number of TKAs performed is increasing rapidly, and is expected to continue to increase [1,2]. Even in young patients, the number of TKAs performed is increasing as the surgical technique and durability of the implant have improved [3].

Although controversy remains over the optimal anesthetic technique in perioperative outcomes following TKA, general anesthesia has historically been used for TKA [4]. There is minimal risk of anesthesia failure with general anesthesia; however, although very rare, neuraxial anesthesia, including spinal anesthesia and epidural anesthesia, is associated with neurologic complications, such as radiculopathy, cauda equina syndrome, and paraplegia [5]. In addition, a meta-analysis showed that general anesthesia had no significant risk on perioperative morbidities and mortality compared to regional anesthesia including neuraxial anesthesia and peripheral nerve block in patients undergoing total joint arthroplasty [6]. Moreover, many surgeons and patients were found to prefer general anesthsia over neuraxial anesthesia because of patient anxiety; anesthesiologists also tend to opt for general anesthesia due to more experience with this technique [7].

However, there is increasing evidence that neuraxial anesthesia has potential advantages over general anesthesia. Several previous studies reported that neuraxial anesthesia can reduce the risk of deep vein thrombosis, surgical site infection, and perioperative blood loss in orthopedic patients [8–10]. A recent study identified that 30-day mortality was also reduced after total joint arthroplasty in patients receiving neuraxial anesthesia [11]. Spinal anesthesia also showed benefits especially in patients with multiple comorbidities [11].

Although various studies have analyzed the effect of anesthetic technique on perioperative morbidity and mortality, little is known about the relationship between acute kidney injury (AKI) after TKA and anesthetic technique. The incidence of AKI in patients undergoing TKA is approximately 4–5% and newly developed AKI after noncardiac surgery was found to lengthen postoperative hospital stay and increase mortality [12–14]. Thus, identification of modifiable factors associated with AKI is important to improve patient outcomes.

The current study aimed to identify the influence of anesthetic technique on the incidence of AKI using propensity score (PS) matching. We also evaluated whether the choice of anesthetic technique affected the occurrence of perioperative complications other than AKI.

## 2. Materials and Methods

This study was approved by the Institutional Review Board of Asan Medical Center (2017-0626; date of approval, 29 May 2017) and written informed consent was waived owing to the retrospective nature of this study. All surgeries were performed by three surgeons at a tertiary center in Seoul, Korea.

### 2.1. *Study Population*

We retrospectively reviewed the medical records of patients who underwent TKA between January 2008 and August 2016. A total of 4702 consecutive TKAs were identified from the electronic medical records system. Of these, 401 TKAs were excluded due to estimated preoperative glomerular filtration rate of less than 60 mL/min/1.73 $m^2$, preoperative serum creatinine (sCr) levels greater than 1.5 mg/dL, or a previous history of renal dysfunction. The remaining 4301 TKAs were performed on 2809 patients. In total, 1317 patients underwent a single TKA surgery. The remaining 1492 patients underwent TKAs on both knees; 555 with staggered operations during one hospitalization, 178 with staged operations at intervals of more than two weeks in two separate hospitalizations, and 759 simultaneous operations.

### 2.2. *Anesthesia*

Standard monitoring was performed in the operating room, including electrocardiogram (ECG), $SpO_2$, non-invasive blood pressure, and body temperature.

In patients receiving TKA under general anesthesia, intravenous propofol (2–3 mL/kg) or thiopental sodium (4–5 mL/kg) with rocuronium (0.6–1.0 mg/kg) was used for induction. After induction, anesthesia was maintained with 1–1.5 minimum alveolar concentration of inhalational agents (sevoflurane or desflurane) with 50% nitrous oxide. Fresh gas flow rate was maintained at 2 L/min and minute ventilation was adjusted with reference to $ETCO_2$. Tidal volume was set at 6–8 mL/kg and respiratory rate was set at 10–12/min without positive end-expiratory pressure (PEEP). In patients with decreased $SpO_2$, recruitment maneuver was performed and 5 cm $H_2O$ PEEP was applied. After the procedure was completed, the inhalation agent and nitrous oxide were turned off and the lung was ventilated with 100% oxygen. When an attempt of self-respiration appeared, sugammadex or a cholinesterase inhibitor with anticholinergics was administered and extubation was performed.

Spinal anesthesia consisted of 10–15 mg bupivacaine and 10–15 mcg of fentanyl intrathecally after a lumbar puncture at the lateral decubitus position. During the intraoperative period, patients were sedated with midazolam and/or dexmedetomidine and breathed 5–6 L/min oxygen via a simple mask.

In both groups, blood pressure was targeted within normal range. If systolic blood pressure dropped below 80 mmHg, ephedrine (5–10 mg) or phenylephrine (50–100 μg) was injected. In the case of persistent hypotension, continuous infusion of phenylephrine was administered. When the blood pressure was high despite the adequate anesthetic depth and sufficient analgesia, calcium channel blocker or beta blocker was administered considering the underlying disease of the patients and other vital signs upon the decision-making of a staff anesthesiologist. When severe bradycardia (HR < 40 BPM/min) was observed, atropine (0.5 mg) or glycopyrrolate (0.2 mg) was applied. Crystalloid and colloid solution was infused by calculating the maintenance volume and bleeding, and by considering the volume status of the patient. Transfusion was carried out based on the amount of hemorrhage, the symptom of anemia including hypotension, tachycardia, or change of ECG, and the hematocrit level. For postoperative pain control, IV patient-controlled analgesia with fentanyl was available to most patients.

### 2.3. *Clinical Data*

We retrospectively obtained demographic, surgical, preoperative, and clinical outcome data of all patients from the electronic medical records system of our institution. The demographic data included age, sex, body mass index (BMI), and the American Society of Anethesiologists' physical status (ASA PS) classification. Surgical data included the operator and the type of surgical strategy. The surgical strategy was classified as surgery on 1) only one knee (single group), 2) both knees simultaneously (simultaneous group), or 3) both knees sequentially. Patients that underwent surgery on both knees sequentially were divided into two groups according to whether the two surgeries were performed during one or two hospitalization periods (staggered group and staged group, respectively). Preoperative clinical data included medical history, including the presence of diabetes, hypertension, ischemic heart disease, cerebrovascular disease, pulmonary disease, adrenal insufficiency, and the use of the following medications: calcium channel blocker, angiotensin converting enzyme inhibitor/angiotensin receptor blocker, beta blocker, aspirin, antiplatelet agent, HMG-CoA reductase inhibitors, antibiotics, non-steroidal anti-inflammatory drugs, selective COX-2 inhibitor, other analgesics, and steroids. In addition, preoperative laboratory findings, including anemia, platelet, white blood cells, blood sodium level, C-reactive protein (CRP), aspartate aminotransferase (AST), alanine aminotransferase (ALT), albumin, and uric acid, as well as transthoracic/transesophageal echocardiographic findings and pulmonary function test (PFT), were also documented.

### 2.4. *Definitions of Outcomes*

The primary outcome of this study was the association of the anesthetic technique with the occurrence of AKI in patients following TKA. AKI was diagnosed based on the Kidney Disease: Improving Global Outcomes (KDIGO) criteria and is described as the change in the sCr level on postoperative days 1 to 7 compared with the baseline sCr level measured before surgery. AKI was defined by alteration of sCr level ≥ 0.3 mg/dL within 48 hours, or a rise in sCr level ≥ 50% within the prior 7 days.

Intraoperative variables including the use of vasopressor, calcium channel blocker, and beta blocker, the total volume of infused crystalloid and colloid, intraoperative packed red blood cell transfusion, and the lowest mean blood pressure (MBP) were evaluated. In addition, the operation time and the tourniquet time were also calculated.

Other outcome variables were classified postoperatively as follows: cardiovascular complications, including hypotension, arrhythmia, ischemic heart disease, and congestive heart failure; pulmonary complications, including pneumonia, pleural effusion and pneumothorax; vascular complications, including deep vein thrombosis (DVT) with or without pulmonary thromboembolism (PTE); delirium; cerebrovascular accident; surgical site infection; gastrointestinal complications, including gastric ulcer, diarrhea, and elevated liver enzymes; and urologic complications, including voiding difficulty and urinary tract infection. Major complications, defined as complications requiring a surgical, endoscopic, or radiologic intervention, or those that were life-threatening (Clavien–Dindo classification ≥ 3), were also analyzed.

### 2.5. Statistical Analysis

The 2809 patients included in this study were classified into four groups based on surgical strategy. Since we aimed to evaluate the risk of AKI during a hospitalization, cases of two TKAs performed on the same patient, staggered and simultaneous, were considered as one case. However, the two TKAs performed on the same patient in the staged group were considered to be two separate cases. Thus, the total number of cases included in the analysis was 2987.

All data are presented as mean ± standard deviation or median (interquartile range) for continuous variables, or number (percentages) for categorical variables. Since the portion of missing data was insignificant, analyses were performed with only the recorded data without any special processing. Demographic characteristics and preoperative laboratory data were compared using Student's t test or the Mann-Whitney U test for continuous variables. Categorical variables were analyzed with Chi-square or Fisher's exact test.

To reduce the influence of potential confounding factors, PS analysis was performed to modify intergroup differences according to the anesthetic technique. Table 1 shows all demographic and perioperative variables used for estimating the PS. Using greedy matching algorithms, we used a caliper of 0.25 standard deviations of the logit of the PS to match patients at a ratio of 1:1. Model discrimination and model calibration were evaluated with c statistics (0.837) and Hosmer-Lemshow statistics (Chi-square = 8.6005, degrees of freedom = 8, $p = 0.377$), respectively. In addition, patients who received both anesthetic techniques were considered self-matching. We evaluated the balance in demographic, surgical, and preoperative covariates of the PS-matched cohort by the standardized mean difference. All absolute standardized differences after PS were less than 0.1. The risk of clinical outcome variables, including occurrence of morbidity, were analyzed by logistic regression using generalized estimating equations in the total and PS-matched cohort. Moreover, hospital stay and postoperative maximum CRP level of each group was compared between the two groups. Statistically significance was set at $p < 0.05$. Statistical analysis was conducted with SAS version 9.4 (SAS Institute Inc., Cary, NC, USA).

**Table 1.** Baseline characteristics of all patients included in the total set.

| Demographic Data | General (N = 2353) | Spinal (N = 634) | $p$-Value | Standardized Difference |
|---|---|---|---|---|
| Age (years) | 68.6 ± 6.6 | 69.3 ± 6.4 | 0.027 | 0.102 |
| Body mass index (kg/m$^2$) | 26.8 ± 3.5 | 26.5 ± 3.2 | 0.048 | 0.090 |
| Sex, Female/male | 2174 / 179 (92.4/7.6) | 568 / 66 (89.6 / 10.4) | 0.022 | 0.092 |
| ASA PS $^{\dagger}$, 1/2/3 | 129/2157/67 (5.5/91.7/2.9) | 21/581/32 (3.3/91.6/5.1) | 0.003 | 0.152 |
| Smoking History Non/current/ex-smoker | 2039/52/262 (86.7/2.2/11.1) | 325/19/290 (51.3/3/45.7) | <0.001 | 0.844 |
| **Surgical Data** | | | | |
| Surgical strategy, Single/staggered/staged_1$^{st}$/ staged_2$^{nd}$/simultaneous | 983/380/149/146/695 (41.8/16.2/6.3/6.2/29.5) | 334/175/29/32/64 (52.7/27.6/4.6/5.1/10.1) | <0.001 | 0.553 |
| Surgeon, B/C/K | 719/1173/461 (30.6/49.9/19.6) | 326/273/35 (51.4/43.1/5.5) | <0.001 | 0.542 |
| **Preoperative Medical History** | | | | |
| Diabetes mellitus | 306 (13.0) | 105 (16.6) | 0.021 | 0.096 |
| Hypertension | 768 (32.6) | 261 (41.2) | <0.001 | 0.173 |
| Ischemic heart disease | 164 (7.0) | 63 (9.9) | 0.012 | 0.099 |
| Cerebrovascular disease | 127 (5.4) | 45 (7.1) | 0.103 | 0.066 |
| Pulmonary disease | 88 (3.7) | 35 (5.5) | 0.045 | 0.078 |
| Adrenal disease | 33 (1.4) | 7 (1.1) | 0.562 | 0.029 |

**Table 1.** *Cont.*

| Demographic Data | General (N = 2353) | Spinal (N = 634) | *p*-Value | Standardized Difference |
|---|---|---|---|---|
| **Preoperative Medication History** | | | | |
| Calcium channel blocker | 927 (39.4) | 243 (38.3) | 0.625 | 0.022 |
| Angiotensin-converting enzyme inhibitor | 803 (34.1) | 220 (34.7) | 0.787 | 0.012 |
| Beta blocker | 360 (15.3) | 106 (16.7) | 0.382 | 0.038 |
| Aspirin | 512 (21.8) | 135 (21.3) | 0.800 | 0.011 |
| Clopidogrel | 150 (6.4) | 58 (9.2) | 0.015 | 0.096 |
| HMG-CoA reductase inhibitors ‡ | 600 (25.5) | 234 (36.9) | <0.001 | 0.236 |
| Antibiotics | 12 (0.5) | 1 (0.2) | 0.323 | 0.089 |
| Nonsteroidal anti-inflammatory drugs | 187 (8.0) | 33 (5.2) | 0.019 | 0.123 |
| Selective cyclooxygenase-2 inhibitor | 408 (17.3) | 140 (22.1) | 0.006 | 0.114 |
| Other analgesics | 356 (15.1) | 116 (18.3) | 0.052 | 0.082 |
| Steroids | 51 (2.2) | 19 (3.0) | 0.220 | 0.049 |
| **Preoperative Laboratory Data** | | | | |
| Anemia | 618 (26.3) | 147 (23.2) | 0.115 | 0.073 |
| Thrombocytopenia/normal/ thrombocytosis | 85/2142/126 (3.6/91.0/5.4) | 19/590/25 (3.0/93.1/3.9) | 0.255 | 0.077 |
| Leukopenia/normal/leukocytosis | 89/2198/66 (3.8/93.4/2.8) | 22/598/14 (3.5/94.3/2.2) | 0.657 | 0.042 |
| Hyponatremia/normal/hypernatremia | 26/2279/48 (1.1/96.9/2.0) | 10/611/13 (1.6/96.4/2.1) | 0.626 | 0.041 |
| Hemoglobin (g/dL) | 12.7 ± 1.1 | 12.8 ± 1.1 | 0.111 | 0.071 |
| C-reactive protein (mg/dL) | 0.23 ± 0.48 | 0.21 ± 0.4 | 0.014 | 0.052 |
| Aspartate aminotransferase (IU/L) | 23.0 ± 8.9 | 22.4 ± 9.0 | 0.008 | 0.064 |
| Alanine aminotransferse (IU/L) | 19.9 ± 11.2 | 20.4 ± 12.0 | 0.569 | 0.039 |
| Albumin (g/dL) | 3.9 ± 0.3 | 3.8 ± 0.3 | <0.001 | 0.418 |
| Uric acid (mg/dL) | 4.6 ± 1.2 | 4.6 ± 1.1 | 0.519 | 0.029 |
| Abnormality on echocardiogram | 279 (11.9) | 48 (7.6) | 0.002 | 0.163 |
| Abnormality on pulmonary function test | 103 (4.4) | 40 (6.4) | 0.041 | 0.081 |

Data are presented as mean ± standard deviation or median (interquartile range (IQR)) for continuous variables, or number (percentages) for categorical variables. † American Society of Anesthesiologists physical status; ‡ 3-hydroxy-3-methyl-glutaryl-coenzyme A reductase inhibitor.

## 3. Results

A total of 2809 patients and 2987 cases of TKA were analyzed in this study. Demographic, surgical, and preoperative data of the general anesthesia and spinal anesthesia group without PS matching are shown in Table 1. Without PS matching, the two groups showed significant differences in age, BMI, sex, ASA PS, smoking history, operator, surgical strategy, DM, HTN, IHD, pulmonary disease, clopidogrel, HMG-CoA reductase, NSAIDs, selective COX-2 inhibitor, CRP, AST, albumin, and echocardiographic/PFT findings. After PS matching, standardized differences of all covariates were less than 0.1 (Table 2) and there were no significant differences between the two groups.

Intraoperative data are shown in Table 3. In the analysis of the matched set, the spinal anesthesia group showed significantly fewer requirements of calcium channel blocker and beta blocker, while the lowest MBP was higher. The infused volume of crystalloid and the infused volume of colloid were significantly different, and the volume of urine output also showed a difference between the two groups.

The incidence of AKI, based on the KDIGO criteria, was 162 (5.4%) in all cases (Table 4). Among these, 143 (6.1%) and 19 (3.0%) cases of AKI occurred in the general anesthesia and spinal anesthesia groups, respectively. In a crude analysis of the total set, the spinal anesthesia group demonstrated a significantly lower risk for AKI than the general anesthesia group (Odds ratio (OR) = 0.477, 95% confidence interval [CI] 0.293–0.778, $p = 0.003$). However, in the PS matched set analysis, a total of 37 cases of AKI were included in the PS matched sets and the spinal anesthesia group showed lower incidence of AKI that was not statistically significant (OR = 0.529, 95% CI 0.273–1.024, $p = 0.059$). There were 33 cases of stage 1 AKI (serum creatinine ≥ 1.5–1.9 times baseline or ≥ 0.3 mg/dL increase), out of which 20 cases occurred in the general anesthesia group. The three cases of stage 2 AKI (serum creatinine ≥ 2.0–2.9 times baseline) and one case of stage 3 AKI (serum creatinine ≥ 3.0 times baseline or ≥ 4.0 mg/dL or requirement of renal replacement therapy) occurred only in the general anesthesia group.

Table 4 shows additional clinical outcomes. Delirium and gastrointestinal complications were significantly more frequent in the spinal versus general anesthesia group in the total set analysis. However, these results were different from the PS-matched set analysis. After PS matching, the general anesthesia group showed a significantly higher risk of pulmonary and vascular complications. Hospital stay was significantly shorter in the spinal anesthesia group compared with the general anesthesia group, in both the total set (spinal anesthesia group 13.6 ± 5.2 days, general anesthesia group 14.0 ± 5.2 days, $p < 0.001$) and the PS matched set (spinal anesthesia group 13.6 ± 5.5 days, general anesthesia group 14.3 ± 5.0 days, $p = 0.0067$). In addition, the patients in the spinal anesthesia group showed significantly lower postoperative maximum CRP levels compared to the general anesthesia group in the total set (spinal anesthesia group 7.1 ± 4.6, general anesthesia group 8.4 ± 5.6, $p < 0.001$) and the PS matched set (spinal anesthesia group 6.9 ± 4.5, general anesthesia group 7.9 ± 5.4, $p = 0.001$).

**Table 2.** Baseline characteristics of the patients included in the propensity score matched set.

| Demographic Data | General (N = 467) | Spinal (N = 467) | Standardized Difference |
|---|---|---|---|
| Age | 69.4 ± 6.5 | 69.3 ± 6.4 | 0.011 |
| Body mass index (kg/m$^2$) | 26.4 ± 3.3 | 26.4 ± 3.3 | 0.017 |
| Sex, Female/male | 423/44 (90.6/9.4) | 416/51 (89.1/10.9) | 0.049 |
| ASA PS †, 1/2/3 | 17/425/25 (3.6/91.0/5.4) | 18/426/23 (3.9/91.2/4.9) | 0.022 |
| Smoking HistoryNon/current/ex-smoker | 340/15/112 (72.8/3.2/24.0) | 320/18/129 (68.5/3.9/27.6) | 0.094 |
| Surgical Data | | | |
| Surgical strategy, Single/staggered/staged_1st/ staged_2nd/simultaneous | 238/120/19/27/63 (51.0/25.7/4.1/5.8/13.5) | 240/110/23/31/63 (51.4/23.6/4.9/6.6/13.5) | 0.069 |
| Surgeon, B/C/K | 216/208/43 (46.3/44.5/9.2) | 204/228/35 (43.7/48.8/7.5) | 0.095 |
| Preoperative Medical History | | | |
| Diabetes mellitus | 74 (15.9) | 70 (15.0) | 0.023 |
| Hypertension | 166 (35.6) | 170 (36.4) | 0.017 |
| Ischemic heart disease | 47 (10.1) | 45 (9.6) | 0.014 |
| Cerebrovascular disease | 29 (6.2) | 30 (6.4) | 0.008 |
| Pulmonary disease | 26 (5.6) | 27 (5.8) | 0.009 |
| Adrenal disease | 7 (1.5) | 6 (1.3) | 0.020 |
| Preoperative Medication History | | | |
| Calcium channel blocker | 186 (39.8) | 178 (38.1) | 0.035 |
| Angiotensin converting enzyme inhibitor | 165 (35.3) | 162 (34.7) | 0.014 |
| Beta blocker | 84 (18.0) | 77 (16.5) | 0.040 |
| Aspirin | 101 (21.6) | 99 (21.2) | 0.010 |
| Clopidogrel | 42 (9.0) | 39 (8.4) | 0.022 |
| HMG-CoA reductase inhibitors ‡ | 160 (34.3) | 150 (32.1) | 0.044 |
| Antibiotics | 0 (0) | 1 (0.2) | 0.054 |
| NSAIDs | 29 (6.2) | 24 (5.1) | 0.048 |
| Selective cyclooxygenase-2 inhibitor | 102 (21.8) | 101 (21.6) | 0.005 |
| Other analgesics | 94 (20.1) | 81 (17.3) | 0.072 |
| Steroids | 13 (2.8) | 11 (2.4) | 0.025 |
| Preoperative Laboratory Data | | | |
| Anemia | 119 (25.5) | 106 (22.7) | 0.066 |
| Thrombocytopenia/normal/thrombocytosis | 18/427/22 (3.9/91.4/4.7) | 17/431/19 (3.6/92.3/4.1) | 0.034 |
| Leukopenia/normal/leukocytosis | 25/432/10 (5.4/92.5/2.1) | 21/437/9 (4.5/93.6/1.9) | 0.043 |
| Hyponatremia/normal/hypernatremia | 7/450/10 (1.5/96.4/2.1) | 4/455/8 (0.9/97.4/1.7) | 0.068 |
| Hemoglobin (g/dL) | 12.7 ± 1.2 | 12.8 ± 1.1 | 0.088 |
| C-reactive protein (mg/dL) | 0.22 ± 0.38 | 0.23 ± 0.45 | 0.008 |
| Aspartate aminotransferase (IU/L) | 22.2 ± 7.7 | 22.6 ± 9.6 | 0.048 |
| Alanine aminotransferse (IU/L) | 20.4 ± 12.2 | 20.5 ± 12.9 | 0.010 |
| Albumin (g/dL) | 3.8 ± 0.3 | 3.8 ± 0.3 | 0.085 |
| Uric acid (mg/dL) | 4.7 ± 1.2 | 4.7 ± 1.1 | 0.003 |
| Abnormality on echocardiogram | 49 (10.5) | 45 (9.6) | 0.032 |
| Abnormality on pulmonary function test | 34 (7.3) | 34 (7.3) | 0.0 |

Data are presented as mean ± standard deviation or median (interquartile range [IQR]) for continuous variables, or number (percentages) for categorical variables. † American Society of Anesthesiologists physical status; ‡ 3-hydroxy-3-methyl-glutaryl-coenzyme A reductase inhibitor.

**Table 3.** Intraoperative data of the study groups by anesthetic technique in total and matched sets.

| Intraoperative Data | Total Set | | | Matched Set | | |
|---|---|---|---|---|---|---|
| | General Group (n = 2353) | Spinal Group (n = 634) | *p*-Value | General Group (n = 467) | Spinal Group (n = 467) | *p*-Value |
| Use of vasopressor | 430 (18.3) | 102 (16.1) | 0.202 | 77 (16.5) | 86 (18.4) | 0.432 |
| Use of calcium channel blocker | 366 (15.6) | 58 (9.2) | <0.001 | 65 (13.9) | 34 (7.3) | 0.001 |
| Use of beta blocker | 516 (21.9) | 8 (1.3) | <0.001 | 95 (20.3) | 5 (1.1) | <0.001 |
| Red blood cell transfusion | 795 (33.8) | 103 (16.3) | <0.001 | 95 (20.3) | 99 (21.2) | 0.730 |
| Infused crystalloid (mL) | 1014.8 ± 600.1 | 961.1 ± 551.2 | 0.016 | 922.4 ± 574.1 | 1013.5 ± 599.9 | 0.012 |
| Infused colloid (mL) | 544.6 ± 305.1 | 382.8 ± 209.0 | <0.001 | 496.7 ± 277.9 | 402.0 ± 215.0 | <0.001 |
| Urine output (mL) | 193.4 ± 230.8 | 379.4 ± 350.6 | <0.001 | 168.0 ± 209.9 | 366.2 ± 341.8 | <0.001 |
| The lowest mean blood pressure (mm Hg) | 69.3 ± 8.5 | 73.1 ± 9.8 | <0.001 | 70.3 ± 8.7 | 72.6 ± 9.9 | <0.001 |
| Operation time (minute) | 133.4 ± 42.3 | 122.5 ± 33.8 | <0.001 | 123.7 ± 34.8 | 124.4 ± 36.9 | 0.731 |
| Tourniquet time (minute) | 123.1 ± 34.5 | 105.3 ±30.6 | <0.001 | 114.0 ± 31.0 | 104.5 ± 31.0 | <0.001 |

**Table 4.** Comparison of postoperative clinical outcomes in the study groups by anesthetic technique.

| Clinical Outcome | Group | Total Set | | | | | Matched Set | | | | |
|---|---|---|---|---|---|---|---|---|---|---|---|
| | | Event | Odds Ratio | 95% Confidence Interval | | *p*-Value | Event | Odds Ratio | 95% Confidence Interval | | *p*-Value |
| Acute kidney injury | General | 143 | 1 | | | | 24 | | | | |
| | Spinal | 19 | 0.477 | 0.293 | 0.778 | 0.003 | 13 | 0.529 | 0.273 | 1.024 | 0.059 |
| Cardiovascular complication | General | 29 | 1 | | | | 10 | | | | |
| | Spinal | 7 | 0.895 | 0.390 | 2.052 | 0.793 | 5 | 0.495 | 0.166 | 1.470 | 0.205 |
| Pulmonary complication | General | 38 | | | | | 14 | | | | |
| | Spinal | 7 | 0.680 | 0.276 | 1.676 | 0.402 | 4 | 0.280 | 0.091 | 0.862 | 0.027 |
| Deep vein thrombosis/Pulmonary thromboembolism | General | 28 | | | | | 11 | | | | |
| | Spinal | 3 | 0.395 | 0.119 | 1.309 | 0.129 | 2 | 0.178 | 0.039 | 0.813 | 0.026 |
| Delirium | General | 32 | | | | | 7 | | | | |
| | Spinal | 19 | 2.241 | 1.254 | 4.004 | 0.006 | 15 | 2.181 | 0.873 | 5.450 | 0.095 |
| Neurologic complication | General | 18 | | | | | 3 | | | | |
| | Spinal | 6 | 1.239 | 0.490 | 3.133 | 0.650 | 6 | 2.013 | 0.497 | 8.146 | 0.327 |
| Surgical site infection | General | 14 | | | | | 4 | | | | |
| | Spinal | 6 | 1.596 | 0.611 | 4.171 | 0.340 | 6 | 1.507 | 0.420 | 5.409 | 0.530 |
| Gastrointestinal complication | General | 58 | | | | | 6 | | | | |
| | Spinal | 26 | 1.692 | 1.060 | 2.701 | 0.028 | 14 | 2.375 | 0.943 | 5.980 | 0.066 |
| Endocrinologic complication | General | 3 | | | | | 2 | | | | |
| | Spinal | 1 | 1.237 | 0.128 | 11.918 | 0.854 | 1 | 0.499 | 0.045 | 5.540 | 0.571 |
| Urologic complication | General | 24 | | | | | 11 | | | | |
| | Spinal | 9 | 1.397 | 0.641 | 3.048 | 0.400 | 4 | 0.358 | 0.122 | 1.053 | 0.062 |
| Major complication | General | 70 | | | | | 18 | | | | |
| | Spinal | 24 | 1.283 | 0.800 | 2.058 | 0.301 | 22 | 1.233 | 0.654 | 2.325 | 0.517 |
| Intensive care unit admission | General | 59 | 1 | | | | 15 | | | | |
| | Spinal | 21 | 1.332 | 0.803 | 2.210 | 0.267 | 19 | 1.278 | 0.647 | 2.526 | 0.480 |

## 4. Discussion

In the current study, we found that spinal anesthesia might be protective for AKI based on KDIGO criteria in patients undergoing TKA. Moreover, spinal anesthesia had lower observable risks of pulmonary and vascular complications compared to general anesthesia. Hospital stay was also reduced in patients receiving spinal anesthesia.

Spinal anesthesia showed a trend for a favorable outcome in the occurrence of AKI compared with general anesthesia, although this effect did not reach statistical significance. The protective mechanism of spinal anesthesia is unclear.

First, we suggest that spinal anesthesia may produce these results through sympathetic nerve blockade. The sympathetic nerve fibers originate from the lower thoracic spinal nerves (T7-11). Sympathetic activity is known to have a significant impact on renal function by altering renal hemodynamics, renin release, and sodium handling [15]. Increased sympathetic tone reduces renal blood flow by stimulation of $\alpha 1$ adrenoceptors on renal vasculature and increasing sodium reabsorption by direct effect on the renal tubules [16]. In addition, increased renal sympathetic nerve activity promotes renin release, which is mediated by $\beta$-1 adrenoceptors on the juxtaglomerular cells [17]. This series of processes acts to reduce renal blood flow and glomerular filtration rate. In this study, we found that intraoperative urine output was higher in the spinal anesthesia group than in general anesthesia group, even though the amount of fluid administered to both groups was similar. We considered the renal sympathetic nerves blocked, and that the blockade of renal sympathetic activity contributed to the greater urine output, thus resulting in a protective effect for AKI under spinal anesthesia.

Acute postoperative pain following orthopedic surgery is known to be more severe under general anesthesia compared with spinal anesthesia, with greater opioid use also observed with general anesthesia [18–20]. Since the duration of local anesthetics for spinal anesthesia was longer than the duration of TKA, patients generally feel comfortable during the immediate postoperative period. In addition, a previous study suggested that spinal anesthesia lowered the postoperative pain score via preemptive inhibition of afferent nociceptive stimuli and improved organ function [21,22]. Greater postoperative pain in patients receiving general anesthesia increases sympathetic nervous system stimulation, and as a result, the general anesthesia group may have showed a tendency for increased risk for AKI.

A second hypothesis in support of our findings is that the systemic inflammatory response to surgical stress is lower in regional anesthesia than in general anesthesia, resulting in less kidney injury with the spinal technique. The postoperative systemic inflammatory response was reported to be associated with any organ dysfunction, including AKI [23,24]. Inflammatory cytokines inducing neutrophil recruitment and accumulation play a key role in the development of AKI [25,26]. Moreover, the integrity of the endothelial glycocalyx layer, which is closely related to AKI, is disrupted by the inflammatory response [27]. Although controversial, some investigators reported that neuraxial anesthesia suppressed the stress response in elective surgical patients by blocking transmission of pain sensation and sympathetic activation [28–30]. In addition, local anesthetics used for neuraxial anesthesia were shown to have intrinsic anti-inflammatory effects [31,32]. In the current study, changes in CRP level revealed that the inflammatory response in the spinal group was reduced compared to the general group, consistent with previous studies. Therefore, we suggest that the reduced inflammatory response to surgical stress by spinal anesthesia might contribute to the trend of decreased risk for AKI.

Moreover, we found some differences in the intraoperative variables between the two groups. These differences seemed to be derived from the anesthetic techniques since PS matching was performed. A previous study showed that prolonged tourniquet time was related to the increased postoperative complications by leading greater ischemic insult [33]. Therefore, the reduced postoperative complications including AKI in the spinal anesthesia group could be seen as an indirect effect of spinal anesthesia by shortening the tourniquet time.

Besides the tourniquet time, the amount of fluid also showed differences between the two groups. The infused volume of crystalloid solution was greater in the spinal anesthesia group, while the infused volume of colloid solution was greater in the general anesthesia group. However, the sum of the crystalloid and colloid solution was similar in both groups, so that it was unlikely that the total volume of infused fluid could have had an impact on the occurrence of AKI. In addition, there was also a difference in the lowest MBP between the two groups. Intraoperative hypotension was known to have an association with AKI [34]. However, in this current study, the difference between the two groups was considered clinically insignificant, as the lowest MBP values in each group were higher than 55–60 mmHg, which was considered as cut-off value of hypotensive MBP.

This study showed that spinal anesthesia has advantages over general anesthesia due to reduced postoperative pulmonary complications after TKA. A recent study using a large national database also demonstrated that neuraxial anesthesia decreased the risk of both pulmonary compromise and pneumonia in TKA patients [7]. Respiratory function is disturbed in many aspects from the start of the general anesthesia, and mechanical ventilation under general anesthesia plays a major role in the occurrence of postoperative pulmonary complications [35]. Therefore, we should consider spinal anesthesia first, then general anesthesia, in patients with risk factors for pulmonary complications.

The beneficial effect of neuraxial anesthesia in vascular complication has been well documented [9,36–39]. Among them, Memtsoudis et al. suggested that neuraxial anesthesia has a beneficial effect itself beyond simply avoiding general anesthesia, and speculated that this result is due to alteration of the coagulation profile, blood flow, and stress responses to the surgery [7]. However, a number of studies have also shown that anesthetic technique was not associated with the risk of vascular complication, or that neuraxial anesthesia rather increased this risk [8,40,41]. An important factor leading to these inconsistent results was prophylactic treatment with chemical antithrombotics [41]. The studies reporting benefits of neuraxial anesthesia generally included patients that did not receive a prophylactic agent. At our institution, chemical antithrombotic prophylaxis was not applied and our results are consistent with those of previous studies. When chemical antithrombotic prophylaxis is not used, neuraxial anesthesia may be a better choice than general anesthesia.

Many studies have investigated whether neuraxial anesthesia can reduce the postoperative hospital stay. Although still controversial, a number of studies reported that the length of hospital stay was shorter with neuraxial anesthesia in orthopaedic patients [7,8,42]. Length of hospital stay is a surrogate marker for postoperative complications and use of resources [43]. Thus, the shorter length in the spinal anesthesia group may reflect a better clinical outcome. However, the length of hospital stay was much longer in both the general and spinal groups in this study compared to other studies [7,8,44,45]. This discrepancy is likely due to differences in management protocol. At our institution, patients are discharged after achieving a certain level of rehabilitation. Nonetheless, the spinal anesthesia group did show a shorter length of hospital stay. That is, spinal anesthesia had a beneficial effect on postoperative outcome.

This study has some limitations. First, there were inevitable flaws due to the nature of the retrospective observational design. We cannot conclude causality between general anesthesia and AKI owing to the characteristics of this study design. Second, there might be other confounding factors that were excluded in the analysis. However, we attempted to include as many factors as possible in the PS matching. Third, our definition of a staged/staggered operation might be different from that of other studies. In the current study, we defined a staggered operation as two operations occurring on two separate days during one hospitalization. However, we focused our investigation on the association of anesthetic technique on AKI, and the surgical strategy was used only for the propensity score matching. Thus, the disparity of the definition of a staged/staggered operation did not likely impact the results. Lastly, since we included patients with normal kidney function in this study, the present findings could not be extrapolated to the patients with decreased renal function. Further studies to evaluate the effect of anesthetic technique on AKI would be required.

In conclusion, the incidence of AKI, based on the KDIGO criteria, in patients who underwent total knee arthroplasty was 5.4%. Spinal anesthesia had a tendency to reduce AKI. In addition, spinal anesthesia reduced vascular and pulmonary complications compared to general anesthesia. Length of hospital stay was also shortened in patients with spinal anesthesia.

**Author Contributions:** H.-J.K. and W.U.K. designed the study, analyzed and interpreted the data, and drafted the manuscript. H.-S.P. and Y.-J.G. contributed to the acquisition of data. H.K., J.-G.S., and Y.-J.R. helped analyze the data. All authors have given approval of the final version of the manuscript.

## References

1. Koh, I.J.; Kim, T.K.; Chang, C.B.; Cho, H.J.; In, Y. Trends in use of total knee arthroplasty in Korea from 2001 to 2010. *Clin. Orthop. Relat. Res.* **2013**, *471*, 1441–1450. [CrossRef] [PubMed]
2. Kurtz, S.; Ong, K.; Lau, E.; Mowat, F.; Halpern, M. Projections of primary and revision hip and knee arthroplasty in the United States from 2005 to 2030. *J. Bone Joint Surg. Am.* **2007**, *89*, 780–785. [PubMed]
3. Kim, Y.H.; Kim, J.S.; Choe, J.W.; Kim, H.J. Long-term comparison of fixed-bearing and mobile-bearing total knee replacements in patients younger than fifty-one years of age with osteoarthritis. *J. Bone Joint Surg. Am.* **2012**, *94*, 866–873. [CrossRef] [PubMed]
4. Turnbull, Z.A.; Sastow, D.; Giambrone, G.P.; Tedore, T. Anesthesia for the patient undergoing total knee replacement: Current status and future prospects. *Local Reg. Anesth.* **2017**, *10*, 1–7. [CrossRef] [PubMed]
5. Brull, R.; McCartney, C.J.; Chan, V.W.; El-Beheiry, H. Neurological complications after regional anesthesia: Contemporary estimates of risk. *Anesth. Analg.* **2007**, *104*, 965–974. [CrossRef] [PubMed]
6. Macfarlane, A.J.; Prasad, G.A.; Chan, V.W.; Brull, R. Does regional anesthesia improve outcome after total knee arthroplasty? *Clin. Orthop. Relat. Res.* **2009**, *467*, 2379–2402. [CrossRef] [PubMed]
7. Memtsoudis, S.G.; Sun, X.; Chiu, Y.-L.; Stundner, O.; Liu, S.S.; Banerjee, S.; Mazumdar, M.; Sharrock, N.E. Perioperative comparative effectiveness of anesthetic technique in orthopedic patients. *Anesthesiology* **2013**, *118*, 1046–1058. [CrossRef]
8. Pugely, A.J.; Martin, C.T.; Gao, Y.; Mendoza-Lattes, S.; Callaghan, J.J. Differences in short-term complications between spinal and general anesthesia for primary total knee arthroplasty. *J. Bone Joint Surg. Am.* **2013**, *95*, 193–199. [CrossRef]
9. Davis, F.M.; Laurenson, V.G.; Gillespie, W.J.; Wells, J.E.; Foate, J.; Newman, E. Deep vein thrombosis after total hip replacement. A comparison between spinal and general anaesthesia. *J. Bone Joint Surg. Br.* **1989**, *71*, 181–185. [CrossRef]
10. Planes, A.; Vochelle, N.; Fagola, M.; Feret, J.; Bellaud, M. Prevention of deep vein thrombosis after total hip replacement. The effect of low-molecular-weight heparin with spinal and general anaesthesia. *J. Bone Joint Surg. Br.* **1991**, *73*, 418–422. [CrossRef]
11. Stundner, O.; Chiu, Y.L.; Sun, X.; Mazumdar, M.; Fleischut, P.; Poultsides, L.; Gerner, P.; Fritsch, G.; Memtsoudis, S.G. Comparative perioperative outcomes associated with neuraxial versus general anesthesia for simultaneous bilateral total knee arthroplasty. *Reg. Anesth. Pain Med.* **2012**, *37*, 638–644. [CrossRef] [PubMed]
12. Kim, H.J.; Koh, W.U.; Kim, S.G.; Park, H.S.; Song, J.G.; Ro, Y.J.; Yang, H.S. Early postoperative albumin level following total knee arthroplasty is associated with acute kidney injury: A retrospective analysis of 1309 consecutive patients based on kidney disease improving global outcomes criteria. *Medicine* **2016**, *95*, e4489. [CrossRef] [PubMed]
13. Warth, L.C.; Noiseux, N.O.; Hogue, M.H.; Klaassen, A.L.; Liu, S.S.; Callaghan, J.J. Risk of acute kidney injury after primary and revision total hip arthroplasty and total knee arthroplasty using a multimodal approach to perioperative pain control including ketorolac and celecoxib. *J. Arthroplasty* **2016**, *31*, 253–255. [CrossRef] [PubMed]
14. Biteker, M.; Dayan, A.; Tekkesin, A.I.; Can, M.M.; Tayci, I.; Ilhan, E.; Sahin, G. Incidence, risk factors, and outcomes of perioperative acute kidney injury in noncardiac and nonvascular surgery. *Am. J. Surg.* **2014**, *207*, 53–59. [CrossRef] [PubMed]
15. Suleiman, M.Y.; Passannante, A.N.; Onder, R.L.; Greene-Helms, W.F.; Perretta, S.G. Alteration of renal blood flow during epidural anesthesia in normal subjects. *Anesth. Analg.* **1997**, *84*, 1076–1080. [CrossRef] [PubMed]
16. DiBona, G.F. Neural control of renal function in health and disease. *Clin. Auton. Res.* **1994**, *4*, 69–74. [CrossRef] [PubMed]
17. Pelayo, J.C.; Tucker, B.J.; Blantz, R.C. Effects of beta-adrenergic stimulation with isoproterenol on glomerular

hemodynamics. *Am. J. Physiol.* **1989**, *257*, F866–F873. [CrossRef] [PubMed]
18. Gonano, C.; Leitgeb, U.; Sitzwohl, C.; Ihra, G.; Weinstabl, C.; Kettner, S.C. Spinal versus general anesthesia for orthopedic surgery: Anesthesia drug and supply costs. *Anesth. Analg.* **2006**, *102*, 524–529. [CrossRef]
19. Jellish, W.S.; Thalji, Z.; Stevenson, K.; Shea, J. A prospective randomized study comparing short-and intermediate-term perioperative outcome variables after spinal or general anesthesia for lumbar disk and laminectomy surgery. *Anesth. Analg.* **1996**, *83*, 559–564. [CrossRef]
20. Korhonen, A.-M.; Valanne, J.V.; Jokela, R.M.; Ravaska, P.; Korttila, K.T. A comparison of selective spinal anesthesia with hyperbaric bupivacaine and general anesthesia with desflurane for outpatient knee arthroscopy. *Anesth. Analg.* **2004**, *99*, 1668–1673. [CrossRef]
21. Carr, D.B.; Goudas, L.C. Acute pain. *Lancet* **1999**, *353*, 2051–2058. [CrossRef]
22. Kehlet, H.; Dahl, J.B. Anaesthesia, surgery, and challenges in postoperative recovery. *Lancet* **2003**, *362*, 1921–1928. [CrossRef]
23. Boehne, M.; Sasse, M.; Karch, A.; Dziuba, F.; Horke, A.; Kaussen, T.; Mikolajczyk, R.; Beerbaum, P.; Jack, T. Systemic inflammatory response syndrome after pediatric congenital heart surgery: Incidence, risk factors, and clinical outcome. *J. Card. Surg.* **2017**, *32*, 116–125. [CrossRef] [PubMed]
24. Park, J.T. Postoperative acute kidney injury. *Korean J. Anesthesiol.* **2017**, *70*, 258–266. [CrossRef] [PubMed]
25. Berry, M.; Clatworthy, M.R. Immunotherapy for acute kidney injury. *Immunotherapy* **2012**, *4*, 323–334. [CrossRef] [PubMed]
26. Nechemia-Arbely, Y.; Barkan, D.; Pizov, G.; Shriki, A.; Rose-John, S.; Galun, E.; Axelrod, J.H. IL-6/IL-6R axis plays a critical role in acute kidney injury. *J. Am. Soc. Nephrol.* **2008**, *19*, 1106–1115. [CrossRef]
27. Song, J.W.; Goligorsky, M.S. Perioperative implication of the endothelial glycocalyx. *Korean J. Anesthesiol.* **2018**, *71*, 92–102. [CrossRef]
28. Milosavljevic, S.B.; Pavlovic, A.P.; Trpkovic, S.V.; Ilić, A.N.; Sekulic, A.D. Influence of spinal and general anesthesia on the metabolic, hormonal, and hemodynamic response in elective surgical patients. *Med. Sci. Monit.* **2014**, *20*, 1833–1840.
29. Buyukkocak, U.; Daphan, C.; Caglayan, O.; Aydinuraz, K.; Kaya, T.; Saygun, O.; Agalar, F. Effects of different anesthetic techniques on serum leptin, C-reactive protein, and cortisol concentrations in anorectal surgery. *Croat. Med. J.* **2006**, *47*, 862–868.
30. Bugada, D.; Ghisi, D.; Mariano, E.R. Continuous regional anesthesia: A review of perioperative outcome benefits. *Minerva Anestesiol.* **2017**, *83*, 1089–1100.
31. Lirk, P.; Picardi, S.; Hollmann, M.W. Local anaesthetics: 10 essentials. *Eur. J. Anaesthesiol.* **2014**, *31*, 575–585. [CrossRef] [PubMed]
32. Lirk, P.; Fiegl, H.; Weber, N.; Hollmann, M. Epigenetics in the perioperative period. *Br. J. Pharmacol.* **2015**, *172*, 2748–2755. [CrossRef] [PubMed]
33. Rasmussen, L.E.; Holm, H.A.; Kristensen, P.W.; Kjaersgaard-Andersen, P. Tourniquet time in total knee arthroplasty. *Knee* **2018**, *25*, 306–313. [CrossRef] [PubMed]
34. Zarbock, A.; Koyner, J.L.; Hoste, E.A.; Kellum, J.A. Update on perioperative acute kidney injury. *Anesth. Analg.* **2018**, *127*, 1236–1245. [CrossRef] [PubMed]
35. Miskovic, A.; Lumb, A.B. Postoperative pulmonary complications. *Br. J. Anaesth.* **2017**, *118*, 317–334. [CrossRef]
36. Turan, A.; Bajracharya, G.R.; Leung, S.; Yazici Kara, M.; Mao, G.; Botsford, T.; Ruetzler, K.; Maheshwari, K.; Ali Sakr Esa, W.; Elsharkawy, H.; et al. Association of neuraxial anesthesia with postoperative venous thromboembolism after noncardiac surgery: A propensity-matched analysis of ACS-NSQIP database. *Anesth. Analg.* **2019**, *128*, 494–501. [CrossRef] [PubMed]
37. Mauermann, W.J.; Shilling, A.M.; Zuo, Z. A comparison of neuraxial block versus general anesthesia for elective total hip replacement: A meta-analysis. *Anesth. Analg.* **2006**, *103*, 1018–1025. [CrossRef]
38. Smith, L.M.; Cozowicz, C.; Uda, Y.; Memtsoudis, S.G.; Barrington, M.J. Neuraxial and combined neuraxial/general anesthesia compared to general anesthesia for major truncal and lower limb surgery: A systematic review and meta-analysis. *Anesth. Analg.* **2017**, *125*, 1931–1945. [CrossRef]
39. Hu, S.; Zhang, Z.Y.; Hua, Y.Q.; Li, J.; Cai, Z.D. A comparison of regional and general anaesthesia for total replacement of the hip or knee: A meta-analysis. *J. Bone Joint Surg. Br.* **2009**, *91*, 935–942. [CrossRef]
40. Walker, J.B.; Nguyen, P.L.; Schmidt, U.H.; Gabriel, R.A. Postoperative outcomes associated with neuraxial vs general anesthesia following bilateral total knee arthroplasty. *J. Arthroplasty* **2017**, *32*, 3632–3636. [CrossRef]
41. Johnson, R.L.; Kopp, S.L.; Burkle, C.M.; Duncan, C.M.; Jacob, A.K.; Erwin, P.J.; Murad, M.H.; Mantilla, C.B.

Neuraxial vs general anaesthesia for total hip and total knee arthroplasty: A systematic review of comparative-effectiveness research. *Br. J. Anaesth.* **2016**, *116*, 163–176. [CrossRef] [PubMed]
42. Helwani, M.A.; Avidan, M.S.; Ben Abdallah, A.; Kaiser, D.J.; Clohisy, J.C.; Hall, B.L.; Kaiser, H.A. Effects of regional versus general anesthesia on outcomes after total hip arthroplasty: A retrospective propensity-matched cohort study. *J. Bone Joint Surg. Am.* **2015**, *97*, 186–193. [CrossRef] [PubMed]
43. Cryer, C.; Gulliver, P.; Langley, J.D.; Davie, G. Is length of stay in hospital a stable proxy for injury severity? *Inj. Prev.* **2010**, *16*, 254–260. [CrossRef] [PubMed]
44. McIsaac, D.I.; McCartney, C.J.; Walraven, C.V. Peripheral Nerve Blockade for Primary Total Knee Arthroplasty: A population-based cohort study of outcomes and resource utilization. *Anesthesiology* **2017**, *126*, 312–320. [CrossRef] [PubMed]
45. El Bitar, Y.F.; Illingworth, K.D.; Scaife, S.L.; Horberg, J.V.; Saleh, K.J. Hospital length of stay following primary total knee arthroplasty: Data from the nationwide inpatient sample database. *J. Arthroplasty* **2015**, *30*, 1710–1715. [CrossRef]

3

# Mitochondrial Dynamics of Proximal Tubular Epithelial Cells in Nephropathic Cystinosis

**Domenico De Rasmo [1,*,†], Anna Signorile [2,†], Ester De Leo [3], Elena V. Polishchuk [4], Anna Ferretta [1], Roberto Raso [3], Silvia Russo [2], Roman Polishchuk [4], Francesco Emma [5] and Francesco Bellomo [3,*]**

1 Institute of Biomembranes, Bioenergetics and Molecular Biotechnology (IBIOM), National Research Council (CNR), 70124 Bari, Italy; a.ferretta@ibiom.cnr.it

2 Department of Basic Medical Sciences, Neurosciences and Sense Organs, University of Bari "Aldo Moro", 70124 Bari, Italy; anna.signorile@uniba.it (A.S.); silvia.russo92@gmail.com (S.R.)

3 Renal Diseases Research Unit, Genetics and Rare Diseases Research Division, Bambino Gesù Children's Hospital—IRCCS, 00146 Rome, Italy; ester.deleo@opbg.net (E.D.L.); roberto.raso@opbg.net (R.R.)

4 Telethon Institute of Genetics and Medicine, 80078 Pozzuoli, Italy; epolish@tigem.it (E.V.P.); polishchuk@tigem.it (R.P.)

5 Division of Nephrology, Department of Pediatric Subspecialties, Bambino Gesù Children's Hospital—IRCCS, 00165 Rome, Italy; francesco.emma@opbg.net

* Correspondence: d.derasmo@ibiom.cnr.it (D.D.R.); francesco.bellomo@opbg.net (F.B.)

† These authors contribute equally to this work.

**Abstract:** Nephropathic cystinosis is a rare lysosomal storage disorder caused by mutations in *CTNS* gene leading to Fanconi syndrome. Independent studies reported defective clearance of damaged mitochondria and mitochondrial fragmentation in cystinosis. Proteins involved in the mitochondrial dynamics and the mitochondrial ultrastructure were analyzed in *CTNS*−/− cells treated with cysteamine, the only drug currently used in the therapy for cystinosis but ineffective to treat Fanconi syndrome. *CTNS*−/− cells showed an overexpression of parkin associated with deregulation of ubiquitination of mitofusin 2 and fission 1 proteins, an altered proteolytic processing of optic atrophy 1 (OPA1), and a decreased OPA1 oligomerization. According to molecular findings, the analysis of electron microscopy images showed a decrease of mitochondrial cristae number and an increase of cristae lumen and cristae junction width. Cysteamine treatment restored the fission 1 ubiquitination, the mitochondrial size, number and lumen of cristae, but had no effect on cristae junction width, making *CTNS*−/− tubular cells more susceptible to apoptotic stimuli.

**Keywords:** Fanconi syndrome; nephropathic cystinosis; mitochondrial dynamics; cysteamine; mitochondrial fusion; mitochondrial fission; mitochondrial cristae

## 1. Introduction

Nephropathic cystinosis (MIM 219800) is a rare inherited metabolic disease characterized by an impaired transport of the amino acid cystine out of lysosomes due to reduced or absent function of the specific carrier cystinosin, which is encoded by *CTNS* gene [1–3]. Kidneys are affected at the initial stage of the disease, leading to early onset Fanconi syndrome, which is characterized by polyuria, glycosuria, phosphaturia, aminoaciduria, and urinary loss of electrolytes and low-molecular-weight proteins [4]. The cystine-depleting agent, cysteamine (MEA), significantly delays symptoms [5,6], but does not treat Fanconi syndrome and is ineffective to prevent the progression of kidney disease. Fanconi syndrome has also been reported in children with specific mitochondrial syndromes [7]. Renal tubular cells are very rich in mitochondria due to the intense reabsorption and excretion processes that occur in this district. We recently reported, in *CTNS−/−* cells derived from proximal tubules, mitochondrial fragmentation associated with respiratory chain dysfunction and low mitochondrial 3′,5′-cyclic adenosine monophosphate (cAMP) levels [8]. Furthermore, enhanced apoptosis [9,10], defect of autophagic flux [11,12], and endo-lysosomal dysfunction [13,14] were observed.

Communication between mitochondria and the endo-lysosomal system is complex. Increasing evidences show close relationship between these two cellular compartments [15,16]. Mitochondria constantly undergo fission and fusion processes to adapt to environmental changes in a continuous and balanced way, in order to maintain morphology and regulate cellular ATP levels. Mitochondrial fission regulates the production of new mitochondria and the segregation of damaged mitochondria. In this process, receptor proteins such as mitochondrial fission factor (Mff), mitochondrial fission 1 protein (Fis1), mitochondrial dynamics protein of 49 kDa (MiD49), and mitochondrial dynamics protein of 51 kDa (MiD51) recruit the large GTPase dynamin-related protein 1 (Drp1) from the cytosol to the outer mitochondrial membrane (OMM), which forms a multimeric complex with mitochondrial membrane adaptors [17,18]. Mitochondrial fusion is mediated by three key regulatory fusion proteins: the dynamin-related GTPases mitofusin 1 (MFN1) and mitofusin 2 (MFN2), responsible for the fusion of OMM and the dynamin-related GTPases optic atrophy 1 (OPA1), which mediates fusion of the inner mitochondrial membrane (IMM) and contributes to the maintenance of mitochondrial potential, to control respiratory chain activity and apoptosis [19,20]. When mitochondrial dynamics are impaired, dysfunctional mitochondria are selectively eliminated through mitophagy, which is initiated by ubiquitin-dependent or ubiquitin-independent signals [21]. The lysosomal alterations in cystinosis lead to defective autophagic clearance of damaged mitochondria [12], therefore the purpose of our study was to investigate mitochondrial dynamics in *CTNS−/−* conditionally immortalized proximal tubular epithelial cells (ciPTEC) carrying the classical homozygous 57-kb deletion in the intent of identifying new therapeutic targets and biomarkers for treatment follow-up.

## 2. Results

### *2.1. CTNS−/− ciPTEC Showed Deregulation of Proteins Involved in Mitochondrial Fission/Fusion Processes*

Recruitment of the GTPase dynamin-related protein 1 (Drp1) to mitochondria is a key step required for mitochondrial fission and its reversible phosphorylation was implicated in the regulation of this process. The analysis of phosphorylated Drp1 at Ser-637 (Drp1$^{pS637}$) showed high variability of protein phosphorylation with no significant differences in wild type and CTNS−/− ciPTEC, also 24 h treatment with 100 μM cysteamine (MEA) did not affect Drp1$^{pS637}$phosphorylation (Figure 1). The western blotting of the pro-fission mitochondrial protein Fis1 revealed the ubiquitinated and not-ubiquitinated forms of protein. *CTNS−/−* ciPTEC showed increased level of Fis1 (2.47 ± 0.27 vs. 1.08 ± 0.08, $p = 0.0027$). Treatment with 100 μM MEA for 24 h further increased total Fis1 protein level (2.47 ± 0.27 vs. 3.59 ± 0.15, $p = 0.011$) but almost completely reduced the ubiquitinated counterpart by 96.3% ($p < 0.001$) (Figure 1). Third key regulatory protein analyzed was mitochondrial fission factor (Mff), which localizes on OMM and promotes the recruitment of DRP1 to the mitochondrial surface. This protein, shown in its four isoforms, was not modified in *CTNS−/−* ciPTEC and the expression was unchanged after MEA treatment (Figure 1).

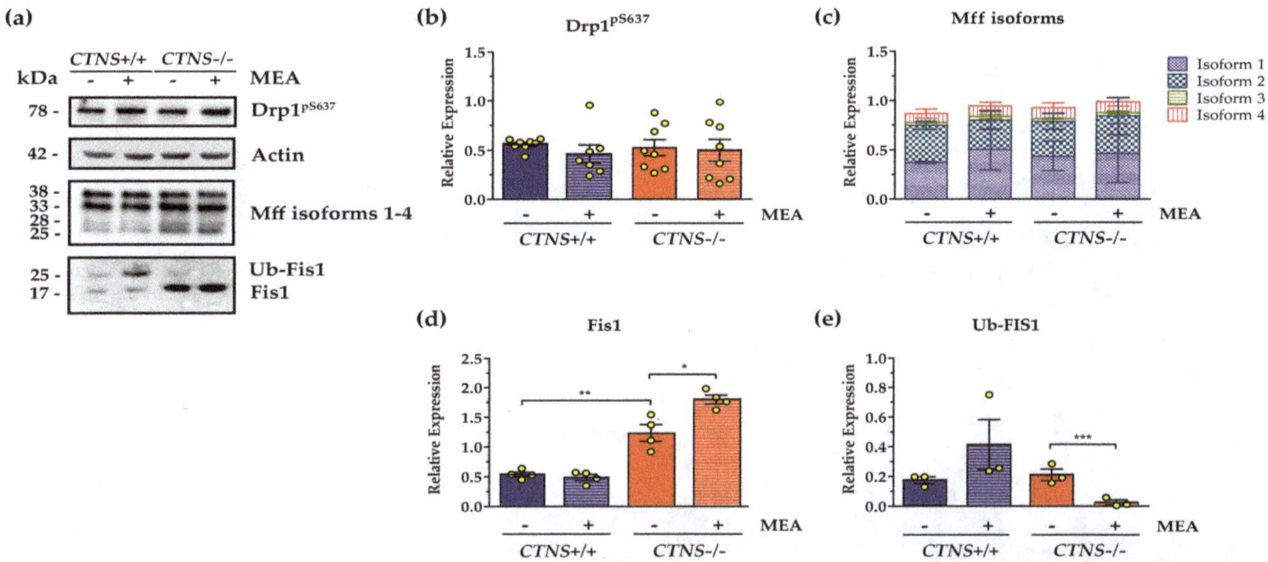


**Figure 1.** Analysis of proteins involved in fission process of mitochondrial dynamics in untreated and cysteamine (MEA)-treated *CTNS−/−*compared to *CTNS+/+*. Cell cultures were treated with 100 μM cysteamine (MEA) or DMSO (vehicle) for 24 h as specified in the figure. (**a**) Representative immunoblotting analysis in cellular lysate of conditionally immortalized proximal tubular epithelial cells (ciPTEC) from a healthy subject (*CTNS+/+*) and cystinotic patient (*CTNS−/−*). (**b**–**e**) The histograms (Drp1$^{pS637}$, panel (**b**), $n = 8$; mitochondrial fission factor (Mff), panel (**c**), $n = 3$; mitochondrial fission 1 protein (Fis1), panel (**d**), $n = 4$; ubiquitinated Fis1 (Ub-Fis1), panel (**e**), $n = 3$) represent the means values ± SEM of the relative expression normalized on actin level. Densitometric analysis was performed by Versa-Doc imaging system BioRad, using Quantity One software. $p$-value less than 0.05 was considered as statistically significant, (Student's $t$ test, *** $p < 0.001$; ** $p < 0.01$; * $p < 0.05$). For further details see under "materials and methods" section.

The inner mitochondrial membrane GTPase OPA1 undergoes constitutive processing leading to the conversion of the un-cleaved long OPA1 (L-OPA1) in cleaved short variants (S-OPA1). Various stress conditions, including apoptotic stimuli, trigger the complete conversion of L-OPA1 into S-OPA1. In this regard, *CTNS−/−* ciPTEC were characterized by a significant increase of short variants (52.4%, $p < 0.05$), but 24 h treatment with 100 μM MEA did not show significant effects (Figure 2). In agreement with higher S-OPA1 levels, we found that the active form of mitochondrial metallo-endopetidase OMA1, which catalyze conversion of OPA1 into short isoforms and triggers mitochondrial fragmentation, was increased by 79.8% in *CTNS−/−* ciPTEC ($p < 0.001$), and not rescued by MEA treatment (Figure 2). OPA1 can oligomerize at the inner mitochondrial membrane to keep the cristae junction tight, therefore cell fresh pellets were treated with the cross-linker bis-maleimidohexane (BMH) 1 mM or with vehicle to test the oligomeric state of OPA1. The OPA1 oligomer, immune-revealed as a high molecular-weight band (≈250 kDa), decreased in *CTNS−/−* cells by 23.5% compared to *CTNS+/+* cells and was not affected by MEA treatment. The absence of OPA1 oligomerization in cells treated with vehicle (DMSO) confirmed the specificity of cross-linking (Figure 2).

The expression of MFN2, an outer mitochondrial membrane GTPase involved in fusion processes, was not changed in *CTNS−/−* ciPTEC with respect to control cells (Figure 3). However, the higher molecular weight band, corresponding to ubiquitinated MFN2, indicated an increase of ubiquitination in *CTNS−/−* ciPTEC by 70.8% ($p < 0.001$). Treatment with MEA showed 37.8% reduction of ubiquitination but the effect was not statistically significant (Figure 3).

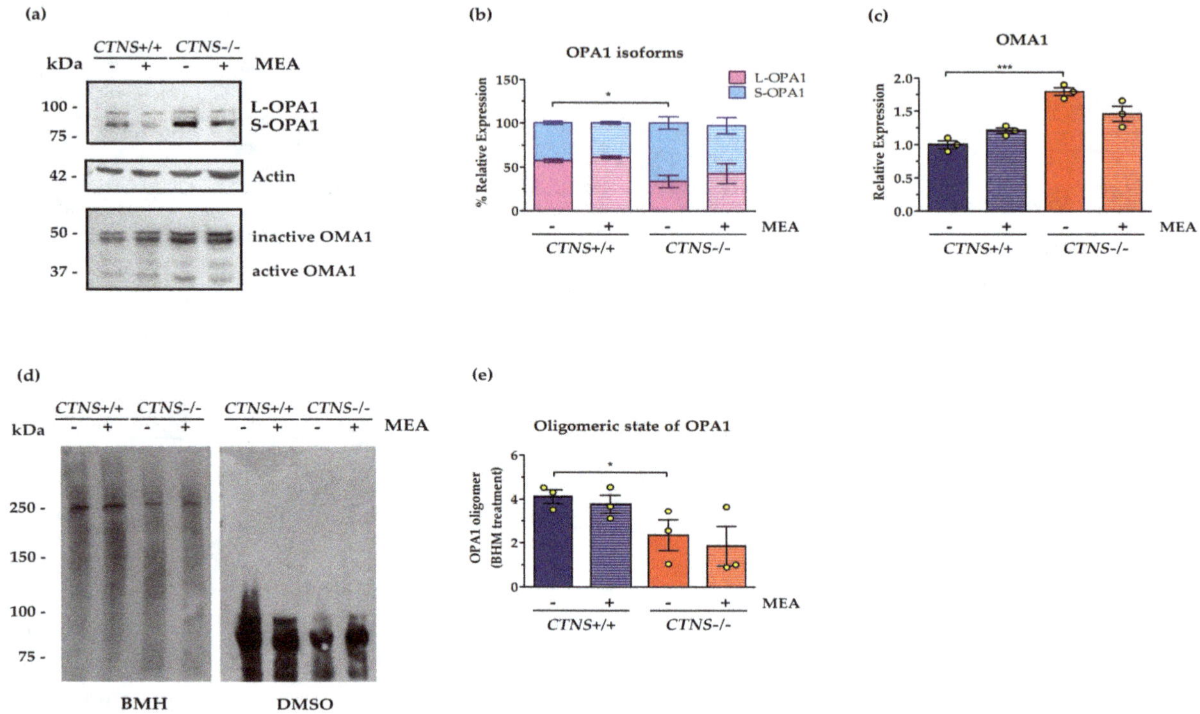


**Figure 2.** Processing and oligomerization of optic atrophy 1 (OPA1) fusion protein in untreated and MEA-treated *CTNS−/−* compared to *CTNS+/+*. (**a**) Representative immunoblotting analysis of ciPTEC obtained from *CTNS+/+* and *CTNS−/−*. Where indicated, the cells were treated with MEA or DMSO (vehicle) for 24 h. The histograms of OPA1 (**b**) represent the percentage of relative expression of L and S forms of OPA1 in each lane ($n = 3$). The histograms of OMA1 (**c**) represent the means values ± SEM of the relative expression normalized on actin level ($n = 3$). (**d**) The fresh collected cells were treated with the cross-linker 1,6-bismaleimidohexane (BMH) 1 mM or with vehicle (DMSO) for 30 min at 37 °C, then centrifuged and resuspended in sodium dodecyl sulfate (SDS) lysis buffer for western blotting analysis with the antibody against OPA1. (**e**) The histograms represent the means values ± SEM of the relative expression of OPA1 oligomers ($n = 3$). Densitometric analysis was performed by Versa-Doc imaging system BioRad, using Quantity One software. Student's *t* test, *** $p < 0.001$; * $p < 0.05$. For further details see under "materials and methods" section.

Numerous mitochondrial outer membrane proteins are modified with K48- and K63-linked ubiquitin chains, including the mitochondrial fusion factors MFN1 and MFN2 and fission factors Fis1 and Drp1, triggering a cascade of events that result in mitophagy. According with previous results, we found in *CTNS−/−* ciPTEC a significant increase in protein levels of the E3 ubiquitin ligase parkin (2.92 ± 0.22 in *CTNS−/−* vs. 1.0 ± 0.04 in *CTNS+/+*, $p = 0.001$). MEA treatment did not change parkin expression (Figure 4A). Ubiquitin carboxyl-terminal hydrolase 30 (USP30) mediates the removal of the ubiquitin chains added by parkin to ubiquitilated forms of mitofusins, such as MFN2, therefore we analyzed the expression of this deubiquitinating enzyme tethered to the OMM and showed in *CTNS−/−* ciPTEC 62.9% decreasing compared to wild type cells ($p < 0.001$). Treatment with MEA rescued USP30 expression in *CTNS−/−* ciPTEC by 87.9% ($p = 0.037$) (Figure 4B).

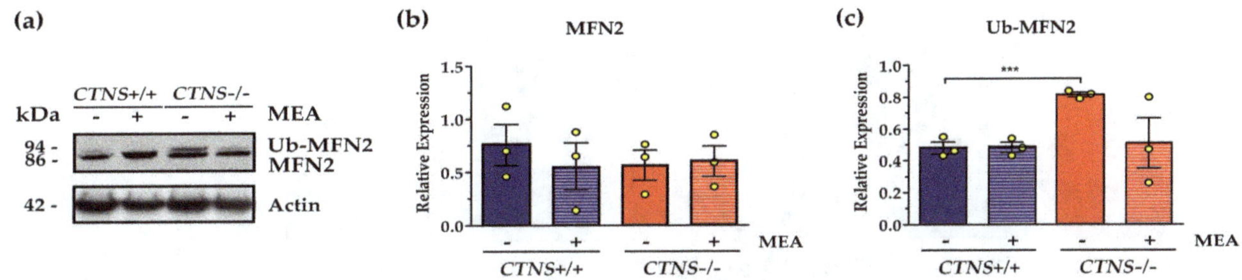


**Figure 3.** Expression and ubiquitination of mitofusin 2 (MFN2) in untreated and MEA-treated *CTNS+/+* and *CTNS−/−*. (**a**) Representative immunoblotting analysis of untreated and MEA-treated ciPTEC *CTNS+/+* and *CTNS−/−*. (**b**) The histogram of MFN2, $n = 3$, and (**c**) the histogram of ubiquitinated MFN2 Ub-MFN2, $n = 3$, represent the mean values ± SEM of the relative expression normalized on actin level. Densitometric analysis was performed by Versa-Doc imaging system BioRad, using Quantity One software. Student's *t* test, *** $p < 0.001$.

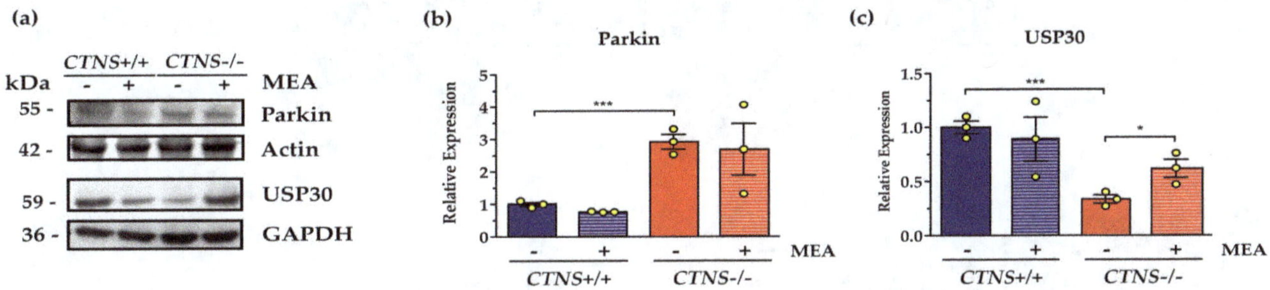


**Figure 4.** Parkin and ubiquitin carboxyl-terminal hydrolase 30 (USP30) proteins levels and MEA effect in *CTNS+/+* and *CTNS−/−*. (**a**) Immunoblotting analysis of untreated and MEA-treated ciPTEC *CTNS+/+* and *CTNS−/−*. (**b**) The histogram represents the means values ± SEM of the relative expression of Parkin normalized on actin level ($n = 3$). (**c**) The histogram represents the means values ± SEM of the relative expression of USP30 normalized on actin level ($n = 3$). Densitometric analysis was performed by Versa-Doc imaging system BioRad, using Quantity One software. Student's *t* test, *** $p < 0.001$; * $p < 0.05$.

### 2.2. *Mitochondrial Cristae Organization Was Impaired in CTNS−/− ciPTEC*

Comparative ultrastructural analysis of mitochondria in ciPTEC, by transmission electron microscopy (TEM), showed the presence of smaller mitochondria in *CTNS−/−* ciPTEC compared to *CTNS+/+* ciPTEC (0.12 ± 0.01 $\mu m^2$ in *CTNS−/−* vs. 0.26 ± 0.01 $\mu m^2$ in *CTNS+/+*, $p < 0.0001$). Mitochondrial area was completely recovered by MEA treatment (0.32 ± 0.04 $\mu m^2$ in *CTNS−/−* + MEA vs. 0.12 ± 0.01 $\mu m^2$ in *CTNS−/−*, $p < 0.0001$). Moreover, TEM showed a substantial reduction in number of cristae per mitochondrial section in *CTNS−/−* (5.1 ± 0.6 in *CTNS+/+* vs. 1.6 ± 0.2 in *CTNS−/−*, $p < 0.0001$). This parameter was rescued by MEA by 167.5% ($p < 0.0001$). Because evidences underlined a critical role of cristae junction in mitochondrial function and organization, we measured them. It was found an increase in cristae junction width (39.65 ± 4.83 nm in *CTNS+/+* vs. 53.21 ± 10.05 nm in *CTNS−/−*, $p < 0.0001$) and cristae lumen width (29.68 ± 3.53 nm in *CTNS+/+* vs. 37.04 ± 6.13 nm in *CTNS−/−*, $p < 0.0003$) partially rescued by cysteamine (Figure 5).

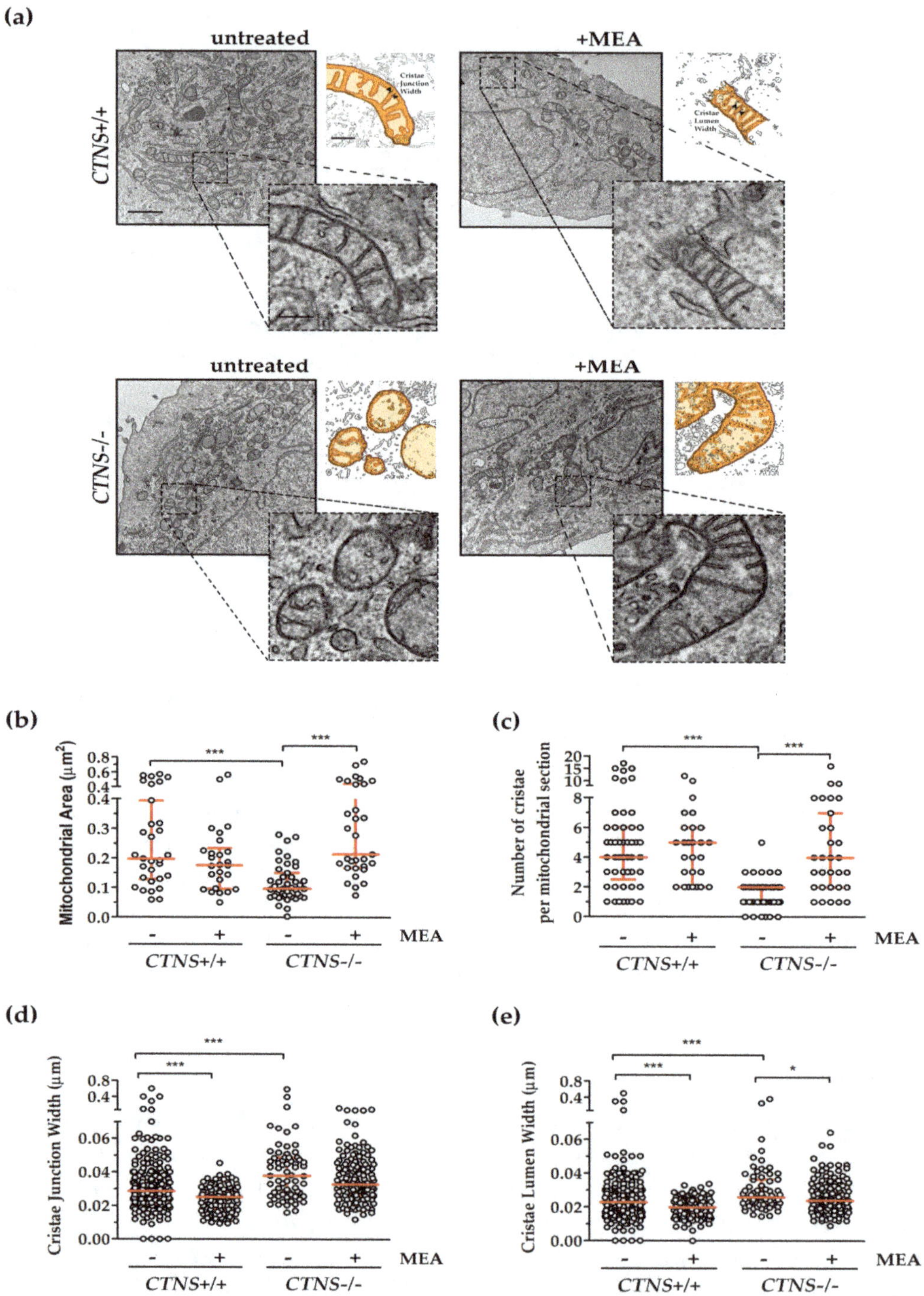


**Figure 5.** Comparative ultrastructural analysis of mitochondria in ciPTEC. (**a**) Representative images of TEM with magnification 16,000× of untreated and MEA-treated ciPTEC *CTNS*+/+ and *CTNS*−/−; scale bar = 1 μm. As shown in high magnification cropped micrographs and in ad hoc schematic reconstruction, mitochondria kept preserved ultrastructure in ciPTEC *CTNS*+/+ and in MEA-treated ciPTEC *CTNS*+/+ and *CTNS*−/−, whereas ciPTEC *CTNS*−/− showed disruption of mitochondrial cristae and the disarrangement of the internal structures; scale bar = 200 nm. (**b**–**e**) Quantitative analysis was performed with ImageJ v.1.52p in $n \geq 5$ double-blind acquisitions for each experimental condition, red lines represent median with interquartile range. (**b**) Evaluation of relative mitochondrial size measured as area of $n \geq 27$ mitochondrial sections. (**c**) Average number of cristae per mitochondrion in each cell ($n \geq 27$ mitochondrial sections). (**d**) The measure of distance of cristae junction near the inner membrane boundary and (**e**) the measure of cristae lumen, assessed on cristae membranes that outline the lumen boundary, were assessed in $n \geq 100$ cristae. Non-parametric Mann-Whitney test was applied, *** $p < 0.001$; * $p < 0.05$.

## 3. Discussion

Nephropathic cystinosis is a rare inherited metabolic disorder, belonging to the group of lysosomal storage diseases (LSD). The disease is the first cause of Fanconi syndrome in children, characterized by loss of electrolytes, glucose, amino acid, low-molecular weight proteins in urine caused by proximal tubule dysfunction [4,22]. The molecular mechanism at the basis of Fanconi syndrome in cystinosis is not completely understood. Several mechanisms have been suggested to contribute to the pathogenesis of cystinosis, including lysosomal overload, endo-lysosomal transport defect, altered chaperone-mediated autophagy, mTOR signaling, transcription factor EB (TFEB) expression [11,13,23–27]. Cysteamine, a cystine-depleting agent, which allows clearance of cystine from lysosomes, represents the only specific treatment for cystinosis. However, cysteamine does not correct the above cited cellular alterations and does not stop the progress of the Fanconi syndrome. Our recent studies have shown in *CTNS−/−* ciPTEC a higher mitochondrial fragmentation index associated with lower mitochondrial potential and mitochondrial cyclic AMP levels, rescued by 24 h treatment with 100 μM cysteamine or with the cell-permeant analogue of cyclic AMP, 8-Br-cAMP [8]. cAMP, in fact, is one of the major regulators of mitochondrial function [28–30] and dynamics [31]. In this contest, it should be noted that MEA has been found to improve mitochondrial function in mitochondrial respiratory chain diseases [32]. Mitochondrial dynamics is balanced between rates of fusion and fission that respond to pathophysiologic signals. This finely regulated equilibrium is closely related to the quality control system, which is mainly ascribed to the ubiquitin protease system (UPS) and to the intra-mitochondrial proteolytic systems [33]. In our experimental model, no significant differences were observed on protein levels of phosphorylated Drp1 at Ser-637. The PKA-dependent phosphorylation of Drp1 at Ser-637 is generally recognized to block Drp1 GTPase activity and to suppress mitochondrial fission. However, and in agreement with data previously reported by Yu et al., Drp1$^{pS637}$ did not contribute substantially to mitochondrial fission regulation in *CTNS−/−* ciPTEC [18]. Several key effector proteins of mitochondrial fusion (MFN1 and MFN2) and fission (Fis1, Mff) are located at the OMM with their domains exposed at the cytosolic side of the membrane. This peculiar topology allows selective removing of fusion or fission components exposed by the UPS, providing fine tuning of this high-level regulatory processes. In mammalian cells, Fis1 accumulates in the mitochondrial outer membrane during the fission process, whereas MFN1 and MFN2 are ubiquitinated and degraded by the proteasome [34]. In this respect, we observed an increase in Fis1, ubiquitinated MFN2 and of the E3 ubiquitin ligase Parkin in *CTNS−/−* ciPTEC, indicating the tendency to mitochondrial fragmentation. The effect of MEA on the reduction of ubiquitilated MFN2 could be ascribed to the modulation of USP30, a mitochondrion-localized deubiquitilase, which counteracts Parkin by deubiquitilating OMM proteins and regulate mitophagy [35]. These findings are consistent with data showing that an increase of parkin expression results in mitochondrial fragmentation [36] and is associated with MFN2 ubiquitination [37]. In addition, the increase of FIS1, in cystinotic cell, might be due to Sirt3 protein [38] that was found downregulated in the same cystinotic cell line [8]. OPA1, an inner mitochondrial membrane GTPase protein, has gained attention because it regulates important mitochondrial functions, including the balance between mitochondrial fusion and fission processes, the stability of the mitochondrial respiratory chain complexes, the proapoptotic release of cytochrome *c* molecules sequestered within the mitochondrial cristae and the maintenance of mitochondrial cristae architecture [39]. The protein expression levels of OPA1 were not significantly changed in mutated cells, compared to control ciPTEC cells (data not shown). However, the activity of OPA1 is also controlled at the post-translational level by proteolytic and acetylation changes [31]. Various stress conditions, including apoptotic stimulation, trigger the complete conversion of L-OPA1 into S-OPA1. The pro-fusion activity of OPA1 depends on the balanced formation of L-OPA1 and S-OPA1 [40]. In this respect, we observed an alteration of OPA1 processing in *CTNS−/−* ciPTEC cells. In particular, cystinotic cells were characterized by a significant increase of S-OPA1, associated with an increase in the protease OMA1 activity, that was not prevented by MEA. In addition to its role as a fusion protein, OPA1 controls the remodeling of mitochondrial cristae. Specifically, OPA1 forms oligomers in the inner mitochondrial membrane that keep the cristae junctions tight. During apoptosis, oligomers are destabilized causing the opening of cristae and release of cytochrome *c* out of the mitochondria. OPA1 oligomers were decreased in cystinotic cells. MEA did not rescue this phenotype. This defect correlates with increased cristae junction width that we observed in our TEM ultrastructural analyses.

In summary, our study shows deregulation of several proteins involved in mitochondrial dynamics in *CTNS−/−* cells. We observed mitochondrial fragmentation in cystinotic cells associated with altered proteolytic processing of OPA1, increased Fis1 and parkin protein levels. The deregulation of parkin could result in increase of ubiquitination of MFN2. The cristae number was decreased while the cristae lumen was increased in cystinotic cells, which parallels the previously reported bioenergetic defects in these cells. The cristae junction width was increased in *CTNS−/−* cells, which is most likely secondary to low OPA1 oligomerization levels. MEA treatment restored mitochondrial size, cristae number, and lumen, but had no effect on cristae junction width, making tubular cells more susceptible to apoptotic stimuli. In this contest, we highlight several cellular mediators of mitochondrial dynamics that could be useful to develop new therapeutic interventions [41].

## 4. Materials and Methods

### 4.1. Cell Culture

Conditionally immortalized proximal tubular epithelial cells (ciPTEC), from healthy donor and cystinotic patients were obtained from Radboud University Medical Center, Nijmegen, The Netherlands and cultured as described in [42]. Cells were grown in a humidified atmosphere with 5% $CO_2$ at 37 °C. Where indicated, the cells were treated with 100 μM MEA or water (vehicle) for 24 h.

### 4.2. SDS-PAGE and Western Blotting

Monolayer cell cultures were harvested with 0.05% trypsin, 0.02% EDTA. After trypsinization, cells were centrifuged at 500× *g* and resuspended in RIPA buffer (150 mM NaCl, 5 mM EDTA, 50 mM Tris/HCl, 0.1% SDS, 1% Triton X-100, pH 7.4), in the presence of a protease inhibitor (0.25 mM PMSF). Cell lysate proteins were subjected to SDS-polyacrylamide gel electrophoresis (PAGE), transferred to a nitrocellulose membrane and immunoblotted with antibodies against OPA1 (Thermo scientific, Waltham, MA, USA; Pierce Antibodies); Fis1, Mfn2 (Merck Millipore, Burlington, MA, USA); parkin, USP30 (Santa Cruz Biotechnology, Dallas, TX, USA); OMA1 (Abcam, Cambridge, UK); Drp1, Mff (Cell Signaling, Danvers, MA, USA) and actin (Merck, Kenilworth, NJ, USA). After being washed in TTBS, the membranes were incubated for 1 h with anti-mouse or anti-rabbit IgG peroxidase-conjugate antibody. Immunodetection was performed with the enhanced chemiluminescence (ECL) (Thermo scientific, Waltham, MA, USA). VersaDoc imaging system (BioRad, Milan, Italy) was used for densitometric analysis.

### 4.3. Analysis of OPA1 Oligomers

To investigate on OPA1 oligomerization, cell fresh pellets were treated with the cross-linker bismaleimidohexane (BMH) 1 mM or with vehicle (DMSO) for 30 min at 37 °C. After incubation, the samples were centrifuged, resuspended in SDS lysis buffer and then subjected to SDS-PAGE and western blotting analysis with the antibody against OPA1.

### 4.4. Electron Microscopy

For routine EM the cells were grown in 12 well plates as a monolayer. At the end of the experiment the cells were fixed with 1% Glutaraldehyde prepared in 0.2 M Hepes buffer. Then the cells were scraped, pelleted, post-fixed in OsO4 and uranyl acetate and embedded in Epon as described previously [43]. From each sample, thin 60 nm sections were cut using Leica EM UC7 (Leica Microsystems, Vienna, Austria). EM images were acquired from thin sections using a FEI Tecnai-12 electron microscope

(FEI, Eindhoven, Netherlands) equipped with a VELETTA CCD digital camera (Soft Imaging Systems GmbH, Munster, Germany).

**Author Contributions:** F.B. and D.D.R. conceptualization; A.S., E.D.L., E.V.P., A.F., R.R., and S.R. investigation; F.B. and D.D.R. writing—original draft preparation; F.B., D.D.R., A.S., R.P., and F.E. writing—review and editing; F.B. and D.D.R. funding acquisition. All authors have read and agreed to the published version of the manuscript.

**Acknowledgments:** We thank Paolo Lattanzio for technical assistance and Manuela Colucci for statistical analysis contribution.

## Abbreviations

| | |
|---|---|
| cAMP | 3′,5′-cyclic adenosine monophosphate |
| Fis1 | Mitochondrial fission 1 protein |
| IMM | Inner Mitochondrial Membrane |
| MEA | β-Mercaptoethylamine (cysteamine) |
| Mff | Mitochondrial fission factor |
| OMM | Outer Mitochondrial Membrane |
| OPA1 | Dynamin-related GTPases Optic Atrophy 1 |
| TEMTFEB | Transmission Electron MicroscopyTranscription factor EB |
| UPS | Ubiquitin Protease System |
| USP30 | Ubiquitin carboxyl-terminal hydrolase 30 |

## References

1. Cherqui, S.; Sevin, C.; Hamard, G.; Kalatzis, V.; Sich, M.; Pequignot, M.O.; Gogat, K.; Abitbol, M.; Broyer, M.; Gubler, M.C.; et al. Intralysosomal Cystine Accumulation in Mice Lacking Cystinosin, the Protein Defective in Cystinosis. *Mol. Cell. Biol.* **2002**, *22*, 7622–7632. [CrossRef] [PubMed]
2. Gahl, W.A.; Bashan, N.; Tietze, F.; Bernardini, I.; Schulman, J.D. Cystine Transport is Defective in Isolated Leukocyte Lysosomes from Patients with Cystinosis. *Science* **1982**, *217*, 1263–1265. [CrossRef] [PubMed]
3. Town, M.; Jean, G.; Cherqui, S.; Attard, M.; Forestier, L.; Whitmore, S.A.; Callen, D.F.; Gribouval, O.; Broyer, M.; Bates, G.P.; et al. A Novel Gene Encoding an Integral Membrane Protein is Mutated in Nephropathic Cystinosis. *Nat. Genet.* **1998**, *18*, 319–324. [CrossRef] [PubMed]
4. Cherqui, S.; Courtoy, P.J. The Renal Fanconi Syndrome in Cystinosis: Pathogenic Insights and Therapeutic Perspectives. *Nat. Rev. Nephrol.* **2017**, *13*, 115–131. [CrossRef] [PubMed]
5. Conforti, A.; Taranta, A.; Biagini, S.; Starc, N.; Pitisci, A.; Bellomo, F.; Cirillo, V.; Locatelli, F.; Bernardo, M.E.; Emma, F. Cysteamine Treatment Restores the in Vitro Ability to Differentiate Along the Osteoblastic Lineage of Mesenchymal Stromal Cells Isolated from Bone Marrow of a Cystinotic Patient. *J. Transl. Med.* **2015**, *13*, 143. [CrossRef] [PubMed]
6. Medic, G.; van der Weijden, M.; Karabis, A.; Hemels, M. A Systematic Literature Review of Cysteamine Bitartrate in the Treatment of Nephropathic Cystinosis. *Curr. Med. Res. Opin.* **2017**, *33*, 2065–2076. [CrossRef] [PubMed]
7. Emma, F.; Montini, G.; Parikh, S.M.; Salviati, L. Mitochondrial Dysfunction in Inherited Renal Disease and Acute Kidney Injury. *Nat. Rev. Nephrol.* **2016**, *12*, 267–280. [CrossRef]
8. Bellomo, F.; Signorile, A.; Tamma, G.; Ranieri, M.; Emma, F.; De Rasmo, D. Impact of Atypical Mitochondrial Cyclic-AMP Level in Nephropathic Cystinosis. *Cell Mol. Life Sci.* **2018**, *75*, 3411–3422. [CrossRef]
9. Park, M.; Helip-Wooley, A.; Thoene, J. Lysosomal Cystine Storage Augments Apoptosis in Cultured Human Fibroblasts and Renal Tubular Epithelial Cells. *J. Am. Soc. Nephrol.* **2002**, *13*, 2878–2887. [CrossRef]
10. Taranta, A.; Bellomo, F.; Petrini, S.; Polishchuk, E.; De Leo, E.; Rega, L.R.; Pastore, A.; Polishchuk, R.; De Matteis, M.A.; Emma, F. Cystinosin-LKG Rescues Cystine Accumulation and Decreases Apoptosis Rate in Cystinotic Proximal Tubular Epithelial Cells. *Pediatr. Res.* **2016**, *81*, 113. [CrossRef]
11. Napolitano, G.; Johnson, J.L.; He, J.; Rocca, C.J.; Monfregola, J.; Pestonjamasp, K.; Cherqui, S.; Catz, S.D. Impairment of Chaperone-Mediated Autophagy Leads to Selective Lysosomal Degradation Defects in the Lysosomal Storage Disease Cystinosis. *EMBO Mol. Med.* **2015**, *7*, 158–174. [CrossRef] [PubMed]
12. Festa, B.P.; Chen, Z.; Berquez, M.; Debaix, H.; Tokonami, N.; Prange, J.A.; Hoek, G.V.; Alessio, C.; Raimondi, A.; Nevo, N.; et al. Impaired Autophagy Bridges Lysosomal Storage Disease and Epithelial Dysfunction in the Kidney. *Nat. Commun.* **2018**, *9*, 161. [CrossRef] [PubMed]

13. Raggi, C.; Luciani, A.; Nevo, N.; Antignac, C.; Terryn, S.; Devuyst, O. Dedifferentiation and Aberrations of the Endolysosomal Compartment Characterize the Early Stage of Nephropathic Cystinosis. *Hum. Mol. Genet.* **2014**, *23*, 2266–2278. [CrossRef] [PubMed]
14. Ivanova, E.A.; De Leo, M.G.; Van Den Heuvel, L.; Pastore, A.; Dijkman, H.; De Matteis, M.A.; Levtchenko, E.N. Endo-Lysosomal Dysfunction in Human Proximal Tubular Epithelial Cells Deficient for Lysosomal Cystine Transporter Cystinosin. *PLoS ONE* **2015**, *10*, 120998. [CrossRef]
15. Soto-Heredero, G.; Baixauli, F.; Mittelbrunn, M. Interorganelle Communication between Mitochondria and the Endolysosomal System. *Front. Cell. Dev. Biol.* **2017**, *5*, 95. [CrossRef]
16. Wong, Y.C.; Ysselstein, D.; Krainc, D. Mitochondria-Lysosome Contacts Regulate Mitochondrial Fission via RAB7 GTP Hydrolysis. *Nature* **2018**, *554*, 382–386. [CrossRef]
17. Koirala, S.; Guo, Q.; Kalia, R.; Bui, H.T.; Eckert, D.M.; Frost, A.; Shaw, J.M. Interchangeable Adaptors Regulate Mitochondrial Dynamin Assembly for Membrane Scission. *Proc. Natl. Acad. Sci. USA* **2013**, *110*, 1342–1351. [CrossRef]
18. Yu, R.; Liu, T.; Ning, C.; Tan, F.; Jin, S.B.; Lendahl, U.; Zhao, J.; Nister, M. The Phosphorylation Status of Ser-637 in Dynamin-Related Protein 1 (Drp1) does Not Determine Drp1 Recruitment to Mitochondria. *J. Biol. Chem.* **2019**, *294*, 17262–17277. [CrossRef]
19. Pernas, L.; Scorrano, L. Mito-Morphosis: Mitochondrial Fusion, Fission, and Cristae Remodeling as Key Mediators of Cellular Function. *Annu. Rev. Physiol.* **2016**, *78*, 505–531. [CrossRef]
20. Zhang, J.; Liu, X.; Liang, X.; Lu, Y.; Zhu, L.; Fu, R.; Ji, Y.; Fan, W.; Chen, J.; Lin, B.; et al. A Novel ADOA-Associated OPA1 Mutation Alters the Mitochondrial Function, Membrane Potential, ROS Production and Apoptosis. *Sci. Rep.* **2017**, *7*, 5704. [CrossRef]
21. Khaminets, A.; Behl, C.; Dikic, I. Ubiquitin-Dependent and Independent Signals in Selective Autophagy. *Trends Cell Biol.* **2016**, *26*, 6–16. [CrossRef] [PubMed]
22. Emma, F.; Nesterova, G.; Langman, C.; Labbe, A.; Cherqui, S.; Goodyer, P.; Janssen, M.C.; Greco, M.; Topaloglu, R.; Elenberg, E.; et al. Nephropathic Cystinosis: An International Consensus Document. *Nephrol. Dial. Transplant.* **2014**, *29*, 87–94. [CrossRef] [PubMed]
23. Gaide Chevronnay, H.P.; Janssens, V.; Van Der Smissen, P.; N'Kuli, F.; Nevo, N.; Guiot, Y.; Levtchenko, E.; Marbaix, E.; Pierreux, C.E.; Cherqui, S.; et al. Time Course of Pathogenic and Adaptation Mechanisms in Cystinotic Mouse Kidneys. *J. Am. Soc. Nephrol.* **2014**, *25*, 1256–1269. [CrossRef] [PubMed]
24. Johnson, J.L.; Napolitano, G.; Monfregola, J.; Rocca, C.J.; Cherqui, S.; Catz, S.D. Upregulation of the Rab27a-Dependent Trafficking and Secretory Mechanisms Improves Lysosomal Transport, Alleviates Endoplasmic Reticulum Stress, and Reduces Lysosome Overload in Cystinosis. *Mol. Cell. Biol.* **2013**, *33*, 2950–2962. [CrossRef] [PubMed]
25. Ivanova, E.A.; van den Heuvel, L.P.; Elmonem, M.A.; De Smedt, H.; Missiaen, L.; Pastore, A.; Mekahli, D.; Bultynck, G.; Levtchenko, E.N. Altered mTOR Signalling in Nephropathic Cystinosis. *J. Inherit. Metab. Dis.* **2016**, *39*, 457–464. [CrossRef]
26. Andrzejewska, Z.; Nevo, N.; Thomas, L.; Chhuon, C.; Bailleux, A.; Chauvet, V.; Courtoy, P.J.; Chol, M.; Guerrera, I.C.; Antignac, C. Cystinosin is a Component of the Vacuolar H+-ATPase-Ragulator-Rag Complex Controlling Mammalian Target of Rapamycin Complex 1 Signaling. *J. Am. Soc. Nephrol.* **2016**, *27*, 1678–1688. [CrossRef]
27. Rega, L.R.; Polishchuk, E.; Montefusco, S.; Napolitano, G.; Tozzi, G.; Zhang, J.; Bellomo, F.; Taranta, A.; Pastore, A.; Polishchuk, R.; et al. Activation of the Transcription Factor EB Rescues Lysosomal Abnormalities in Cystinotic Kidney Cells. *Kidney Int.* **2016**, *89*, 862–873. [CrossRef]
28. De Rasmo, D.; Signorile, A.; Santeramo, A.; Larizza, M.; Lattanzio, P.; Capitanio, G.; Papa, S. Intramitochondrial Adenylyl Cyclase Controls the Turnover of Nuclear-Encoded Subunits and Activity of Mammalian Complex I of the Respiratory Chain. *Biochim. Biophys. Acta* **2015**, *1853*, 183–191. [CrossRef]
29. Papa, S.; Scacco, S.; De Rasmo, D.; Signorile, A.; Papa, F.; Panelli, D.; Nicastro, A.; Scaringi, R.; Santeramo, A.; Roca, E. cAMP-Dependent Protein Kinase Regulates Post-Translational Processing and Expression of Complex I Subunits in Mammalian Cells. *Biochim. Biophys. Acta* **2010**, *1797*, 649–658. [CrossRef]
30. Signorile, A.; Micelli, L.; De Rasmo, D.; Santeramo, A.; Papa, F.; Ficarella, R.; Gattoni, G.; Scacco, S.; Papa, S. Regulation of the Biogenesis of OXPHOS Complexes in Cell Transition from Replicating to Quiescent State: Involvement of PKA and Effect of Hydroxytyrosol. *Biochim. Biophys. Acta* **2014**, *1843*, 675–684. [CrossRef]
31. Signorile, A.; Santeramo, A.; Tamma, G.; Pellegrino, T.; D'Oria, S.; Lattanzio, P.; De Rasmo, D. Mitochondrial

cAMP Prevents Apoptosis Modulating Sirt3 Protein Level and OPA1 Processing in Cardiac Myoblast Cells. *Biochim. Biophys. Acta* **2017**, *1864*, 355–366. [CrossRef] [PubMed]

32. Guha, S.; Konkwo, C.; Lavorato, M.; Mathew, N.D.; Peng, M.; Ostrovsky, J.; Kwon, Y.J.; Polyak, E.; Lightfoot, R.; Seiler, C.; et al. Pre-Clinical Evaluation of Cysteamine Bitartrate as a Therapeutic Agent for Mitochondrial Respiratory Chain Disease. *Hum. Mol. Genet.* **2019**, *28*, 1837–1852. [CrossRef]
33. Ali, S.; McStay, G.P. Regulation of Mitochondrial Dynamics by Proteolytic Processing and Protein Turnover. *Antioxidants* **2018**, *7*, 15.
34. Bragoszewski, P.; Turek, M.; Chacinska, A. Control of Mitochondrial Biogenesis and Function by the Ubiquitin-Proteasome System. *Open Biol.* **2017**, *7*, 170007. [CrossRef] [PubMed]
35. Liang, J.R.; Martinez, A.; Lane, J.D.; Mayor, U.; Clague, M.J.; Urbe, S. USP30 Deubiquitylates Mitochondrial Parkin Substrates and Restricts Apoptotic Cell Death. *EMBO Rep.* **2015**, *16*, 618–627. [CrossRef] [PubMed]
36. Yu, W.; Sun, Y.; Guo, S.; Lu, B. The PINK1/Parkin Pathway Regulates Mitochondrial Dynamics and Function in Mammalian Hippocampal and Dopaminergic Neurons. *Hum. Mol. Genet.* **2011**, *20*, 3227–3240. [CrossRef] [PubMed]
37. Tanaka, A.; Cleland, M.M.; Xu, S.; Narendra, D.P.; Suen, D.F.; Karbowski, M.; Youle, R.J. Proteasome and p97 Mediate Mitophagy and Degradation of Mitofusins Induced by Parkin. *J. Cell Biol.* **2010**, *191*, 1367–1380. [CrossRef]
38. Zhou, J.; Shi, M.; Li, M.; Cheng, L.; Yang, J.; Huang, X. Sirtuin 3 Inhibition Induces Mitochondrial Stress in Tongue Cancer by Targeting Mitochondrial Fission and the JNK-Fis1 Biological Axis. *Cell Stress Chaperones* **2019**, *24*, 369–383. [CrossRef]
39. Burte, F.; Carelli, V.; Chinnery, P.F.; Yu-Wai-Man, P. Disturbed Mitochondrial Dynamics and Neurodegenerative Disorders. *Nat. Rev. Neurol.* **2015**, *11*, 11–24. [CrossRef]
40. Lee, H.; Smith, S.B.; Yoon, Y. The Short Variant of the Mitochondrial Dynamin OPA1 Maintains Mitochondrial Energetics and Cristae Structure. *J. Biol. Chem.* **2017**, *292*, 7115–7130. [CrossRef]
41. Bellomo, F.; Medina, D.L.; De Leo, E.; Panarella, A.; Emma, F. High-Content Drug Screening for Rare Diseases. *J. Inherit. Metab. Dis.* **2017**, *40*, 601–607. [CrossRef] [PubMed]
42. Wilmer, M.J.; Emma, F.; Levtchenko, E.N. The Pathogenesis of Cystinosis: Mechanisms beyond Cystine Accumulation. *Am. J. Physiol. Renal Physiol.* **2010**, *299*, 905–916. [CrossRef] [PubMed]
43. Polishchuk, E.V.; Polishchuk, R.S. Pre-Embedding Labeling for Subcellular Detection of Molecules with Electron Microscopy. *Tissue Cell* **2019**, *57*, 103–110. [CrossRef] [PubMed]

4

# Acute Kidney Injury and Septic Shock—Defined by Updated Sepsis-3 Criteria in Critically Ill Patients

**Vin-Cent Wu [1], Shih-Chieh Jeff Chueh [2], Jui-Ting Chang [3], Bang-Gee Hsu [4], Marlies Ostermann [5,*] and Tzong-Shinn Chu [1,6,7,*]**

1 Division of Nephrology, National Taiwan University Hospital, No. 7 Chung-Shan South Road, Zhong-Zheng District, Taipei 100, Taiwan; q91421028@ntu.edu.tw
2 Glickman Urological and Kidney Institute, Cleveland Clinic Lerner College of Medicine, Cleveland Clinic, Cleveland, 9500 Euclid Ave., Cleveland, OH 44195, USA; jeffchueh@gmail.com
3 Division of Nephrology, Department of Internal Medicine, Shin Kong Memorial Wu Ho-Su Hospital, Taipei 111, Taiwan; skhnephropgy@gmail.com
4 Division of Nephrology, Hualien Tzu Chi Hospital, Buddhist Tzu Chi Medical Foundation; and School of Medicine, Tzu Chi University, Hualien 970, Taiwan; gee.lily@msa.hinet.net
5 Department of Critical Care and Nephrology, King's College London, Guy's and St Thomas Hospital, London SE1 7EH, UK
6 NSARF group (National Taiwan University Hospital Study Group of ARF), Zhong-Zheng District, Taipei 100, Taiwan
7 CAKS group (Taiwan Consortium for Acute Kidney Injury and Renal Diseases), Guishan District, Taoyuan City 333, Taiwan
* Correspondence: Marlies.Ostermann@gstt.nhs.uk (M.O.); tschu@ntu.edu.tw (T.S.-C.)

**Abstract:** Sepsis is commonly associated with acute kidney injury (AKI), particularly in those requiring dialysis (AKI-D). To date, Sepsis-3 criteria have not been applied to AKI-D patients. We investigated sepsis prevalence defined by Sepsis-3 criteria and evaluated the outcomes of septic-associated AKI-D among critically ill patients. Using the data collected from a prospective multi-center observational study, we applied the Sepsis-3 criteria to critically ill AKI-D patients treated in intensive care units (ICUs) in 30 hospitals between September 2014 and December 2015. We described the prevalence, outcomes, and characteristics of sepsis as defined by the screening Sepsis-3 criteria among AKI-D patients, and compared the outcomes of AKI-D patients with or without sepsis using the Sepsis-3 criteria. A total of 1078 patients (median 70 years; 673 (62.4%) men) with AKI-D were analyzed. The main etiology of AKI was sepsis (71.43%) and the most frequent indication for acute dialysis was oliguria (64.4%). A total of 577 (53.3% of 1078 patients) met the Sepsis-3 criteria, and 206 among the 577 patients (19.1%) had septic shock. Having sepsis and septic shock were independently associated with 90-day mortality among these ICU AKI-D patients (hazard ratio (HR) 1.23 ($p = 0.027$) and 1.39 ($p = 0.004$), respectively). Taking mortality as a competing risk factor, AKI-D patients with septic shock had a significantly reduced chance of weaning from dialysis at 90 days than those without sepsis (HR 0.65, $p = 0.026$). The combination of the Sepsis-3 criteria with the AKI risk score led to better performance in forecasting 90-day mortality. Sepsis affects more than 50% of ICU AKI patients requiring dialysis, and one-fifth of these patients had septic shock. In AKI-D patients, coexistent with or induced by sepsis (as screened by the Sepsis-3 criteria), there is a significantly higher mortality and reduced chance of recovering sufficient renal function, when compared to those without sepsis.

**Keywords:** Sepsis-3; acute dialysis; qSOFA; acute kidney injury

## 1. Introduction

Sepsis is considered the most frequent cause of acute kidney injury (AKI) in critically ill patients in the intensive care unit (ICU) [1]. It is a heterogeneous syndrome caused by an unbalanced host response to an infection, often resulting in variable clinical signs and symptoms. Until the early 1990s, sepsis was not formally defined, and numerous different criteria were used in research and clinical practice. In 2016, the 'Sepsis-3' consensus definition was published. Accordingly, sepsis constitutes life-threatening organ dysfunction that is caused by a dysregulated host response to infection and defined by an acute change in total Sequential Organ Failure Assessment (SOFA) score by ≥2 points (delta SOFA). In addition, the concept of the quick SOFA (qSOFA) was introduced as a possible tool to identify patients with sepsis outside the ICU [2]. The qSOFA describes the presence of any two of the following three factors: Respiratory rate ≥ 22/min, altered mentation or systolic blood pressure ≤ 100 mmHg. Septic shock is recognized as a subset of sepsis with profound circulatory, cellular, and metabolic abnormalities as evidenced by a serum lactate concentration >2 mmol/L and vasopressor requirement to maintain a mean arterial pressure (MAP) of at least 65 mmHg in the absence of hypovolemia. Of note, the terms systemic inflammatory response syndrome (SIRS) and severe sepsis were removed.

An analysis of data from a large cohort of patients admitted to 409 hospitals in the USA in 2004–2009 revealed that more than 40% of patients with sepsis, as defined by the Sepsis-3 criteria, also had AKI [3]. In patients with AKI, mortality and long-term outcomes are worst in those treated with renal replacement (RRT), also known as 'AKI with dialysis' (AKI-D) [2,4]. To date, the prevalence and outcomes of sepsis defined by the Sepsis-3 criteria among AKI-D patients has not been well reported. It is unclear whether the two criteria of the Sepsis-3 definition are equally predictive when used in association with AKI-D patients.

The aims of our project were: (i) To describe the incidence, outcomes, and characteristics of sepsis, as defined by the screening Sepsis-3 criteria, among AKI-D patients; and (ii) to show the outcomes of AKI-D patients without or with sepsis.

## 2. Methods

### 2.1. Study Population

We analyzed data of the Taiwan Consortium for Acute Kidney Injury and Renal Diseases (CAKs) study. The CAKS study was approved by the institutional review boards of the participating institutions. The need for informed consent was waived because all personal data was fully de-identified and only data that were routinely collected for clinical purposes were analyzed (approval number NRPB2014050014). The CAKs study has been extensively described previously [5,6]. In brief, it is a prospective observational study of ICU patients with AKI-D admitted to one of 30 hospitals in Taiwan. The hospitals are distributed widely through the various geographical regions of Taiwan (north, middle, south, and east) and there is a 1:1 ratio of tertiary medical centers to regional hospitals in each region. We analyzed patients who had been enrolled in four distinct months (October 2014, January 2015, April 2015 and July 2015) and were followed-up for at least three months after hospital discharge. Patients receiving chronic dialysis before the index hospitalization were excluded.

### 2.2. Dialysis Initiation

The pre-determined indications for RRT protocol or algorithm or simply clinician judgement were: (1) Presence of azotemia (blood urea nitrogen (BUN) > 80 mg/dL and serum creatinine (sCr) > 2 mg/dL) and uremic symptoms (encephalopathy, pericarditis or pleurisy); (2) oliguria (urine output < 400 mL/24 h) or anuria refractory to fluid challenges and diuretics; (3) fluid overload refractory to diuretics with a central venous pressure (CVP) > 12 mmHg or pulmonary edema with a $PaO2/FiO2$ < 300 mmHg; (4) hyperkalemia (serum potassium > 5.5 mmol/L) refractory to medical treatment, and/or (5) metabolic acidosis (arterial pH < 7.2) [7–9].

### 2.3. *Infection and Sepsis*

The medical records of all patients were independently reviewed by two investigators to identify AKI-D patients who met the Sepsis-3 criteria at initiation of RRT. In case of any discordance, a third investigator (VCW) acted as an adjudicator.

To be classified as having sepsis, patients with a suspected or confirmed infection had to have at least two qSOFA criteria [10] or an acute increase in total SOFA score by ≥2 within the 24 h period before acute RRT was started (distribution as Figure S1). Infection was defined as body fluids with positive culture or antibiotics started as a criterion of suspected infection. In patients with a nosocomial infection in whom a pre-admission SOFA score was not available, the first SOFA value at hospital admission qualified as baseline score (1). Patients with hepatic dysfunction who received acute RRT within 24 h of ICU admission, were assigned a baseline SOFA score of four, and in case of chronic respiratory impairment, a baseline score of two was assigned [11]. In all other cases, the baseline SOFA score was considered to be zero [2]. Consistent with previous studies, missing values were considered to be normal [10].

### 2.4. *Outcomes*

The primary study outcome was 90-day mortality after hospital discharge. Secondary outcomes were inability to wean from acute RRT and/or a composite outcome of mortality or RRT dependence at 90 days after hospital discharge [12].

### 2.5. *Clinical Data Collection*

In patients with AKI-D at initiation of RRT, we extracted the following data: Baseline characteristics and demographics, severity of illness scores including SOFA score, acute physiology and chronic health evaluation II (APACHE II) score and multiple organ dysfunction syndrome (MODS) score, comorbidities and the presumed etiology of AKI. AKI was defined by the serum creatinine criteria of the Kidney Disease Improving Global Outcome classification [13]. We also calculated the AKI risk prediction score as proposed by Demirjian et al. [14] (Table S1). The worst physiological and biochemical values during the initial 24-h period before RRT were recorded, together with the severity of illness scores and vasopressor administration at initiation of RRT [15].

The pre-determined indications for RRT were mentioned above and as in supplemental methods.

### 2.6. *Statistical Analyses*

Continuous data were expressed as mean ± standard deviation (SD) and group comparisons were conducted using $\chi$ 2 tests for equal proportions, t tests for normally distributed data, and Wilcoxon rank sum tests otherwise.

We performed multivariable analyses of all factors that were significant in univariate analyses, including age, sex, baseline comorbidities, indication for RRT, etiology of AKI, renal parameters and SOFA score at initiation of RRT and modality of RRT. The significance levels for entry (SLE) and for stay (SLS) were set at a conservative level of 0.15. The best candidate final logistic regression model was identified manually by dropping the covariates with a $p$ value > 0.05 one at a time until all regression coefficients were significantly different from zero.

Net reclassification improvement (NRI) and integrated discrimination improvement (IDI) analysis were used to examine the role of the Sepsis-3 criteria to stratify individuals into higher or lower risk categories (reclassification) [16,17]. Focusing on 90-day mortality, an increase in NRI was calculated in a model containing the Sepsis-3 criteria in combination with the AKI risk prediction or SOFA score. The results were compared with the individual criteria of the Sepsis-3 definition. We distinguished between three risk categories (0%–40%, 40%–80%, and >80%) and reclassified the patients who died from all-causes or were still dialysis dependent at 90 days after hospital discharge (according to decision curve analysis, Figure S2).

All analyses were performed with R software, version 3.2.2 (Free Software Foundation, Inc., Boston, MA, USA), MedCalc Statistical Software, version 15.11.3 (MedCalc Software bvba, Ostend, Belgium; https://www.medcalc.org; 2015) and Stata version 12 (StataCorp LP, College Station, TX, USA) for competing-risk analysis. A $p$-value < 0.05 was considered significant.

## 3. Results

### 3.1. Patient Cohort

We enrolled a total of 1078 critically ill patients with AKI-D (median age 70 years; 673 (62.4%) male). At initiation of RRT, their median SOFA score was 12, APACHE II score 24 and MODS score was 11. A total of 577 (53.5%) patients had sepsis, of whom 206 (19.1%) met the criteria for septic shock (Figure 1). Supplementary Figure S1 shows the distribution of the qSOFA and SOFA scores. The main source of infection was the respiratory tract (53.6%), followed by the genitourinary tract (31.4%). The missing data were mainly come from bilirubin ($n$ = 4, 3.7%) and coagulation INR (5, 4.6%).

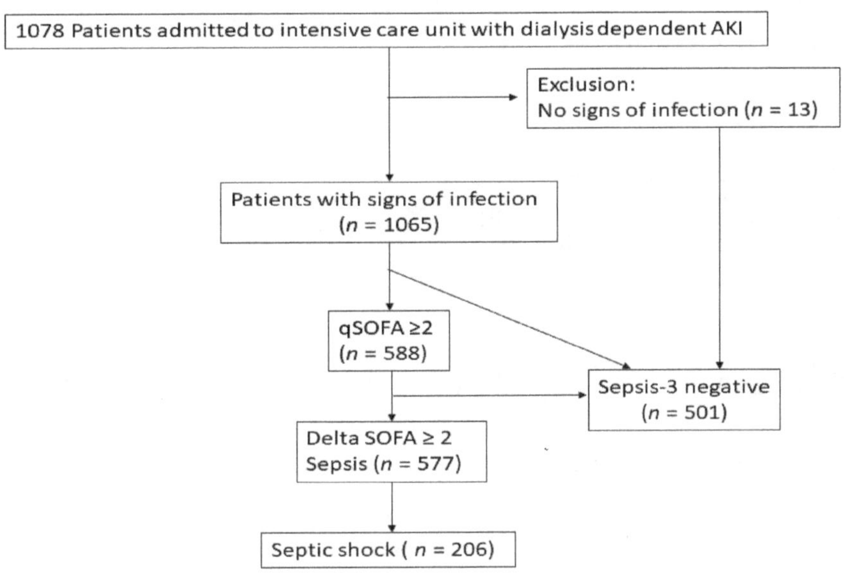


**Figure 1.** Algorithm of enrollee.

Based on judgment by the clinicians treating the patients, the main etiologies of AKI were sepsis (71.4%), shock (57.1%) and rhabdomyolysis (14.4%). The most frequent indication for acute RRT was oliguria (64.4%), followed by fluid overload (56.0%), azotemia (54.4%) and metabolic acidosis (49.6%).

### 3.2. Impact of Sepsis

Patients with AKI-D who had sepsis (53.5%) or septic shock (19.1%) at initiation of RRT were significantly older, had better baseline renal function and a higher serum lactate result on admission to ICU compared to AKI-D patients without sepsis (Table 1).

### 3.3. Comparison between 90-Day Survivors and Non-Survivors

Mortality and composite outcome (mortality or RRT dependence) at 90 days were 62.3%, and 76.4% in the 1078 AKI-D patients, respectively (Table 2). Sepsis and septic shock were more common among non-survivors compared to survivors (63.2% and 25.6% versus 37.4% and 8.4%, respectively). Other significant differences between 90-day survivors and non-survivors were older age, a higher comorbidity score, lower baseline serum creatinine and a higher prevalence of liver cirrhosis and cancer in non-survivors.

**Table 1.** Clinical characteristics of patients with and without sepsis.

| | Non-Sepsis ($n$ = 501) | Sepsis ($n$ = 371) | Septic Shock ($n$ = 206) | $p$ Value |
|---|---|---|---|---|
| Patient characteristics | | | | |
| Age, median (range) | 71.8 (60.6–80.3) | 69.3 (57.6–79.7) | 65.8 (54.3–76.3) | 0.011 |
| Male gender, $n$ (%) | 299 (59.68%) | 228 (61.46%) | 146 (70.87%) | 0.018 |
| BMI, median (range) | 23.9 (21.4–27.2) | 24 (21–27.2) | 23.9 (21–26.9) | 0.579 |
| Charlson comorbidity index | 7 (5–9) | 7 (5–9) | 6 (5–8) | 0.020 |
| Baseline sCr (mg/dL), median (range) | 1.7 (1–3.3) | 1.4 (0.9–2.4) | 1 (0.8–1.7) | <0.001 |
| eGFR (ml/min/1.73 $m^2$), median (range) | 32.5 (15.5–63.3) | 44 (21.9–73.8) | 63.9 (35.2–88) | <0.001 |
| Comorbidities, $n$ (%) | | | | |
| Diabetes mellitus, $n$ (%) | 276 (55.09%) | 189 (50.94%) | 97 (47.09%) | 0.131 |
| Liver cirrhosis, $n$ (%) | 56 (11.18%) | 58 (15.63%) | 40 (19.42%) | 0.011 |
| COPD, $n$ (%) | 43 (8.58%) | 29 (7.82%) | 12 (5.83%) | 0.462 |
| CAD, $n$ (%) | 156 (31.14%) | 102 (27.49%) | 52 (25.24%) | 0.233 |
| CVA, $n$ (%) | 78 (15.57%) | 59 (15.90%) | 22 (10.68%) | 0.185 |
| Hemiplegia, $n$ (%) | 22 (4.39%) | 20 (5.39%) | 6 (2.91%) | 0.383 |
| GI bleeding, $n$ (%) | 129 (25.75%) | 109 (29.38%) | 58 (28.16%) | 0.479 |
| Dementia, $n$ (%) | 11 (2.20%) | 12 (3.23%) | 9 (4.37%) | 0.282 |
| Cancer, $n$ (%) | 86 (17.17%) | 79 (21.29%) | 63 (30.58%) | <0.001 |
| Congestive heart failure, $n$ (%) | 194 (48.7%) | 159 (58.49%) | 68 (44.66%) | <0.001 |
| Laboratory data at ICU admission | | | | |
| BUN (mg/dL), median (range) | 61 (34.5–95.9) | 57.7 (27–92) | 42 (23.2–68.8) | <0.001 |
| sCr (mg/dL), median (range) | 3.7 (2–6.4) | 2.7 (1.4–5) | 2.3 (1.3–3.8) | <0.001 |
| Lactate (mmol/L), median (range) | 2.5 (1.4–5.6) | 2.4 (1.3–4.8) | 6.3 (2.9–10) | <0.001 |
| Etiology of AKI (except sepsis), $n$ (%) | | | | |
| Shock | 225 (44.91%) | 203 (54.72%) | 188 (91.26%) | <0.001 |
| Cardiorenal syndrome | 206 (41.12%) | 134 (36.12%) | 53 (25.73%) | <0.001 |
| Drug nephrotoxicity | 26 (5.19%) | 18 (4.85%) | 10 (4.85%) | 0.969 |
| Rhabdomyolysis | 34 (6.79%) | 24 (6.47%) | 23 (11.17%) | 0.086 |
| Intravascular hemolysis | 16 (3.19%) | 10 (2.70%) | 8 (3.88%) | 0.735 |
| Hepatorenal | 26 (5.19%) | 22 (5.93%) | 21 (10.19%) | 0.043 |
| ATIN | 4 (0.80%) | 5 (1.35%) | 0 (0%) | 0.276 |
| Contrast | 38 (7.58%) | 24 (6.47%) | 13 (6.31%) | 0.750 |
| Obstructive | 8 (1.60%) | 3 (0.81%) | 1 (0.49%) | 0.472 |
| Others | 117 (23.35%) | 56 (15.09%) | 24 (11.65%) | <0.001 |

**Table 1.** *Cont.*

| | Non-Sepsis | Sepsis | Septic Shock | *p* Value |
|---|---|---|---|---|
| At initiation of RRT | | | | |
| Urine output (mL/24 h), median (range) | 450 (150–1095) | 250 (70–620) | 130 (50–418) | <0.001 |
| AKI risk prediction score, median (range) | 22 (17–28) | 27 (21–33) | 33.5 (26–40) | <0.001 |
| Lactate (mmol/L), median (range) | 2.2 (1.3–5.2) | 1.6 (1–3.1) | 6.6 (3.4–10.7) | <0.001 |
| SOFA score, median (range) | 10 (7–13) | 12 (10–15) | 15 (13–17) | <0.001 |
| qSOFA, median (range) | 1 (1–1) | 2 (2-3) | 2 (2–3) | <0.001 |
| APACHE II score, median (range) | 20 (16–25) | 25 (21–30) | 27 (22.8–33) | <0.001 |
| MODS score, median (range) | 9 (7–11) | 12 (10–14) | 12 (10–15) | <0.001 |
| Site of infection, *n* (%) | | | | |
| Respiratory | 227 (45.31%) | 237 (63.88%) | 114 (55.34%) | <0.001 |
| GU | 156 (31.14%) | 129 (34.77%) | 53 (25.73%) | 0.080 |
| Bacteremia | 96 (19.16%) | 84 (22.64%) | 57 (27.67%) | 0.043 |
| Abdomen | 41 (8.18%) | 40 (10.78%) | 33 (16.02%) | 0.009 |
| Others | 56 (11.18%) | 38 (10.24%) | 21 (10.19%) | 0.880 |
| Indication for dialysis, *n* (%) | | | | |
| Azotemia | 291 (58.08%) | 225 (60.65%) | 70 (33.98%) | <0.001 |
| Fluid overload | 245 (48.90%) | 225 (60.65%) | 134 (65.05%) | <0.001 |
| Electrolyte imbalance | 190 (37.92%) | 148 (39.89%) | 79 (38.35%) | 0.835 |
| Metabolic acidosis | 210 (41.92%) | 192 (51.75%) | 133 (64.56%) | <0.001 |
| Oliguria | 275 (54.89%) | 255 (68.73%) | 164 (79.61%) | <0.001 |
| Uremic encephalopathy | 46 (9.18%) | 26 (7.01%) | 6 (2.91%) | 0.014 |
| Dialysis modality, *n* (%) | | | | <0.001 |
| CVVH | 128 (25.55%) | 110 (29.65%) | 133 (64.56%) | |
| IHD | 334 (66.67%) | 252 (67.92%) | 58 (28.16%) | |
| SLEDD | 39 (7.78%) | 9 (2.43%) | 15 (7.28%) | |
| Outcomes of interest | | | | |
| Dialysis days in hospital, median (range) | 12 (4–26) | 10 (4–27) | 6 (3–15) | 0.012 |
| Hospital mortality, *n* (%) | 221 (44.11%) | 228 (61.46%) | 167 (81.07%) | <0.001 |
| 90-day ICU free days | 63 (0–85) | 1 (0–78) | 0 (0–0) | <0.001 |
| 90-day hospital free days | 30 (0–70) | 0 (0–53) | 0 (0–0) | <0.001 |
| 90-day mortality, *n* (%) | 246 (49.10%) | 253 (68.19%) | 172 (83.49%) | <0.001 |
| 90-day composite outcome, *n* (%) | 352 (70.26%) | 296 (79.78%) | 175 (84.95%) | <0.001 |

Paired comparison between the groups. Abbreviations: AKI, acute kidney injury; APACHE; acute physiology and chronic health evaluation; ATIN, acute tubule-interstitial nephritis; BMI, body mass index; BUN, blood urea nitrogen; CAD, coronary artery disease; CABG, coronary artery bypass graft; COPD, chronic obstructive pulmonary disease; CPB, cardiopulmonary bypass; CVA, cerebrovascular accident; CVVH, continuous veno-venous hemofiltration; CPR, cardio-pulmonary resuscitation; eGFR, estimated glomerular filtration rate; GSC, Glasgow Coma Scale; GI, gastrointestinal; GU, genitourinary; IABP, intra-aortic balloon pump; ICU, intensive care unit; IHD, intermittent hemodialysis; IQR, interquartile range; MODS, multiple organ dysfunction; RRT, renal replacement therapy; sCr, serum creatinine; SLEDD, sustained low efficiency daily dialysis; SOFA, Sequential Organ Failure Assessment.

**Table 2.** Clinical characteristics of survivors and non-survivors.

| | All | 90 Day Survivors | 90 Day Mortality | $p$ Value | No Dialysis Dependence or Mortality at 90 Days | Dialysis Dependence or Mortality at 90 Days | $p$ Value |
|---|---|---|---|---|---|---|---|
| | ($n$ = 1078) | ($n$ = 406) | ($n$ = 672) | | ($n$ = 254) | ($n$ = 824) | |
| Baseline characteristics | | | | | | | |
| Age, median (range) | 70 (57.8–79.5) | 69 (56.7–77.4) | 71 (58.9–81) | 0.014 | 67.7 (53.9–76.8) | 70.9 (59.8–80.4) | <0.001 |
| Male gender, $n$ (%) | 673 (62.43%) | 247 (60.84%) | 426 (63.39%) | 0.401 | 158 (62.20%) | 515 (62.50%) | 0.932 |
| BMI, median (range) | 23.95 (21.2–27.1) | 24.2 (21.5–27.6) | 23.7 (21–26.8) | 0.870 | 24.6 (22–27.9) | 23.7 (21–26.8) | 0.598 |
| Charlson comorbidity index, median (range) | 7 (5–9) | 7 (5–8.3) | 7 (5–9) | 0.001 | 6 (4–8) | 7 (5–9) | <0.001 |
| Baseline sCr (mg/dL), median (range) | 1.4 (0.9–2.7) | 1.8 (1–3.6) | 1.3 (0.9–2.3) | <0.001 | 1.2 (0.9–2.1) | 1.5 (0.9–2.8) | <0.001 |
| eGFR (mL/min/1.73 $m^2$), median (range) | 41.79 (20.4–73.6) | 31.9 (14.6-64.3) | 48.2 (24.4-77.1) | <0.001 | 49.9 (25.3-78) | 40.5 (18.2-71.7) | 0.040 |
| Comorbidities | | | | | | | |
| Diabetes mellitus, $n$ (%) | 562 (52.13%) | 228 (56.16%) | 334 (49.70%) | 0.040 | 139 (54.72%) | 423 (51.33%) | 0.344 |
| Liver cirrhosis, $n$ (%) | 154 (14.29%) | 26 (6.40%) | 128 (19.05%) | <0.001 | 19 (7.48%) | 135 (16.38%) | <0.001 |
| COPD, $n$ (%) | 84 (7.79%) | 31 (7.64%) | 53 (7.89%) | 0.881 | 19 (7.48%) | 65 (7.89%) | 0.832 |
| CAD, $n$ (%) | 310 (28.76%) | 130 (32.02%) | 180 (26.79%) | 0.066 | 77 (30.31%) | 233 (28.28%) | 0.530 |
| CVA, $n$ (%) | 159 (14.75%) | 61 (15.02%) | 98 (14.58%) | 0.843 | 30 (11.81%) | 129 (15.66%) | 0.131 |
| Hemiplegia, $n$ (%) | 48 (4.45%) | 19 (4.68%) | 29 (4.32%) | 0.779 | 11 (4.33%) | 37 (4.49%) | 0.914 |
| GI bleeding, $n$ (%) | 296 (27.46%) | 89 (21.92%) | 207 (30.80%) | 0.002 | 53 (20.87%) | 243 (29.49%) | 0.007 |
| Dementia, $n$ (%) | 32 (2.97%) | 7 (1.72%) | 25 (3.72%) | 0.061 | 6 (2.36%) | 26 (3.16%) | 0.515 |
| Cancer, $n$ (%) | 228 (21.15%) | 60 (14.78%) | 168 (25.00%) | <0.001 | 40 (15.75%) | 188 (22.82%) | 0.016 |
| Congestive heart failure, $n$ (%) | 553 (51.30%) | 205 (50.49%) | 348 (50.79%) | 0.787 | 122 (48.41%) | 431 (52.31%) | 0.019 |
| Parameters at ICU admission | | | | | | | |
| BUN (mg/dL), median (range) | 56 (29.2–89) | 63 (35–91) | 50.5 (26.4–88) | 0.001 | 51 (26–80.5) | 57.7 (30–91.6) | 0.192 |
| sCr (mg/dL), median (range) | 3 (1.7–5.5) | 4.1 (2.2–6.9) | 2.6 (1.4–4.5) | <0.001 | 3 (1.9–5.3) | 3 (1.6–5.6) | 0.984 |
| Lactate (mmol/L), median (range) | 3.1 (1.7–7) | 2.6 (1.3–5.2) | 3.7 (2–8.6) | <0.001 | 3 (1.6–6.1) | 3.2 (1.7–7.3) | 0.030 |
| Etiology of AKI, $n$ (%) | | | | | | | |
| Shock, $n$ (%) | 616 (57.14%) | 165 (40.64%) | 451 (67.11%) | <0.001 | 132 (51.97%) | 484 (58.74%) | 0.057 |
| Sepsis, $n$ (%) | 770 (71.43%) | 242 (59.61%) | 528 (78.57%) | <0.001 | 153 (60.24%) | 617 (74.88%) | <0.001 |
| Cardiorenal syndrome, $n$ (%) | 393 (36.46%) | 170 (41.87%) | 223 (33.18%) | 0.010 | 93 (36.61%) | 300 (36.41%) | 0.952 |
| Nephrotoxic drugs, $n$ (%) | 54 (5.01%) | 27 (6.65%) | 27 (4.02%) | 0.055 | 22 (8.66%) | 32 (3.88%) | 0.002 |
| Rhabdomyolysis, $n$ (%) | 81 (7.51%) | 33 (8.13%) | 48 (7.14%) | 0.552 | 28 (11.02%) | 53 (6.43%) | 0.015 |
| Intravascular hemolysis, $n$ (%) | 34 (3.15%) | 14 (3.45%) | 20 (2.98%) | 0.667 | 11 (4.33%) | 23 (2.79%) | 0.220 |
| Hepatorenal syndrome, $n$ (%) | 69 (6.40%) | 4 (0.99%) | 65 (9.67%) | <0.001 | 4 (1.57%) | 65 (7.89%) | <0.001 |
| ATIN, $n$ (%) | 9 (0.83%) | 5 (1.23%) | 4 (0.60%) | 0.309 | 2 (0.79%) | 7 (0.85%) | 0.999 |
| Contrast exposure, $n$ (%) | 75 (6.96%) | 33 (8.13%) | 42 (6.25%) | 0.240 | 22 (8.66%) | 53 (6.43%) | 0.222 |
| Obstruction, $n$ (%) | 12 (1.11%) | 6 (1.48%) | 6 (0.89%) | 0.375 | 3 (1.18%) | 9 (1.09%) | 1.000 |
| Others, $n$ (%) | 197 (18.27%) | 103 (25.37%) | 94 (13.99%) | <0.001 | 61 (24.02%) | 136 (16.50%) | 0.007 |

**Table 2.** *Cont.*

| | All | 90 Day Survivors | 90 Day Mortality | $p$ Value | No Dialysis Dependence or Mortality at 90 Days | Dialysis Dependence or Mortality at 90 Days | $p$ Value |
|---|---|---|---|---|---|---|---|
| | ($n$ = 1078) | ($n$ = 406) | ($n$ = 672) | | ($n$ = 254) | ($n$ = 824) | |
| Parameters at RRT initiation | | | | | | | |
| Urine output (mL/24 h), median (range) | 300 (90–822.5) | 490 (160–1223) | 204 (70–595) | <0.001 | 520 (180–1305) | 250 (75–670) | <0.001 |
| AKI risk prediction score | 25 (19–33) | 21 (16–28.3) | 27.5 (22–35) | <0.001 | 22 (17–29.3) | 26 (21–34) | <0.001 |
| Lactate (mmol/L), median (range) | 3.2 (1.6–7.6) | 2.3 (1.2–5.4) | 3.9 (1.9–9.1) | <0.001 | 2.8 (1.4–6.5) | 3.3 (1.6–8.2) | 0.090 |
| SOFA score, median (range) | 12 (8–15) | 9 (7–12) | 13 (10–16) | <0.001 | 10 (7–13) | 12 (9–15) | <0.001 |
| qSOFA, median (range) | 2 (1–2) | 1 (1–2) | 2 (1–2) | <0.001 | 1 (1–2) | 2 (1–2) | <0.001 |
| qSOFA ≥ 2, $n$ (%) | 582 (53.99%) | 153 (37.66%) | 429 (63.84%) | <0.001 | 107 (42.13%) | 475 (57.65%) | <0.001 |
| APACHE II score, median (range) | 24 (19–28) | 20 (16–25) | 25 (21–30) | <0.001 | 21 (16–26) | 24 (20–29) | <0.001 |
| MODS score, median (range) | 11 (9–13) | 10 (7–12) | 11 (9–14) | <0.001 | 10 (7.5–13) | 11 (9–13) | 0.008 |
| Sepsis 3 criteria | | | | | | | |
| Sepsis, $n$ (%) | 577 (53.53%) | 152 (37.44%) | 425 (63.24%) | <0.001 | 106 (41.73%) | 471 (57.16%) | <0.001 |
| Septic shock, $n$ (%) | 206 (19.11%) | 34 (8.37%) | 172 (25.60%) | <0.001 | 31 (12.20%) | 175 (21.24%) | 0.001 |
| Site of infection, $n$ (%) | | | | | | | |
| Respiratory | 578 (53.62%) | 188 (46.31%) | 390 (58.04%) | <0.001 | 1113 (44.49%) | 465 (56.43%) | 0.001 |
| GU | 338 (31.35%) | 134 (33.00%) | 204 (30.36%) | 0.364 | 83 (32.68%) | 255 (30.95%) | 0.603 |
| Bacteremia | 237 (21.99%) | 60 (14.78%) | 177 (26.34%) | <0.001 | 43 (16.93%) | 194 (23.54%) | 0.026 |
| Abdomen | 114 (10.58%) | 39 (9.61%) | 75 (11.16%) | 0.421 | 32 (12.60%) | 82 (9.95%) | 0.230 |
| Others | 115 (10.67%) | 37 (9.11%) | 78 (11.61%) | 0.199 | 25 (9.84%) | 90 (10.92%) | 0.626 |
| Indication for RRT | | | | | | | |
| Azotemia, $n$ (%) | 586 (54.36%) | 220 (54.19%) | 366 (54.46%) | 0.929 | 113 (44.49%) | 473 (57.40%) | <0.001 |
| Fluid overload, $n$ (%) | 604 (56.03%) | 200 (49.26%) | 404 (60.12%) | 0.001 | 132 (51.97%) | 472 (57.28%) | 0.136 |
| Electrolyte imbalance, $n$ (%) | 417 (38.68%) | 160 (39.41%) | 257 (38.24%) | 0.704 | 108 (42.52%) | 309 (37.50%) | 0.151 |
| Metabolic acidosis, $n$ (%) | 535 (49.63%) | 180 (44.33%) | 355 (52.83%) | 0.007 | 114 (44.88%) | 421 (51.09%) | 0.084 |
| Oliguria, $n$ (%) | 694 (64.38%) | 205 (50.49%) | 489 (72.77%) | <0.001 | 122 (48.03%) | 572 (69.42%) | <0.001 |
| Uremic encephalopathy, $n$ (%) | 78 (7.24%) | 38 (9.36%) | 40 (5.95%) | 0.036 | 16 (6.30%) | 62 (7.52%) | 0.510 |
| First Dialysis modality, $n$ (%) | | | | <0.001 | | | 0.239 |
| CVVH | 371 (34.42%) | 97 (23.89%) | 274 (40.77%) | | 79 (31.10%) | 292 (35.44%) | |
| IHD | 644 (59.74%) | 289 (71.18%) | 355 (52.83%) | | 163 (64.17%) | 481 (58.37%) | |
| SLEDD | 63 (5.84%) | 20 (4.93%) | 43 (6.40%) | | 12 (4.72%) | 51 (6.19%) | |
| Outcomes of interest | | | | | | | |
| 90-day ICU free days | 7 (0–81) | 81 (69–86) | 0(0–1) | <0.001 | 80 (68–86) | 0 (0–54.5) | <0.001 |
| 90-day hospital free days | 0 (0–59.25) | 63 (44.5–76) | 0(0–0) | <0.001 | 63 (42–76) | 0 (0–2.5) | <0.001 |
| Days of RRT in hospital, median (range) | 10 (4–24) | 11 (3–26) | 9.5 (4–22.8) | 0.461 | 5.5 (2–13.3) | 12 (4–27.8) | <0.001 |

Abbreviations: AKI, acute kidney injury; APACHE; acute physiology and chronic health evaluation; ATIN, acute tubule-interstitial nephritis; BMI, body mass index; BUN, blood urea nitrogen; CAD, coronary artery disease; CABG, coronary artery bypass graft; COPD, chronic obstructive pulmonary disease; CPB, cardiopulmonary bypass; CVA, cerebrovascular accident; CVVH, continuous veno-venous hemofiltration; CPR, cardio-pulmonary resuscitation; eGFR, estimated glomerular filtration rate; GSC, Glasgow Coma Scale; GI, gastrointestinal; GU, genitourinary; IABP, intra-aortic balloon pump; ICU, intensive care unit; IHD, intermittent hemodialysis; IQR, interquartile range; MODS, multiple organ dysfunction; RRT, renal replacement therapy; sCr, serum creatinine; SLEDD, sustained low efficiency daily dialysis; SOFA, Sequential Organ Failure Assessment.

### 3.4. Sepsis-3 Criteria versus 90-Day Outcomes

Multivariable analysis showed that AKI-D patients with sepsis or septic shock at initiation of RRT had a significantly higher risk of mortality at 90 days compared to AKI-D patients without sepsis (Table 3 and Figure 2a). There was a positive correlation between the Sepsis-3 criteria and APACHE II score ($r = 0.385$, $p < 0.001$), SOFA score ($r = 0.391$, $p < 0.001$) and AKI risk prediction score ($r = 0.359$, $p < 0.001$). AKI-D patients with septic shock had a greater incremental increase in 90-day mortality across all deciles of APACHE II at initiation of RRT compared to AKI-D patients with qSOFA ≥ 2 (Figure S4, Table S2).

**Table 3.** Multivariable risk model for hospital mortality or composite outcome at discharge.

| Sepsis | Non-Shock Sepsis vs Non-Sepsis | | | Septic Shock vs. Non-Sepsis | | |
|---|---|---|---|---|---|---|
| Outcome of interests | Hazard Ratio | 95% CI | *p* | Hazard Ratio | 95% CI | *p* |
| Hospital mortality | 1.12 | 0.91–1.37 | 0.276 | 1.48 | 1.17–1.88 | 0.001 |
| Hospital composite outcomes | 0.97 | 0.80–1.17 | 0.732 | 1.24 | 1.08–1.47 | 0.047 |
| For 90-day mortality | 1.23 | 1.02–1.47 | 0.027 | 1.39 | 1.11–1.75 | 0.004 |
| For 90-day composite outcome | 1.26 | 1.03–1.53 | 0.022 | 1.45 | 1.15–1.83 | 0.002 |
| For 90-day weaning from dialysis | 0.96 | 0.76–1.22 | 0.760 | 0.65 | 0.45–0.95 | 0.026 |

*p*; paired comparison between the groups. All relevant covariates included in the multi-variable analysis, including age, sex, baseline comorbidities, indication for dialysis, etiology of AKI, kidney profile and SOFA score at dialysis initiation, dialysis modality, and some of their interactions. Abbreviations: AKI, acute kidney injury; CI, confidence interval.

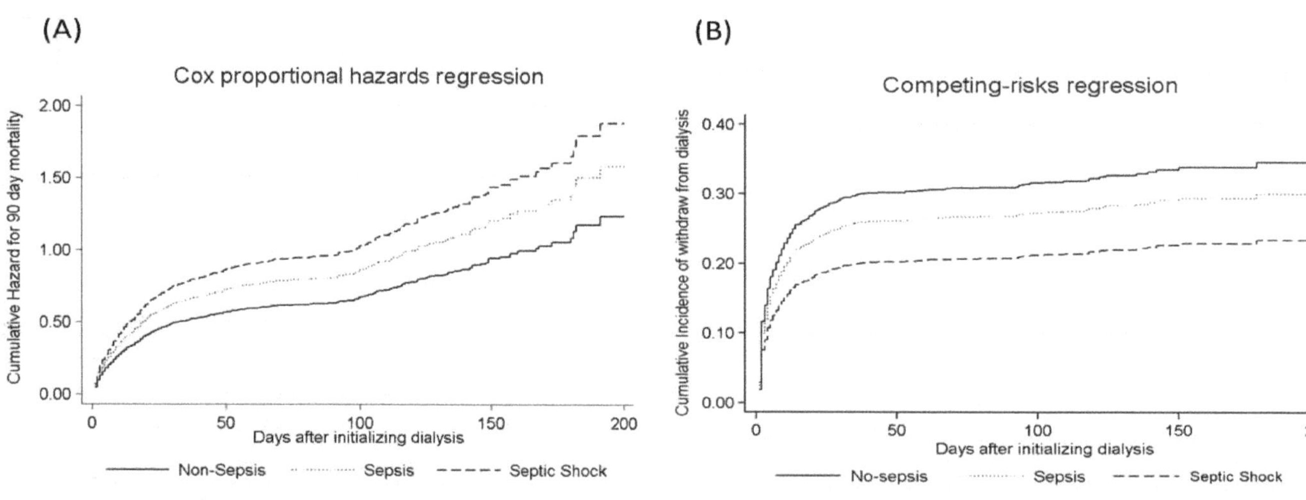


**Figure 2.** Cox proportional hazards models. (**A**) Cox proportional hazards models are plotted to model the probability of free from 90 days mortality, stratified by Sepsis-3 status. (**B**) Model the risk of chronic dialysis, taking mortality as a competing risk.

### 3.5. Sepsis per Sepsis-3 Criteria versus the Risk of Dialysis Dependence

Multivariable analysis showed that after controlling for mortality, AKI-D patients with septic shock who survived had a significantly lower likelihood of weaning from dialysis, when compared to AKI-D patients without sepsis (hazard ratio (HR), 0.65, $p = 0.026$) (Table 3). There was no significant difference in likelihood of weaning from dialysis at 90 days between AKI-D patients without sepsis and AKI-D patients with sepsis but without septic shock (HR 0.96, $p = 0.760$) (Table 3, Figure 2b).

### 3.6. Evaluation of Sepsis-3 Criteria in Combination with AKI Risk Prediction Score and SOFA Score versus the 90 Days Mortality

Combining the Sepsis-3 criteria with the AKI risk prediction score at initiation of RRT led to a significant increase in risk stratification (total NRI = 0.07; 95% CI, 0.02–0.11; $p < 0.01$). The majority of this effect came from those without death (NRI event = 0.04; 95% CI, 0.01–0.07; $p = 0.039$). Likewise, the total IDI was significant (0.02, 95% CI, 0.01–0.02; $p < 0.001$).

In case of sequential diagnosis of sepsis according to the Sepsis-3 criteria, we added Sepsis-3 to the qSOFA criteria in estimating the risk of 90-day mortality after initiation of dialysis. This led to a significant increase in risk stratification (total NRI = 0.11; 95% CI, 0.04–0.19; $p = 0.004$). The majority of this effect came from those without death (NRI event = 0.07; $p = 0.03$), whereas the NRI with death was 0.05 (NRI non-event = 0.04, $p = 0.049$) (Figure S3). Similarly, the total integrated discrimination improvement (IDI) was significant at 0.06 (95% CI, 0.03 to 0.05; $p < 0.001$).

## 4. Discussion

To our best knowledge, this is the first study that applied the most recent Sepsis-3 screening criteria to the patients with AKI-D. The key findings of this large multi-center prospective study are that sepsis affects 53.5% of patients with AKI-D, and that at time of RRT 19.1% of patients had septic shock. The chances of renal recovery at 90 days were significantly lower in AKI-D patients with septic shock compared to those without sepsis. Presence of sepsis per Sepsis-3 criteria in AKI-D patients is associated with higher mortality rate and composite outcome at 90 days. Combining the Sepsis-3 criteria with the AKI risk score or SOFA criteria led to a further improvement in risk identification.

A 53.5% prevalence of sepsis among AKI-D patients is slightly higher than previously reported [18]. This may be a reflection of our specific patient cohort of critically ill ICU patients or a result of using the Sepsis-3 criteria. Similarly, in-hospital mortality rate of this cohort was high, including its non-septic controls (44.1%), which again may be explained by the characteristics of our patient population (older age, high comorbidity and acute severity of illness scores) and the criteria used to identify patients.

### *4.1. Association of Mortality and Non-Recovery from Dialysis*

Patients with AKI requiring RRT constitute a high-risk group. An accurate prognostic assessment is crucial for clinical management and planning of future care. The Sepsis-3 criteria identified AKI-D patients with a suspected or confirmed infection who were at increased risk of mortality, and a combo endpoint of mortality or dialysis dependence at 90 days. Our data also showed that the criteria to define septic shock (i.e., a raised serum lactate level and the need for inotropic support) indeed identified the subgroup of patients with the highest mortality (>80%).

The Sepsis-3 criteria correlated with SOFA and APACHE II scores at initiation of dialysis which underpins the potential use of Sepsis-3 in a critical care setting. It can be hypothesized that a higher Sepsis-3 score also reflects a higher degree of systemic inflammation.

Data on the risk of long-term dialysis dependence in AKI-D patients with sepsis are conflicting [18, 19], similar to a French multicentric study [19]. We found a statistically significant trend towards reduced likelihood of recovery from dialysis in AKI-D patients with septic shock compared to those without sepsis. In contrast, Bagshaw and colleagues analyzed data from 2000/2001 and reported improved renal recovery in patients with septic AKI compared to patients without sepsis [18]. It is important to note that there were differences in patient characteristics, criteria to define sepsis and clinical care. Moreover, our analysis has extra strength by including mortality as a competing outcome for analysis of dialysis dependence.

### *4.2. Sepsis-3 Criteria and Outcome*

It is important to emphasize that most AKI patients already had a SOFA score of two or more at the time when RRT was initiated simply as a result of AKI and oliguria. It is possible that different delta SOFA cut-off points are necessary for this patient cohort to differentiate sepsis from non-sepsis (Figure S6). As such, our results provide confirmation that AKI-D patients with sepsis, as defined by Sepsis-3 criteria, had higher mortality and less withdraw from dialysis in AKI-D patients with septic shock.

Combining the Sepsis-3 criteria with a clinical AKI risk prediction score resulted in greater IDI and NRI, and improved the ability associating subsequent death. Given the lack of appropriate risk stratification tools for septic AKI patients requiring RRT, the new Sepsis-3 criteria may associate patients outcome (Figures S3 and S5).

*4.3. Strengths and Limitations*

This is the first study that applied the new consensus criteria for sepsis to AKI-D patients, a cohort of patients that is known to have a high risk of sepsis and also a high risk of poor outcomes. Using a large multi-center national database with prospectively collected representative data from 30 ICUs, we showed for the first time that the Sepsis-3 criteria identified a group of patients that were at higher risk of dying or remaining dialysis dependent after discharge. With complete follow-up for 90 days after discharge from hospital, we focused on patient-centered outcomes (mortality and long-term dialysis dependence) and provide important data for a group of patients that is commonly seen in ICUs worldwide. Further in-depth studies are mandatory before we can make any positive comment on this issue.

The limitations of our study are related to any observational cohort study and include the possibility of both unmeasured and residual confounding factors. We could not identify how many patients received early goal-directed therapy in our cohort, however the nationwide education program instituted in Taiwan is able to positively change critical-care physician behavior in sepsis care following the Surviving Sepsis Campaign guidelines. We also acknowledge that we recorded the worst value of SOFA criteria within 24 h before initiation of dialysis. Although this approach is consistent with clinical practice, the daily SOFA score or qSOFA value may not reflect the value immediately before initiation of RRT.

## 5. Conclusions

More than half of the critically ill AKI patients treated with dialysis had sepsis, as defined by the Sepsis-3 criteria, at dialysis initiation, and one-fifth of AKI-D patients had septic shock screened by Sepsis-3 criteria. Having sepsis and septic shock were independently associated with 90-day mortality among these ICU AKI-D patients. Among survivors, AKI-D patients with septic shock had a significantly reduced chance of recovering sufficient renal function to wean-off dialysis, when compared to those without sepsis. These findings provide support for the use of Sepsis-3 criteria in the AKI-D patients.

**Supplementary Materials:**
Figure S1: Distribution of Patients by SOFA Score, and qSOFA Score at initiation of acute dialysis ($n$ = 1,078), X axis is %, Figure S2: Prognostic Accuracy of Sepsis-3 components among AKI-D patients with suspected or confirmed infection at dialysis initiation. a) 90 day mortality Receiver-operator characteristic curves discriminate (denoted area under the receiver operating characteristic curve): Sepsis-3, (0.650), qSOFA score ≥ 2 (0.631), AKI risk prediction score (0.688) and increased SOFA ≥ 2 (0.520). b) 90 day composite outcome. Receiver-operator characteristic curves discriminate (denoted area under the receiver operating characteristic curve): Sepsis-3, (0.587), qSOFA score ≥ 2 (0.578), AKI risk prediction score (0.596) and increased SOFA ≥ 2 (0.501), Figure S3: Decision curve analysis (DCA) plot to assess the clinical consequences of screening AKI-D patients for risk of 90 day mortality using sepsis-3 score in addition to AKI risk prediction score. *Y*-axis is the net benefit of the decision strategy. Net benefit is the net proportion of patients with 90 day mortality in whom a prediction model would provide benefit without applying a prediction model to patients with good outcomes. For AKI patients initiated on dialysis, forecasting with the AKI predicting model and Sepsis-3 criteria in combination would yield no net benefit. For risk thresholds between 30 and 80% the superior strategy, forecasting with the AKI risk prediction score and Sepsis-3 is beneficial. For moderate to high-risk thresholds (80 to 100%), there is no net benefit from using the AKI risk prediction score together with the Sepsis-3 model, Figure S4. Hazard Ratios for 90-day Mortality comparing different criteria of Sepsis-3 definition, Figure S5: Scatter plot of AKI risk prediction forecasted probabilities without and with the Sepsis-3 score. Note that some AKI-D patients have higher predicted risks in the model with Sepsis-3 values than in the model without Sepsis-3 (dots in right lower corner of the graph), Figure S6. Generalized additive model (GAM) plot for the probability of 90-day mortality against delta SOFA, in term of the difference of SOFA at initializing dialysis and ICU admission, initiating the subject-specific (longitudinal) random effects expressed as the logarithm of the odds (logit). The relationship of delta SOFA with these variables was further illustrated by GAM analysis, adjusted for Acute Physiology and Chronic Health Evaluation (APACHEII) at ICU admission, sex and age, showing that qSOFA levels at dialysis initializing could predict risk of mortality. GAM results showed the best cut-off points predicting 90 day mortality were a change of SOFA score by more than 10, Table S1: Integer risk score for prediction of 60-day mortality in critically ill patients with AKI requiring dialysis, Table S2. Diagnostic performance of Sepsis-3 criteria in prediction of 90-day hospital mortality.

**Author Contributions:** Study selection and analysis, writing up of the first draft of the paper, critical revision, and final approval of the article: V.-C.W. Data curation and investigation: S.-C.J.C. Study selection and analysis, critical revision, and final approval of the article: J.-S.C., J.-T.C. and B.-G.H. Data interpretation, critical revisions, and final approval of the article: M.O. and T.-S.C.

**Acknowledgments:** We would like to thank the National Taiwan University Hospital, Taiwan's National Health Research Institutes and Taiwan's Ministry of Science and Technology. And we would like to express our sincere gratitude to all staff of the Taiwan Clinical Trial Consortium, TR15, TCTC. We also express our sincere gratitude to all the staff of the Taiwan Clinical Trial Consortium, TCTC. The authors appreciate and thank all the members of the CAKS and NSARF, which are listed in alphabetical order of their affiliation names: (Fu Jen Catholic University Hospital): Kuo-Cheng Lu. (Chi-Mei Medical Center, Liouying): Jian-Jhong Wang. (Chi-Mei Medical Center, Yongkang): Wei-Chih Kan. (China Medical University Hospital): Chiu-Ching Huang, Che-Yi Chou, Ya-Fei Yang. (Dalin Tzu-Chi Hospital): Jen-Pi Tsai. (International-Harvard Statistical Consulting Company): Fu-Chang Hu. (Kaohsiung Chang Gung Memorial Hospital): Chien-Te Lee, Jin-Bor Chen, Chih-Hsiung Lee, Wen-Chin Lee, Lung-Chih Li, Te-Chuan Chen. (Kaohsiung Municipal Ta-Tung Hospital): Hugo You-Hsien Lin. (Keelung Chang Gung Memorial Hospital): Yung-Chang Chen, Chin-Chan Lee, Chiao-Yin Sun, Heng-Chih Pan. (Linkou Chang Gung Memorial Hospital): Ming-Yang Chang, Chang-Chyi Jenq, Chan-Yu Lin, Chih-Hsiang Chang, Tsung-Yu Tsai. (Lin-Shin Hospital): Cheng-Min Chen. (Lotung Poh-Ai Hospital): En-Tzu Lin. (Saint Mary's Hospital Luodong): Chih-Chung Shiao. (Mackay Memorial Hospital): Chih-Jen Wu, Cheng-Jua Lin, Pei-Chen Wu. (Mackay Memorial Hospital Taitung Branch): Feng-Chi Kuo. (Min-Sheng General Hospital): Chih-Jen Weng. (National Health Research Institutes): Li-Kwang Chen. (National Taiwan University Hospital): Kwan-Dun Wu, Tzong-Shinn Chu, Yung-Ming Chen, Shuei-Liong Lin, Vin-Cent Wu, Tao-Min Huang, Yu-Feng Lin, Chun-Fu Lai. Tai-Shuan Lai. (National Taiwan University Hospital Hsin Chu Branch): Wei-Shun Yang. (New Taipei City Hospital Sanchong Branch): Wen-Ding Hsu. (Shin-Kong Wo Ho-Su Memorial Hospital): Jyh-Gang Leu, Jui-Ting Chang. (Sin-Ren Hospital): Hung-Hsiang Liou. (Taichung Veteran General Hospital): Kuo-Hsiung Hsu, Ming-Ju Wu, Chun-Te Huang. (Taichung Veteran General Hospital Chiayi Branch): Zi-hong You. (Taipei City Hospital Heping Branch): Chao-Fu Chang. (Taipei Medical University Hospital): Tzen-Wen Chen, Hsi-Hsien Chen, Fan-Chi Chang, Yen- Chung Lin, Mai-Szu Wu, Chih-Chin Kao. (Taipei Tzu Chi Hospital): Szu-Chun Hung, Ko-Lin Kuo, Che-Hsiung Wu. (Taipei Veterans General Hospital): Der-Cherng Tarng, Jinn-Yang Chen, Chih-Yu Yang, Kuo-Hua Lee. (Taoyuan General Hospital, Ministry of Health and Welfare): Wei-Jie Wang, Sheng-Wen Ko, Jui-Hsiang Lin. The authors thank the English editing by Eric B. Chueh of Case Western University, Cleveland, Ohio, USA.

## Abbreviations

| | |
|---|---|
| APACHEII | Acute Physiology and Chronic Health Evaluation II |
| AKI | acute kidney injury |
| AKI-D | acute kidney injury with dialysis |
| MODS | multiple organ dysfunction syndrome |
| qSOFA | quick Sequential Organ Failure Assessment |
| RRT | renal replacement therapy |
| SOFA | Sequential Organ Failure Assessment |
| ICU | intensive care units |

## References

1. Hoste, E.A.; Bagshaw, S.M.; Bellomo, R.; Cely, C.M.; Colman, R.; Cruz, D.N.; Edipidis, K.; Forni, L.G.; Gomersall, C.D.; Govil, D.; et al. Epidemiology of acute kidney injury in critically ill patients: The multinational AKI-EPI study. *Intensive Care Med.* **2015**, *41*, 1411–1423. [CrossRef] [PubMed]
2. Singer, M.; Deutschman, C.S.; Seymour, C.W.; Shankar-Hari, M.; Annane, D.; Bauer, M.; Bellomo, R.; Bernard, G.R.; Chiche, J.D.; Coopersmith, C.M.; et al. The Third International Consensus Definitions for Sepsis and Septic Shock (Sepsis-3). *JAMA* **2016**, *315*, 801–810. [CrossRef] [PubMed]
3. Rhee, C.; Dantes, R.; Epstein, L.; Murphy, D.J.; Seymour, C.W.; Iwashyna, T.J.; Kadri, S.S.; Angus, D.C.; Danner, R.L.; Fiore, A.E.; et al. Incidence and Trends of Sepsis in US Hospitals Using Clinical vs Claims Data, 2009–2014. *JAMA* **2017**, *318*, 1241–1249. [CrossRef] [PubMed]
4. Hsu, C.Y.; McCulloch, C.E.; Fan, D.; Ordonez, J.D.; Chertow, G.M.; Go, A.S. Community-based incidence of acute renal failure. *Kidney Int.* **2007**, *72*, 208–212. [CrossRef] [PubMed]
5. Shiao, C.C.; Wu, P.C.; Wu, V.C.; Lin, J.H.; Pan, H.C.; Yang, Y.F.; Lai, T.S.; Huang, T.M.; Wu, C.H.; Yang, W.S.; et al. Nationwide epidemiology and prognosis of dialysis-requiring acute kidney injury (NEP-AKI-D) study: Design and methods. *Nephrology (Carlton)* **2016**, *21*, 758–764. [CrossRef] [PubMed]
6. Chen, Y.Y.; Wu, V.C.; Huang, W.C.; Yeh, Y.C.; Wu, M.S.; Huang, C.C.; Wu, K.D.; Fang, J.T.; Wu, C.J.; CAKS Group. Norepinephrine Administration Is Associated with Higher Mortality in Dialysis Requiring Acute

Kidney Injury Patients with Septic Shock. *J. Clin. Med.* **2018**, *7*, 274. [CrossRef] [PubMed]

7. Wu, V.C.; Ko, W.J.; Chang, H.W.; Chen, Y.S.; Chen, Y.W.; Chen, Y.M.; Hu, F.C.; Lin, Y.H.; Tsai, P.R.; Wu, K.D. Early renal replacement therapy in patients with postoperative acute liver failure associated with acute renal failure: Effect on postoperative outcomes. *J. Am. Coll. Surg.* **2007**, *205*, 266–276. [CrossRef] [PubMed]
8. Lin, Y.F.; Ko, W.J.; Wu, V.C.; Chen, Y.S.; Chen, Y.M.; Hu, F.C.; Shiao, C.C.; Wu, M.S.; Chen, Y.W.; Li, W.Y.; et al. A modified sequential organ failure assessment score to predict hospital mortality of postoperative acute renal failure patients requiring renal replacement therapy. *Blood Purif.* **2008**, *26*, 547–554. [CrossRef] [PubMed]
9. Shiao, C.C.; Ko, W.J.; Wu, V.C.; Huang, T.M.; Lai, C.F.; Lin, Y.F.; Chao, C.T.; Chu, T.S.; Tsai, H.B.; Wu, P.C.; et al. U-curve association between timing of renal replacement therapy initiation and in-hospital mortality in postoperative acute kidney injury. *PLoS ONE* **2012**, *7*, e42952. [CrossRef] [PubMed]
10. Seymour, C.W.; Liu, V.X.; Iwashyna, T.J.; Brunkhorst, F.M.; Rea, T.D.; Scherag, A.; Rubenfeld, G.; Kahn, J.M.; Shankar-Hari, M.; Singer, M.; et al. Assessment of Clinical Criteria for Sepsis: For the Third International Consensus Definitions for Sepsis and Septic Shock (Sepsis-3). *JAMA* **2016**, *315*, 762–774. [CrossRef] [PubMed]
11. Raith, E.P.; Udy, A.A.; Bailey, M.; McGloughlin, S.; MacIsaac, C.; Bellomo, R.; Pilcher, D.V. Prognostic Accuracy of the SOFA Score, SIRS Criteria, and qSOFA Score for In-Hospital Mortality Among Adults With Suspected Infection Admitted to the Intensive Care Unit. *JAMA* **2017**, *317*, 290–300. [CrossRef] [PubMed]
12. Wu, V.C.; Ko, W.J.; Chang, H.W.; Chen, Y.W.; Lin, Y.F.; Shiao, C.C.; Chen, Y.M.; Chen, Y.S.; Tsai, P.R.; Hu, F.C.; et al. Risk factors of early redialysis after weaning from postoperative acute renal replacement therapy. *Intensive Care Med.* **2008**, *34*, 101–108. [CrossRef] [PubMed]
13. Bellomo, R.; Kellum, J.A.; Ronco, C.; Wald, R.; Martensson, J.; Maiden, M.; Bagshaw, S.M.; Glassford, N.J.; Lankadeva, Y.; Vaara, S.T.; et al. Acute kidney injury in sepsis. *Intensive Care Med.* **2017**, *43*, 816–828. [CrossRef] [PubMed]
14. Demirjian, S.; Chertow, G.M.; Zhang, J.H.; O'Connor, T.Z.; Vitale, J.; Paganini, E.P.; Palevsky, P.M.; VA/NIH Acute Renal Failure Trial Network. Model to predict mortality in critically ill adults with acute kidney injury. *Clin. J. Am. Soc. Nephrol.* **2011**, *6*, 2114–2120. [CrossRef] [PubMed]
15. Chen, Y.S.; Ko, W.J.; Lin, F.Y.; Huang, S.C.; Chou, T.F.; Chou, N.K.; Hsu, R.B.; Wang, S.S.; Chu, S.H. Preliminary result of an algorithm to select proper ventricular assist devices for high-risk patients with extracorporeal membrane oxygenation support. *J. Heart Lung Transplant.* **2001**, *20*, 850–857. [CrossRef]
16. Shu, K.H.; Wang, C.H.; Wu, C.H.; Huang, T.M.; Wu, P.C.; Lai, C.H.; Tseng, L.J.; Tsai, P.R.; Connolly, R.; Wu, V.C. Urinary pi-glutathione S-transferase Predicts Advanced Acute Kidney Injury Following Cardiovascular Surgery. *Sci. Rep.* **2016**, *6*, 26335. [CrossRef] [PubMed]
17. Wang, J.J.; Chi, N.H.; Huang, T.M.; Connolly, R.; Chen, L.W.; Chueh, S.J.; Kan, W.C.; Lai, C.C.; Wu, V.C.; Fang, J.T.; et al. Urinary biomarkers predict advanced acute kidney injury after cardiovascular surgery. *Crit. Care* **2018**, *22*, 108. [CrossRef] [PubMed]
18. Bagshaw, S.M.; Uchino, S.; Bellomo, R.; Morimatsu, H.; Morgera, S.; Schetz, M.; Tan, I.; Bouman, C.; Macedo, E.; Gibney, N.; et al. Septic acute kidney injury in critically ill patients: Clinical characteristics and outcomes. *Clin. J. Am. Soc. Nephrol.* **2007**, *2*, 431–439. [CrossRef] [PubMed]
19. Venot, M.; Weis, L.; Clec'h, C.; Darmon, M.; Allaouchiche, B.; Goldgran-Toledano, D.; Garrouste-Orgeas, M.; Adrie, C.; Timsit, J.F.; Azoulay, E. Acute Kidney Injury in Severe Sepsis and Septic Shock in Patients with and without Diabetes Mellitus: A Multicenter Study. *PLoS ONE* **2015**, *10*, e0127411. [CrossRef] [PubMed]

# 5

# Long-Term Outcomes in Patients with Incident Chronic Obstructive Pulmonary Disease after Acute Kidney Injury: A Competing-Risk Analysis of a Nationwide Cohort

**Che-Hsiung Wu [1,2,†], Huang-Ming Chang [3,†], Cheng-Yi Wang [4], Likwang Chen [5], Liang-Wen Chen [6], Chien-Heng Lai [6], Shuenn-Wen Kuo [6], Hao-Chien Wang [3], Vin-Cent Wu [3,*] and The National Taiwan University Study Group on Acute Renal Failure [‡]**

1 Division of Nephrology, Taipei Tzu Chi Hospital, Buddhist Tzu Chi Medical Foundation, New Taipei City 231, Taiwan; tcubear@gmail.com
2 School of Medicine, Tzu Chi University, Hualien 970, Taiwan
3 Department of Internal Medicine, National Taiwan University Hospital, Taipei 100, Taiwan; eddie925@ms33.hinet.net (H.-M.C.); haochienwang@gmail.com (H.-C.W.)
4 Department of Internal Medicine, College of Medicine, Fu Jen Catholic University, New Taipei City 242, Taiwan; cywang@mospital.com
5 Institute of Population Health Sciences, National Health Research Institutes, Zhunan 350, Taiwan; likwang.chen@gmail.com
6 Department of Surgery, National Taiwan University Hospital, National Taiwan University, Taipei 100, Taiwan; liangwenyumin@gmail.com (L.-W.C.); b8805007@gmail.com (C.-H.L.); shuenn8@gmail.com (S.-W.K.)
* Correspondence: q91421028@ntu.edu.tw
† These authors contribute equally to this article.
‡ Membership of National Taiwan University Study Group on Acute Renal Failure is provided in the Acknowledgments.

**Abstract:** Both acute kidney injury (AKI) and chronic obstructive pulmonary disease (COPD) are associated with increased morbidity and mortality. However, the incidence of de novo COPD in patients with AKI, and the impact of concurrent COPD on the outcome during post-AKI care is unclear. Patients who recovered from dialysis-requiring AKI (AKI-D) during index hospitalizations between 1998 and 2010 were identified from nationwide administrative registries. A competing risk analysis was conducted to predict the incidence of adverse cardiovascular events and mortality. Among the 14,871 patients who recovered from temporary dialysis, 1535 (10.7%) were identified as having COPD (COPD group) one year after index discharge and matched with 1473 patients without COPD (non-COPD group) using propensity scores. Patients with acute kidney disease superimposed withs COPD were associated with a higher risk of incident ischemic stroke (subdistribution hazard ratio (sHR), 1.52; 95% confidence interval (95% CI), 1.17 to 1.97; $p = 0.002$) and congestive heart failure (CHF; sHR, 1.61; (95% CI), 1.39 to 1.86; $p < 0.001$). The risks of incident hemorrhagic stroke, myocardial infarction, end-stage renal disease, and mortality were not statistically different between the COPD and non-COPD groups. This observation adds another dimension to accumulating evidence regarding pulmo-renal consequences after AKI.

**Keywords:** acute kidney injury; chronic obstructive pulmonary disease; congestive heart failure; stroke

## 1. Introduction

The incidence of acute kidney injury (AKI) in hospitalized patients is increasing [1] and has been associated with high mortality and morbidity worldwide over the past decade [2]. The incidence of AKI requiring dialysis (AKI-D) is increasing by 10% per year in the United States and is higher than that of end-stage renal disease (ESRD) [3]. Patient survival from an episode of AKI has been improved by advances in critical care medicine and dialysis technology increasing the survival rate of hospitalized patients discharged after temporary dialysis [4]. Previous studies showed that patients with a history of AKI have a higher incidence of coronary events [5], stroke [6], congestive heart failure (CHF) [7], ESRD, and mortality [8] than individuals without AKI. The American Society of Nephrology AKI Advisory Group has highlighted the transition of care as a potential opportunity to reduce the long-term impact of AKI [9]. To improve the situation of dialysis patients, novel renal replacement therapies, such as an implantable artificial renal assist device, are under development. The artificial renal assist device strategy utilizes micromachining techniques to fabricate a biohybrid system able to mimic renal morphology and function [10]. Chronic obstructive pulmonary disease (COPD) is a chronic inflammatory lung disease characterized by airflow limitations. Comorbidities are common in COPD, including cardiovascular [11], cerebrovascular [12], and chronic kidney diseases [13]. These comorbidities are possibly attributed to a chronic inflammatory state in COPD and are increasingly recognized as important determinants of COPD prognosis [13].

Each injured organ can initiate various complex pathways affecting distant organs through hemodynamic, neurohormonal, and cell signaling feedback mechanisms [14]. The kidney plays a key role in fluid, electrolyte, acid-base and clearance homeostasis so that AKI provides a significant impulse for the initiation of organ crosstalk. At the cellular level, the renal tubular epithelium plays a fundamental role in regulating the inflammatory processes [7]. A study has shown that lung inflammation is a consistent finding after ischemic AKI [15]. Nonetheless, there is no study addressing the incidence of COPD in patients with AKI-D. In addition, metabolic and respiratory acidosis is a common and severe complication observed in patients with AKI-D and COPD. When COPD occurs in patients with renal failure, the compensatory role of the kidneys and lungs in acidosis may be less effective, resulting in a more severe acidosis status. The recent Kidney Disease Improving Global Outcomes (KDIGO) guideline introduced a new conceptual model, called acute kidney disease (AKD), to emphasize the need to follow patients who survived AKI episodes. The AKD period, linking AKI to chronic kidney disease (CKD), requires intensive care to manage possible hypertension and cardiovascular disease [16]. However, no study has ascertained the contributing role of COPD in patients with a history of AKI in aggravating subsequent morbidity and mortality. With the increasing recognition that COPD and kidney disease extend beyond the pulmo-renal syndrome, interest in lung–kidney–cardiovascular interactions has increased. Using the Taiwan National Health Insurance research dataset, we designed a nationwide, population-based cohort study to examine the long-term risk of adverse cardiovascular incidents, chronic dialysis events, and mortality in patients with COPD during the AKD period.

## 2. Methods

### *2.1. Data Sources*

This population-based cohort study used medical information from Taiwan's National Health Insurance (NHI) database, a compulsory universal health insurance program that covers outpatient visits, hospital admissions, prescriptions, interventions, disease profiles, and vital status of nearly all 23.7 million Taiwan residents. The NHI database is one of the largest and most comprehensive health-care registries worldwide. Patients were anonymous in our study; thus, informed consent was not required. Additionally, since the identification numbers of all individuals in the database were encrypted to protect their privacy, this study was exempt from a full ethical review by the National Taiwan University Hospital institutional review board (201212021RINC).

### 2.2. Study Group

The first AKI-D after hospitalization was defined as the index hospitalization for each individual. AKI was defined using the International Classification of Diseases-9 (ICD-9) codes 584.X, 634.3, 635.3, 636.3, 637.3, 638.3, 639.3, 669.3, and 958.5 and procedure codes for acute dialysis. Dialysis certificate data in Taiwan are highly reliable because they are used for insurance payments [17]. We extracted all newly diagnosed AKI patients with de novo AKI-D (identified using the procedure codes) during their index hospitalizations who subsequently recovered from AKI-D (dialysis withdrawal) at least 30 days after discharge between 1 January 1998 and 31 December 2010. Pre-admission comorbidities were identified during at least three outpatient visits or during one inpatient claim within 1 year preceding the index admission. In Taiwan's National Health Insurance Research Database, ICD-9 codes are used to define diseases. We excluded individuals who had a previous diagnosis of AKI; received a kidney transplant; undergone creation of hemodialysis vascular accesses, peritoneal dialysis catheter implantation, or any form of dialysis preceding the index hospitalization; hospitalizations >180 days with AKI; or those who died during the index hospitalization. Our study enrolled only patients who survived the index hospitalization and had no re-dialysis 30 days after discharge. This identification procedure avoided selective bias [18,19].

The COPD group comprised patients with AKI who recovered from dialysis and incidental COPD within 1 year after the index hospitalization. To ensure accuracy, the diagnosis of COPD was validated based on one inpatient or three outpatient records with ICD-9-CM codes 490–492, 494, and 496 [20,21] and received at least one bronchodilator during the follow-up period [22]. Patients without COPD and no recorded previous asthma or COPD medication prescriptions were included in the control (non-COPD) group (Figure 1).

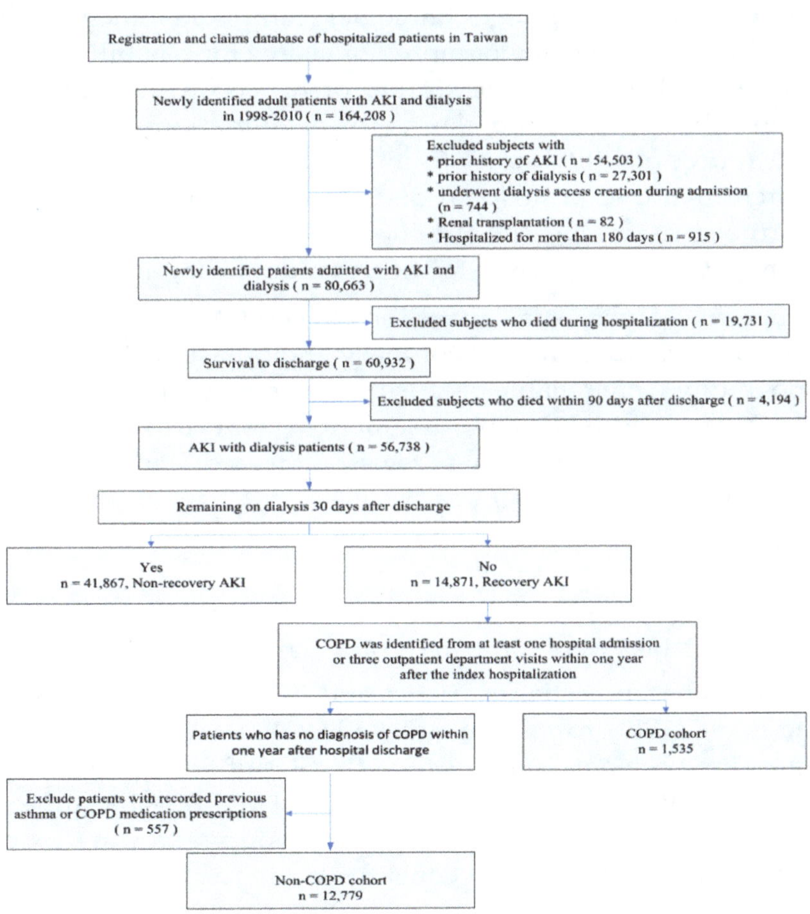


**Figure 1.** Flow Chart of the enrollee.

### 2.3. Baseline Characteristics

The baseline comorbidities were identified from at least three outpatient visits or one inpatient claim within one year preceding the index hospitalization. This identification method has been well validated with good predictive power [18,23–26]. The Charlson comorbidity index (CCI) was calculated by weighting baseline comorbidities. We collected concomitant medication data associated with the outcomes of interest. According to the Taiwan NHI reimbursement policy, erythropoiesis-stimulating agents may only be prescribed for pre-dialysis chronic kidney disease (CKD) patients with anemia, hematocrits ≤28%, and serum creatinine levels >6 mg/dL (equivalent to an estimated glomerular filtration rate of <15 mL/min/1.73 $m^2$, CKD stage 5). We defined this combination of CKD diagnosis codes and pre-dialysis patients using erythropoiesis-stimulating agents as having "advanced CKD" [27].

### 2.4. Outcomes

In order to avoid immortal time bias, the observation period began one year after the index hospitalization discharge and continued until the first documented outcome of interest or the end of the study (31 December 2010), whichever occurred first. The outcomes of interest included all-cause mortality, hospitalization, or death with a principal diagnosis of ischemic stroke (ICD-9-CM code 433.x, 434.x, or 436), hemorrhagic stroke (ICD-9-CM code 431 or 432) [6], CHF (ICD-9-CM code 428.x), major adverse cardiovascular events (MACE), and ESRD [28].

Stroke was defined as one of the following conditions [29]: (a) records of emergency room service or hospitalization claims for >1 day or records of emergency room service with ICD-9-CM codes followed by claims for various brain-imaging technologies (computed tomography, magnetic resonance imaging, transcranial or carotid Doppler sonography) or claims for rehabilitation and anti-coagulation prescriptions customarily used for ischemic stroke; or (b) records of three or more consecutive outpatient visits with the above codes and claims for examinations, services, or prescriptions as described in (a) [24]. A reproducibility study found that the ICD-9 stroke codes from the Taiwan National Health Research Institutes at hospital discharge were highly accurate with a substantial kappa test [26]. Furthermore, prior studies have shown that the algorithms using ICD-9 diagnostic codes have a positive predictive value (>95%) for heart failure hospitalizations [26,30].

MACE included nonfatal myocardial infarction (ICD-9-CM code 410.x) [26], coronary artery bypass grafts, and percutaneous transluminal coronary angioplasty [31]. Records of coronary artery bypass grafts and angiography were reliable because they were constructed based on NHI procedure codes that were tied to the audited NHI reimbursement system. In Taiwan, patients who continue dialysis for >90 days receive a catastrophic illness registration card, which ensures the accuracy of our dialysis continuation definition.

### 2.5. Statistical Analysis

Continuous variables were compared using an unpaired t-test and are expressed as a mean ± standard deviation (SD). Categorical variables were compared using the $\chi^2$ test and expressed as a percentage.

Given the differences in baseline characteristics and the risk of cardiovascular disease between the incident COPD and non-COPD groups, we matched COPD patients to non-COPD patients using a greedy matching algorithm with a caliper width of 0.2 SDs of the log of the odds of the estimated propensity score with a 1:1 ratio (Supplementary Table S1). Crude hazard ratios (HR) with 95% confidence intervals (CIs) for the outcomes of interest were derived from Cox proportional hazards models. Matched individuals without COPD constituted the reference group. Because of the high mortality rate in patients with COPD after AKI-D, competing risk regression was also performed using the Fine and Gray model considering the subdistribution hazard [32,33]. We used R software version 2.8.1 (Free Software Foundation, Inc., Boston, MA, USA) for the time-varying Cox model and Stata/MP version 14 (Stata Corporation, Lakeway Drive College Station, TX, USA) for the competing risk analysis. Two-sided $p$ values <0.05 were considered statistically significant.

## 3. Results

### 3.1. Characteristics of the Study Population

A total of 14,871 individuals after short-term dialysis who survived after hospital discharge were eligible. Among these patients, incident COPD was identified in 1535 (10.7%); 557 with recorded previous asthma or COPD medication prescriptions were excluded. The remaining 12,779 patients were non-COPD controls (Figure 1). The mean age of the COPD group was 73.91 ± 11.25 years, and the proportion of men was 66.94%. After propensity score matching, we identified 1473 patients with COPD and 1473 matched controls with similar baseline characteristics. Detailed demographic information of the individuals with or without COPD before and after propensity score matching is shown in Table 1 and Supplementary Figure S1.

**Table 1.** AKI patients after temporary dialysis with and without COPD, before and after propensity score matching.

| | **Before Matching** | | | **After Matching** | | |
|---|---|---|---|---|---|---|
| | **Non COPD (*n* = 12,779)** | **COPD (*n* = 1535)** | ***p*-Value** | **Non COPD (*n* = 1473)** | **COPD (*n* = 1473)** | ***p*-Value** |
| Age (year, SD) | 63.63 ± 16.39 | 74.02 ± 11.31 | <0.001 | 73.95 ± 11.28 | 73.91 ± 11.25 | 0.888 |
| Male gender | 6715 (52.55%) | 1044 (68.01%) | <0.001 | 960 (65.17%) | 986 (66.94%) | 0.331 |
| Monthly income, US dollars | | | | | | |
| <600 | 7865 (61.55%) | 923 (60.13%) | | 903 (61.30%) | 890 (60.42%) | |
| 600–1300 | 4484 (35.09%) | 581 (37.85%) | 0.004 | 530 (35.98%) | 554 (37.61%) | 0.304 |
| ≥1300 | 430 (3.36%) | 31 (2.02%) | | 40 (2.72%) | 29 (1.97%) | |
| Hospital location | | | | | | |
| Urban | 5276 (41.29%) | 604 (39.35%) | | 559 (37.95%) | 579 (39.31%) | |
| Suburban | 2947 (23.06%) | 320 (20.85%) | 0.005 | 311 (21.11%) | 312 (21.18%) | 0.696 |
| Rural | 4556 (35.65%) | 611 (39.80%) | | 603 (40.94%) | 582 (39.51%) | |
| Baseline comorbidities | | | | | | |
| Charlson comorbidity index | 2.17 ± 2.03 | 2.61 ± 2.06 | <0.001 | 2.59 ± 2.09 | 2.61 ± 2.08 | 0.736 |
| Myocardial infarction | 542 (4.24%) | 75 (4.89%) | 0.232 | 68 (4.62%) | 75 (5.09%) | 0.607 |
| Congestive heart failure | 1956 (15.31%) | 349 (22.74%) | <0.001 | 326 (22.13%) | 336 (22.81%) | 0.691 |
| Peripheral vascular disease | 244 (1.91%) | 25 (1.63%) | 0.487 | 29 (1.97%) | 25 (1.70%) | 0.681 |
| Cerebrovascular disease | 1382 (10.81%) | 276 (17.98%) | <0.001 | 246 (16.70%) | 256 (17.38%) | 0.659 |
| Dementia | 315 (2.46%) | 98 (6.38%) | <0.001 | 91 (6.18%) | 91 (6.18%) | 0.999 |
| Reumatologic disease | 243 (1.90%) | 18 (1.17%) | 0.043 | 16 (1.09%) | 18 (1.22%) | 0.863 |
| Peptic ulcer disease | 1791 (14.02%) | 273 (17.79%) | <0.001 | 265 (17.99%) | 259 (17.58%) | 0.81 |
| Hemiplegia or paraplegia | 117 (0.92%) | 26 (1.69%) | 0.006 | 16 (1.09%) | 26 (1.77%) | 0.161 |
| Diabetes | 4956 (38.78%) | 582 (37.92%) | 0.524 | 544 (36.93%) | 569 (38.63%) | 0.362 |
| Moderate or severe liver disease | 1036 (8.11%) | 98 (6.38%) | 0.019 | 89 (6.04%) | 94 (6.38%) | 0.76 |
| Chronic kidney disease | 4034 (31.57%) | 445 (28.99%) | 0.041 | 447 (30.35%) | 437 (29.67%) | 0.718 |
| Hypertension | 6630 (51.88%) | 950 (61.89%) | <0.001 | 889 (60.35%) | 911 (61.85%) | 0.427 |
| Dyslipidemia | 1765 (13.81%) | 167 (10.88%) | 0.001 | 185 (12.56%) | 164 (11.13%) | 0.254 |
| Medication for hypertension before index hospitalization | | | | | | |
| Alpha-blocker | 1326 (10.38%) | 206 (13.42%) | <0.001 | 201 (13.65%) | 201 (13.65%) | 0.999 |
| Beta-blocker | 4696 (36.75%) | 509 (33.16%) | 0.006 | 507 (34.42%) | 494 (33.54%) | 0.641 |
| CCB | 6807 (53.27%) | 946 (61.63%) | <0.001 | 881 (59.81%) | 903 (61.30%) | 0.429 |
| Diuretic | 6657 (52.09%) | 926 (60.33%) | <0.001 | 859 (58.32%) | 887 (60.22%) | 0.311 |
| ACEI or ARB | 5577 (43.64%) | 767 (49.97%) | <0.001 | 719 (48.81%) | 744 (50.51%) | 0.376 |
| Other medication | | | | | | |
| Aspirin | 1107 (8.66%) | 163 (10.62%) | 0.013 | 171 (11.61%) | 156 (10.59%) | 0.412 |
| Clopidogrel | 640 (5.01%) | 107 (6.97%) | 0.002 | 97 (6.59%) | 105 (7.13%) | 0.61 |
| Ticlopidine | 471 (3.69%) | 76 (4.95%) | 0.017 | 70 (4.75%) | 74 (5.02%) | 0.798 |
| Dipyridamole | 2851 (22.31%) | 357 (23.26%) | 0.4 | 358 (24.30%) | 348 (23.63%) | 0.698 |
| Nitrate | 93 (0.73%) | 22 (1.43%) | 0.006 | 19 (1.29%) | 19 (1.29%) | 0.999 |
| Statin | 2009 (15.72%) | 191 (12.44%) | 0.001 | 209 (14.19%) | 184 (12.49%) | 0.193 |
| NSAID | 6375 (49.89%) | 859 (55.96%) | <0.001 | 822 (55.80%) | 819 (55.60%) | 0.941 |
| PPI | 1214 (9.50%) | 201 (13.09%) | <0.001 | 165 (11.20%) | 191 (12.97%) | 0.158 |

**Table 1.** *Cont.*

| | Before Matching | | | After Matching | | |
|---|---|---|---|---|---|---|
| | Non COPD (*n* = 12,779) | COPD (*n* = 1535) | *p*-Value | Non COPD (*n* = 1473) | COPD (*n* = 1473) | *p*-Value |
| Index hospital comorbidity | | | | | | |
| Cardiovascular | 1148 (8.98%) | 150 (9.77%) | 0.301 | 153 (10.39%) | 142 (9.64%) | 0.539 |
| Respiratory | 2819 (22.06%) | 635 (41.37%) | <0.001 | 602 (40.87%) | 582 (39.51%) | 0.475 |
| Hepatic | 267 (2.09%) | 15 (0.98%) | 0.002 | 22 (1.49%) | 14 (0.95%) | 0.24 |
| Neurologic | 250 (1.96%) | 37 (2.41%) | 0.247 | 35 (2.38%) | 35 (2.38%) | 0.999 |
| Hematologic | 201 (1.57%) | 16 (1.04%) | 0.121 | 17 (1.15%) | 15 (1.02%) | 0.859 |
| Metabolic | 365 (2.86%) | 35 (2.28%) | 0.219 | 41 (2.78%) | 35 (2.38%) | 0.561 |
| ICU admission | 8492 (66.45%) | 1189 (77.46%) | <0.001 | 1141 (77.46%) | 1130 (76.71%) | 0.661 |
| Operation | 1314 (10.28%) | 151 (9.84%) | 0.624 | 136 (9.23%) | 139 (9.44%) | 0.899 |
| Renal function status at AKD periods (1 year after index hospitalization) | | | | | | |
| CKD | 4958 (38.80%) | 642 (41.82%) | 0.023 | 532 (36.12%) | 622 (42.23%) | 0.001 |
| Advanced CKD | 2410 (18.86%) | 206 (13.42%) | <0.001 | 199 (13.51%) | 201 (13.65%) | 0.957 |

All data were descripted as number (%), except mean age. Abbreviations: ACEI, angiotensin-converting-enzyme inhibitors; AKD, acute kidney disease; ARB, Angiotensin II receptor blockers; CCB, calcium channel blocker; CKD, chronic kidney disease; COPD, chronic obstructive pulmonary disease; GI, gastrointestinal; ICU, intensive care unit; NSAIDs, Non-steroidal anti-inflammatory drugs; PPI, proton-pump inhibitor; SD, standard deviation.

### *3.2. Long-Term Risks of Death, Stroke, and CHF*

After a mean follow-up period of 3.32 years, a total of 1050 (71.28%) and 971 (65.92%) patients in the COPD and the non-COPD groups, respectively, died (Table 2). The incidences of all-cause mortality were 226.6 per 1000 person-years in the COPD group and 188.2 per 1000 person-years in the non-COPD group (Table 3). The disparity in all-cause mortality between the two groups was not statistically significant after adjusting the propensity score and renal function status during the AKD period (adjusted HR, 1.04; 95% CI, 0.96–1.14; $p = 0.331$).

**Table 2.** Long-term outcomes the first year after index hospitalization discharge.

| Events | Before Matching | | | After Matching | | |
|---|---|---|---|---|---|---|
| | Non-COPD (*n* = 12,779) | COPD (*n* = 1535) | *p*-Value | Non-COPD (*n* = 1473) | COPD (*n* = 1473) | *p*-Value |
| All-cause death | 6931 (54.24%) | 1096 (71.40%) | <0.001 | 971 (65.92%) | 1050 (71.28%) | 0.002 |
| Stroke | 1044 (8.17%) | 172 (11.21%) | <0.001 | 121 (8.21%) | 170 (11.54%) | 0.003 |
| Ischemic stroke | 774 (6.06%) | 144 (9.38%) | <0.001 | 95 (6.45%) | 143 (9.71%) | 0.001 |
| Hemorrhagic stroke | 327 (2.56%) | 36 (2.35%) | 0.668 | 30 (2.04%) | 35 (2.38%) | 0.616 |
| CHF | 2541 (19.88%) | 458 (29.84%) | <0.001 | 296 (20.10%) | 448 (30.41%) | <0.001 |
| MACE * | 802 (6.28%) | 96 (6.25%) | 0.999 | 87 (5.91%) | 95 (6.45%) | 0.592 |
| ESRD | 3362 (26.31%) | 311 (20.26%) | <0.001 | 299 (20.30%) | 302 (20.50%) | 0.927 |

CHF, congestive heart failure; COPD, chronic obstructive pulmonary disease; ESRD, end-stage renal disease; MACE, major adverse cardiovascular events; SD, standard deviation; * MACE includes myocardial infarction, coronary artery bypass graft, and percutaneous transluminal coronary angioplasty.

**Table 3.** Incidence and risk of outcomes of interest among patients after temporary dialysis with and without chronic obstructive pulmonary disease.

| | COPD | | | Non-COPD | | | Crude | | Adjusted † | | Compete Risk †† | |
|---|---|---|---|---|---|---|---|---|---|---|---|---|
| | Event | Person-Year | Incidence Rate (per 1000 Person-Years) | Event | Person-Year | Incidence Rate (per 1000 Person-Years) | HR (95%CI) | *p* Value | HR (95%CI) | *p* Value | sHR (95%CI) | *p* Value |
| Before Propensity Score Matching | | | | | | | | | | | | |
| All-cause death | 1096 | 4848.71 | 226.0 | 6931 | 57,368.8 | 120.8 | 1.55 [1.45,1.65] | <0.001 | 0.96 [0.90,1.04] | 0.323 | NA | NA |
| Stroke | 172 | 4368.39 | 39.4 | 1044 | 53,890 | 19.4 | 1.70 [1.45,2.00] | <0.001 | 1.27 [1.06,1.53] | 0.009 | 1.30 [1.07,1.56] | 0.007 |
| Ischemic stroke | 144 | 4413.14 | 32.6 | 774 | 54,369.5 | 14.2 | 1.88 [1.57,2.24] | <0.001 | 1.33 [1.09,1.63] | 0.006 | 1.37 [1.11,1.69] | 0.004 |
| Hemorrhagic stroke | 36 | 4783.3 | 7.5 | 327 | 56,658.6 | 5.8 | 1.18 [0.84,1.67] | 0.349 | 1.08 [0.74,1.57] | 0.691 | 1.05 [0.72,1.54] | 0.8 |
| CHF | 458 | 3769.6 | 121.5 | 2541 | 50,533.8 | 50.3 | 1.89 [1.71,2.09] | <0.001 | 1.37 [1.22,1.53] | <0.001 | 1.39 [1.24,1.56] | <0.001 |
| MACE | 127 | 4595.71 | 27.6 | 1127 | 54,737.5 | 20.6 | 1.20 [1.00,1.44] | 0.055 | 0.89 [0.73,1.09] | 0.270 | 0.89 [0.72,1.08] | 0.240 |
| ESRD | 311 | 4073.25 | 76.4 | 3362 | 45,620.2 | 73.7 | 0.81 [0.72,0.91] | <0.001 | 0.90 [0.80,1.02] | 0.102 | 0.91 [0.80,1.03] | 0.120 |
| After Propensity Score Matching | | | | | | | | | | | | |
| All-cause death | 1050 | 4633.13 | 226.6 | 971 | 5159.11 | 188.2 | 1.08 [0.99,1.17] | 0.104 | 1.04 [0.96,1.14] | 0.331 | NA | NA |
| Stroke | 170 | 4156.28 | 40.9 | 121 | 4788.18 | 25.3 | 1.45 [1.14,1.83] | 0.002 | 1.42 [1.12,1.79] | 0.004 | 1.43 [1.13,1.81] | 0.003 |
| Ischemic stroke | 143 | 4201.03 | 34.0 | 95 | 4831.49 | 19.7 | 1.52 [1.17,1.97] | 0.002 | 1.48 [1.14,1.92] | 0.003 | 1.52 [1.17,1.97] | 0.002 |
| Hemorrhagic stroke | 35 | 4567.72 | 7.7 | 30 | 5107.35 | 5.9 | 1.26 [0.77,2.05] | 0.362 | 1.26 [0.77,2.05] | 0.361 | 1.19 [0.73,1.96] | 0.480 |
| CHF | 448 | 3583.99 | 125.0 | 296 | 4547.46 | 65.1 | 1.62 [1.40,1.88] | <0.001 | 1.59 [1.37,1.84] | <0.001 | 1.61 [1.39,1.86] | <0.001 |
| MACE * | 126 | 4391.31 | 28.7 | 116 | 4871.23 | 23.8 | 1.13 [0.87,1.45] | 0.357 | 1.12 [0.87,1.44] | 0.396 | 1.09 [0.84,1.40] | 0.520 |
| ESRD | 302 | 3870.54 | 78.0 | 299 | 4367.31 | 68.5 | 0.97 [0.83,1.14] | 0.695 | 0.96 [0.81,1.12] | 0.579 | 0.95 [0.81,1.12] | 0.550 |

CHF, congestive heart failure; CI, confidence interval; ESRD, end stage renal disease; HR, hazard ratio; MACE, major adverse cardiovascular events, NA, not available; sHR, subdistribution hazard ratio; * MACE includes myocardial infarction, coronary artery bypass graft, and percutaneous transluminal coronary angioplasty. † Adjusted for propensity score and renal function status 1 year after index hospitalization. †† Death was calculated as a competing risk, adjusted for propensity score and renal function status 1 year after index hospitalization.

In contrast to the non-COPD group, the COPD group had a higher long-term risk of incident CHF (sHR, 1.61; 95% CI, 1.39–1.86; $p < 0.001$; Figure 2a) and ischemic stroke (sHR, 1.52; 95% CI, 1.17–1.97; $p = 0.002$; Figure 2b), but had a similar risk of hemorrhagic stroke (sHR, 1.19; 95% CI, 0.73–1.96; $p = 0.480$; Figure 2c) after considering mortality as a competing risk.

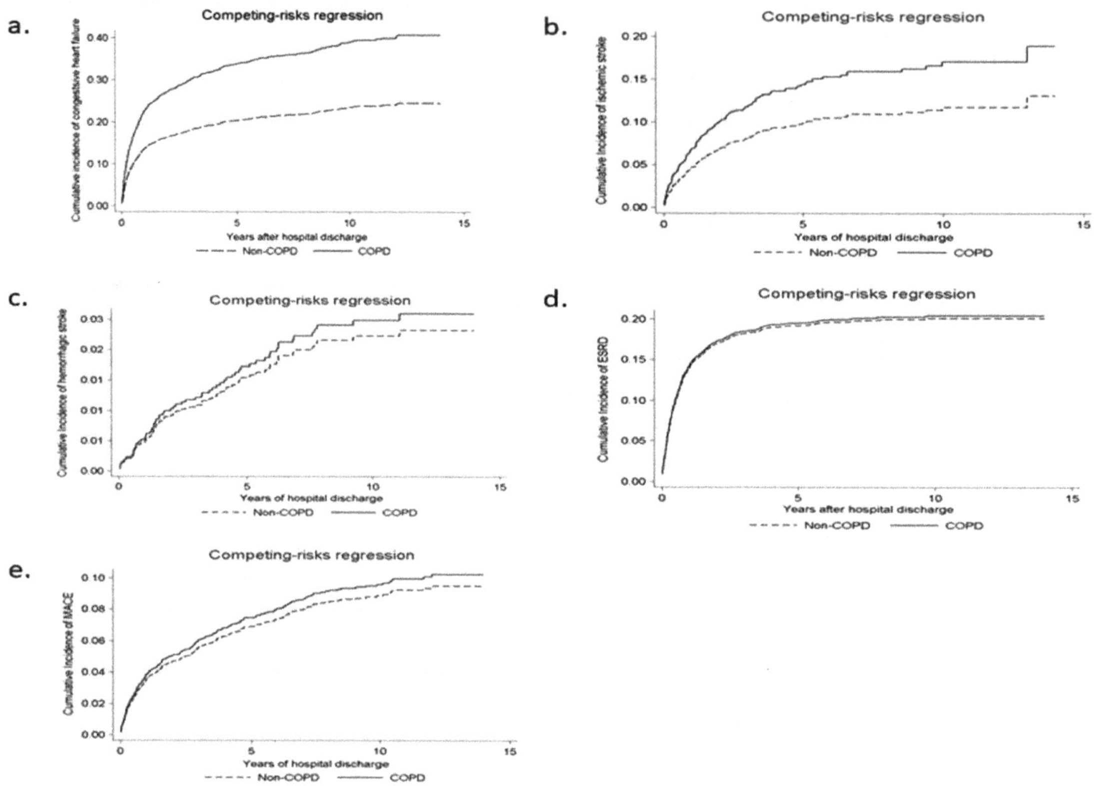


**Figure 2.** Cumulative probability of (**a**) congestive heart failure (HR 1.61; $p < 0.001$), (**b**) ischemic stroke (HR 1.52; $p = 0.002$), (**c**) hemorrhagic stroke (HR 1.19; $p = 0.480$), (**d**) end- stage renal disease (HR 0.95; $p = 0.550$), and (**e**) major adverse cardiovascular events (HR 1.09; $p = 0.520$) in the matched patients after acute kidney injury with or without chronic obstructive pulmonary disease, using mortality as a competing risk.

### *3.3. Long-Term Risks of MACE and ESRD*

A total of 95 (6.45%) patients in the COPD group and 87 (5.91%) in the non-COPD group experienced MACE, but the difference was not statistically significant (Table 2; $p = 0.592$). The COPD group had similar risks of ESRD compared with the matched non-COPD group ($p = 0.927$). After adjusting for in-hospital death as a competing risk, the analysis yielded consistent results (Figure 2d,e). The subdistribution hazard ratio for MACE was 1.09 (95% CI, 0.84–1.40; $p = 0.520$) and 0.95 (95% CI, 0.81–1.12; $p = 0.550$) for ESRD (Table 3).

### *3.4. Subgroup Analysis with Comorbidities*

A subgroup analysis of baseline characteristics and comorbidities was performed to investigate whether the COPD group consistently had a higher long-term risk of ischemic stroke and CHF compared to the non-COPD group. Using participant characteristics, we found that COPD was associated with a higher risk of ischemic stroke and CHF in most patients after AKI regardless of any prior history of COPD (Figure 3a,b).

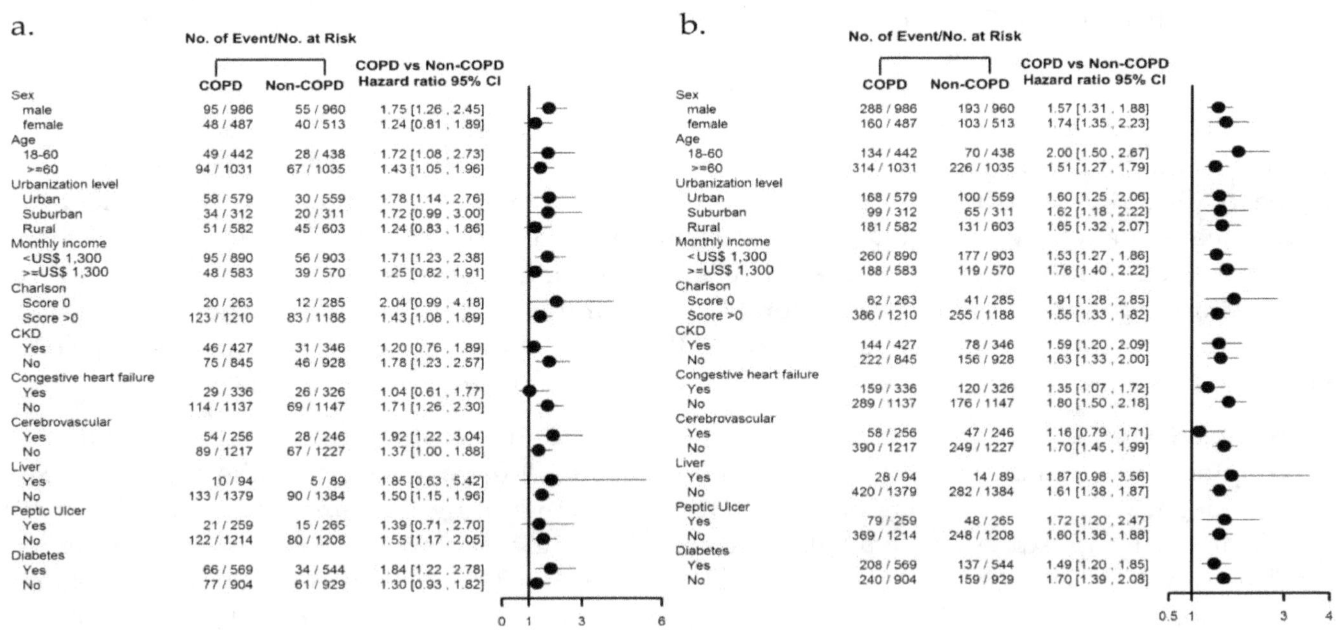


**Figure 3.** Risk of (**a**) ischemic stroke, and (**b**) congestive heart failure in matched patients after AKI with or without COPD using participant characteristics.

## 4. Discussion

In this large population-based group study, we found that more than one-tenth of patients were likely to have COPD early after temporary dialysis. In patients who recovered from AKI-D, concomitant COPD was associated with a higher risk of incident ischemic stroke and CHF; however, the risks of all-cause mortality, MACE, and ESRD were similar to those who did not have COPD. These results remained constant even after the identification of severe kidney sequelae during the AKD period and when accounting for death as a competing risk.

### *4.1. Risk of COPD after AKI-D*

The current study revealed that 10.7% of patients who recovered from temporary dialysis were concomitantly diagnosed with COPD one year after index hospitalization. To our knowledge, this is the first study addressing the incidence of COPD after AKI-D. The age-standardized reported prevalence of COPD was 3.2% in males and 2.0% in females [34]. A population-based study demonstrated that the diagnosis of COPD was recorded in 2.6% of hospitalized patients [35]. The incidence of COPD in patients with AKI-D is much higher than in the general population. Data from animal models support the supposition that cardiogenic pulmonary edema and non-cardiogenic pulmonary edema (from endothelial injury due to inflammation and apoptosis) can occur in AKI [36]. Lung inflammation is a consistent finding after ischemic AKI, especially after prolonged AKI with more than 7 days of dialysis [15]. Accumulated evidence from animal models and patients with AKI suggests that IL-6, IL-8, TNF, and caspase-3-mediated apoptosis are mediators of lung injury after AKI [36–38]. These cytokines play an important role in many immunopathological processes of COPD [39,40] and could lead to the development of COPD [40,41].

### *4.2. Stroke Risk in Patients with COPD after AKI-D*

Our results further showed that patients with COPD after recovery from AKI-D, compared to those without COPD, have an approximately 52% increased risk of ischemic stroke. According to the results of our specificity analysis (Figure 3a), the incidence is especially high for male patients and for those with diabetes.

In patients with COPD, systemic inflammation secondary to pulmonary inflammation can elicit unstable atherosclerotic plaques and a pro-thrombotic status, with an eventual ischemic stroke [42,43]. Our findings raise the possibility that in AKI patients, COPD may further trigger a cascade of perturbations that never completely resolve. Some nontraditional risk factors such as endothelial dysfunction, impaired endothelial progenitor cells, oxidative stress, and inflammation during AKI may be involved in the pathogenic mechanisms of lung–kidney–brain interactions [44–46]. Acid–base disturbances in patients with COPD after AKI-D may also contribute to the increased risk of ischemic stroke. Acidemia fully protonates free fatty acids forming an oil phase that may fuse with the endothelium and initiate plaque formation [47]. Respiratory acidosis could further serve as a risk factor for thrombus formation [48] and involves the accumulation of serum calcium and phosphate ions which has a major influence on the vascular endothelium [49].

Soluble Klotho could exert multiple actions, including anti-oxidation, anti-senescence, autophagy, anti-apoptosis, and anti-fibrosis [50]. AKI is a state of acute Klotho deficiency. Klotho deficiency exerts multiple negative systemic effects on numerous organs including the cardiovascular system [51]. Importantly, Klotho expression was also reduced in lung alveolar macrophages and peripheral blood mononuclear cells of COPD patients [52]. The enhanced deficiency of Klotho in AKI patients superimposed with COPD will further lead to impaired endothelium-dependent vasodilation and impaired angiogenesis and is related to ischemic stroke [53] and cardiomyopathy [54].

### *4.3. CHF Risk in Patients with COPD after AKI-D*

Our results also showed that patients with COPD after recovery from AKI-D have an approximately 61% increased risk of CHF compared with those without COPD. AKI itself could cause a number of systemic vascular endothelial alterations that impact cardiovascular health [55]. In type 3 cardiorenal syndrome, AKI can lead to cardiac dysfunction by fluid overload, electrolytes, acid–base shift, and renin-angiotensin-aldosterone system or central nervous system activation [7]. Among COPD patients, the prevalence of ventricular dysfunction was 12–17% [56,57]. Patients with COPD were more likely to develop new-onset heart failure during their hospital stay [58]. In addition, pulmonary hypertension is common in severe COPD and can lead to heart failure. Chronic severe hypoxia, on the other hand, increases plasma norepinephrine and aldosterone, but suppresses renin activity and causes salt and water retention in humans [59]. When COPD occurs in AKI-D patients, the compensatory role of the kidney and lung in acidosis is less effective, resulting in a more severe acidosis state which is known to reduce left ventricle contractility [60]. These are possible mechanisms by which COPD confers additional risks to CHF among AKI survivors.

Human neutrophil gelatinase-associated lipocalin (NGAL), initially identified as a protein isolated from the secondary granules of human neutrophils, is actively secreted by certain cells such as respiratory epithelial cells and renal tubule cells [61]. It was reported to be an important player in vascular remodeling, atherosclerotic plaque stability, and thrombus formation [62]. NGAL from neutrophils may drive COPD epithelial mesenchymal transitions [63] and could reflect the state of systemic inflammation in COPD. In light of this, plasma NGAL which supposedly accumulates in AKI patients with COPD during the AKD period, could serve as a predictor of stroke [64] and heart failure [65].

### *4.4. Risk of MI and ESRD in Patients with COPD after AKI-D*

AKI as well as COPD increases the risk of MI [5,66]. However, our study showed that the incidence of MI was not further increased in AKI-D patients with COPD, as compared to those without COPD. This finding implies that shared risk factors of AKI and COPD accounts for much of the elevated risk, and that COPD does not confer a large additional risk. Similarly, previous research suggested that AKI is associated with an increased risk of ESRD [3]. Since AKI already has a strong association with MACE and ESRD, the presence of COPD adds little attributable risk of MACE and ESRD in the nationwide population.

### 4.5. Care of Patients with COPD after AKI-D

Clinicians should be alert to the presence of COPD among patients with AKI-D. AKI and COPD are now global health problems; however, the AKD period has not been listed as a clinically important consequence in clinical guidelines of lung diseases [67]. Findings of the current study are noteworthy from the perspective of a clinician caring for a patient with COPD after recovery from AKI-D. Attention should be given to the importance of raising awareness about the co-existence of COPD with AKI and cardiovascular risks. A public health initiative is needed to monitor and control subsequent adverse cardiovascular events, including ischemic stroke and CHF, among AKI-D patients with COPD especially after discharge. Optimizing the control of respiratory and uremic conditions, early detection of cardiovascular complications, and decreasing inflammatory status may be the best strategies for improving the quality of health care. Additionally, the pathophysiologic link between kidney and lung disease deserves further investigation, particularly during AKD care.

### 4.6. Limitation and Strength

A few clinical and research implications emerged from our study. The NHI database has a large national sample size, a long follow-up, and we used a propensity score method to reduce imbalances in key characteristics between COPD and non-COPD groups. The ICD-9-CM codes and procedure codes for AKI and COPD were well validated. Although smaller studies would need to rely on changes in estimated glomerular filtration rates or albuminuria as kidney end points, the availability of incident ESRD, major adverse cardiac events, and mortality as primary outcomes in this study is a notable strength. However, the present study has some limitations that should also be acknowledged. First, like all claims databases, the data describing lifestyle factors such as body mass index and smoking are not available, and residual confounding may be contributing to the association of COPD with outcomes. However, these missing confounding factors were adjusted by obesity and smoking-related disorders such as hyperlipidemia, hypertension, and ischemic heart disease. Second, the NHI research database does not contain information on several potential confounders, including nutritional conditions, proteinuria data, and the adequacy of glycemic, lipid, and blood pressure control. Finally, certain medications used by COPD patients may serve as potential confounders. For example, combined inhalers, containing a long-acting β2-agonist and an anticholinergic, when compared to monotherapy, were associated with an increased risk of heart failure [68].

## 5. Conclusions

In a large cohort study, more than one-tenth of the patients who recovered from AKI-D were diagnosed with COPD at their one-year follow-up. Adverse cardiovascular events including CHF and ischemic stroke are more prevalent in these patients; however, the risk of ESRD, myocardial infarction, or mortality are not different in patients with or without COPD. A public health initiative is needed to monitor and control subsequent adverse cardiovascular events among COPD patients during the AKD period, even those who have recovered from temporary dialysis.

**Author Contributions:** C.-H.W., C.-Y.W., L.C., H.-C.W data curation; C.-H.W., V.-C.W. initial analysis; H.-M.C., L.-W.C., C.-H.L.do the revised analysis, C.-Y.W., L.C., S.-W.K. writing—review & editing; C.-H.W., H.-M.C. drafted the manuscript; V.-C.W. conceptualization and methodology.

**Acknowledgments:** The study was partly based on data provided by National Health Insurance Administration, Ministry of Health and Welfare, Taiwan. The interpretation and conclusions shown in this paper do not represent those of National Health Insurance Administration, Ministry of Health and Welfare, National Health Research Institutes, or National Taiwan University Hospital. We also express our sincere gratitude to all staff of the Taiwan Clinical Trial Consortium, TCTC. The following are members of NSARF Group: Vin-Cent Wu, Tai-Shuan Lai, Yu-Feng Lin, I-Jung Tsai, Chun-Fu Lai, Tao-Min Huang, Tzong-Shinn Chu, Yung-Ming Chen, Yu-hsing Chang, Yu-Chang Yeh, Chien-Heng Lai, Li-Jung Tseng, and Kwan-Dun Wu, in the National Taiwan University Hospital. Che-Hsiung Wu, in the Taipei Tzu Chi Hospital, Buddhist Tzu Chi Medical Foundation. Chih-Chung Shiao, in the Saint Mary's Hospital Luodong. Chih-Jen Wu, in the Mackay Memorial Hospital. Jian-Jhong Wang, in the Chi Mei Medical Center, Liouying. Wei-Jie Wang, and Jui-Hsiang Lin, in the Taoyuan General Hospital, Ministry of Health and Welfare. Cheng-Yi Chen, in the Mackay Memorial Hospital, Hsinchu.

## References

1. Ali, T.; Khan, I.; Simpson, W.; Prescott, G.; Townend, J.; Smith, W.; Macleod, A. Incidence and outcomes in acute kidney injury: A comprehensive population-based study. *J. Am. Soc. Nephrol.* **2007**, *18*, 1292–1298. [CrossRef] [PubMed]
2. Liangos, O.; Wald, R.; O'Bell, J.W.; Price, L.; Pereira, B.J.; Jaber, B.L. Epidemiology and outcomes of acute renal failure in hospitalized patients: A national survey. *Clin. J. Am. Soc. Nephrol.* **2006**, *1*, 43–51. [CrossRef] [PubMed]
3. Ishani, A.; Xue, J.L.; Himmelfarb, J.; Eggers, P.W.; Kimmel, P.L.; Molitoris, B.A.; Collins, A.J. Acute kidney injury increases risk of ESRD among elderly. *J. Am. Soc. Nephrol.* **2009**, *20*, 223–228. [CrossRef] [PubMed]
4. Waikar, S.S.; Winkelmayer, W.C. Chronic on acute renal failure: Long-term implications of severe acute kidney injury. *JAMA* **2009**, *302*, 1227–1229. [CrossRef] [PubMed]
5. Wu, V.C.; Wu, C.H.; Huang, T.M.; Wang, C.Y.; Lai, C.F.; Shiao, C.C.; Chang, C.H.; Lin, S.L.; Chen, Y.Y.; Chen, Y.M.; et al. Long-term risk of coronary events after AKI. *J. Am. Soc. Nephrol.* **2014**, *25*, 595–605. [CrossRef] [PubMed]
6. Wu, V.C.; Wu, P.C.; Wu, C.H.; Huang, T.M.; Chang, C.H.; Tsai, P.R.; Ko, W.J.; Chen, L.; Wang, C.Y.; Chu, T.S.; et al. The impact of acute kidney injury on the long-term risk of stroke. *J. Am. Heart Assoc.* **2014**, *3*, e000933. [CrossRef] [PubMed]
7. Husain-Syed, F.; McCullough, P.A.; Birk, H.W.; Renker, M.; Brocca, A.; Seeger, W.; Ronco, C. Cardio-pulmonary-renal interactions: A multidisciplinary approach. *J. Am. Coll. Cardiol.* **2015**, *65*, 2433–2448. [CrossRef] [PubMed]
8. Wu, V.C.; Shiao, C.C.; Chang, C.H.; Huang, T.M.; Lai, C.F.; Lin, M.C.; Chiang, W.C.; Chu, T.S.; Wu, K.D.; Ko, W.J.; et al. Long-term outcomes after dialysis-requiring acute kidney injury. *Biomed. Res. Int.* **2014**, *2014*, 365186. [CrossRef] [PubMed]
9. Goldstein, S.L.; Jaber, B.L.; Faubel, S.; Chawla, L.S.; Acute Kidney Injury Advisory Group of American Society of Nephrology. AKI transition of care: A potential opportunity to detect and prevent CKD. *Clin. J. Am. Soc. Nephrol.* **2013**, *8*, 476–483. [CrossRef] [PubMed]
10. Attanasio, C.; Latancia, M.T.; Otterbein, L.E.; Netti, P.A. Update on renal replacement therapy: Implantable artificial devices and bioengineered organs. *Tissue Eng. Part B Rev.* **2016**, *22*, 330–340. [CrossRef] [PubMed]
11. Anthonisen, N.R.; Connett, J.E.; Enright, P.L.; Manfreda, J.; Lung Health Study Research Group. Hospitalizations and mortality in the lung health study. *Am. J. Respir. Crit. Care Med.* **2002**, *166*, 333–339. [CrossRef] [PubMed]
12. Hansell, A.L.; Walk, J.A.; Soriano, J.B. What do chronic obstructive pulmonary disease patients die from? A multiple cause coding analysis. *Eur. Respir. J.* **2003**, *22*, 809–814. [CrossRef] [PubMed]
13. Chen, C.Y.; Liao, K.M. Chronic obstructive pulmonary disease is associated with risk of chronic kidney disease: A nationwide case-cohort study. *Sci. Rep.* **2016**, *6*, 25855. [CrossRef] [PubMed]
14. Virzi, G.; Day, S.; de Cal, M.; Vescovo, G.; Ronco, C. Heart-kidney crosstalk and role of humoral signaling in critical illness. *Crit. Care* **2014**, *18*, 201. [CrossRef] [PubMed]
15. Andres-Hernando, A.; Altmann, C.; Bhargava, R.; Okamura, K.; Bacalja, J.; Hunter, B.; Ahuja, N.; Soranno, D.; Faubel, S. Prolonged acute kidney injury exacerbates lung inflammation at 7 days post-acute kidney injury. *Physiol. Rep.* **2014**, *2*, e12084. [CrossRef] [PubMed]
16. Chawla, L.S.; Bellomo, R.; Bihorac, A.; Goldstein, S.L.; Siew, E.D.; Bagshaw, S.M.; Bittleman, D.; Cruz, D.; Endre, Z.; Fitzgerald, R.L.; et al. Acute kidney disease and renal recovery: Consensus report of the acute disease quality initiative (ADQI) 16 workgroup. *Nat. Rev. Nephrol.* **2017**, *13*, 241–257. [CrossRef] [PubMed]
17. Chao, C.T.; Hou, C.C.; Wu, V.C.; Lu, H.M.; Wang, C.Y.; Chen, L.; Kao, T.W. The impact of dialysis-requiring acute kidney injury on long-term prognosis of patients requiring prolonged mechanical ventilation: Nationwide population-based study. *PLoS ONE* **2012**, *7*, e50675. [CrossRef] [PubMed]
18. Wang, W.J.; Chao, C.T.; Huang, Y.C.; Wang, C.Y.; Chang, C.H.; Huang, T.M.; Lai, C.F.; Huang, H.Y.; Shiao, C.C.; Chu, T.S.; et al. The impact of acute kidney injury with temporary dialysis on the risk of fracture. *J. Bone Miner. Res.* **2013**, *29*, 676–684. [CrossRef] [PubMed]
19. Wu, P.C.; Wu, C.J.; Lin, C.J.; Wu, V.C.; National Taiwan University Study Group on Acute Renal Failure Group. Long-term risk of upper gastrointestinal hemorrhage after advanced AKI. *Clin. J. Am. Soc. Nephrol.* **2015**, *10*, 353–362. [CrossRef] [PubMed]
20. Li, C.H.; Chen, W.C.; Liao, W.C.; Tu, C.Y.; Lin, C.L.; Sung, F.C.; Chen, C.H.; Hsu, W.H. The association

between chronic obstructive pulmonary disease and Parkinson's disease: A nationwide population-based retrospective cohort study. *QJM* **2015**, *108*, 39–45. [CrossRef] [PubMed]

21. Huang, J.Y.; Jian, Z.H.; Nfor, O.N.; Ku, W.Y.; Ko, P.C.; Lung, C.C.; Ho, C.C.; Pan, H.H.; Huang, C.Y.; Liang, Y.C.; et al. The effects of pulmonary diseases on histologic types of lung cancer in both sexes: A population-based study in Taiwan. *BMC Cancer* **2015**, *15*, 834. [CrossRef] [PubMed]
22. Liao, K.M.; Chen, C.Y. Incidence and risk factors of atrial fibrillation in Asian COPD patients. *Int. J. Chron. Obstruct. Pulmon. Dis.* **2017**, *12*, 2523–2530. [CrossRef] [PubMed]
23. Wu, V.C.; Hu, Y.H.; Wu, C.H.; Kao, C.C.; Wang, C.Y.; Yang, W.S.; Lee, H.H.; Chang, Y.S.; Lin, Y.H.; Wang, S.M.; et al. Administrative data on diagnosis and mineralocorticoid receptor antagonist prescription identified patients with primary aldosteronism in Taiwan. *J. Clin. Epidemiol.* **2014**, *67*, 1139–1149. [CrossRef] [PubMed]
24. Wu, C.S.; Lai, M.S.; Gau, S.S.; Wang, S.C.; Tsai, H.J. Concordance between patient self-reports and claims data on clinical diagnoses, medication use, and health system utilization in Taiwan. *PLoS ONE* **2014**, *9*, e112257. [CrossRef] [PubMed]
25. Chu, Y.T.; Wu, S.C.; Lee, Y.C.; Lai, M.S.; Tam, S.C. Assessing measures of comorbidity using national health insurance databases. *Taiwan J. Public Health* **2010**, *29*, 191–200.
26. Cheng, C.L.; Kao, Y.H.; Lin, S.J.; Lee, C.H.; Lai, M.L. Validation of the national health insurance research database with ischemic stroke cases in Taiwan. *Pharmacoepidemiol. Drug Saf.* **2011**, *20*, 236–242. [CrossRef] [PubMed]
27. Wu, C.H.; Yang, Y.W.; Hung, S.C.; Kuo, K.L.; Wu, K.D.; Wu, V.C.; Hsieh, T.C.; National Taiwan University Study Group on Acute Renal Failure. Ketoanalogues supplementation decreases dialysis and mortality risk in patients with anemic advanced chronic kidney disease. *PLoS ONE* **2017**, *12*, e0176847.
28. Ou, S.M.; Chen, Y.T.; Chao, P.W.; Lee, Y.J.; Liu, C.J.; Yeh, C.M.; Chen, T.J.; Chen, T.W.; Yang, W.C.; Li, S.Y. Nonsteroidal anti-inflammatory drug use is associated with cancer risk reduction in chronic dialysis patients. *Kidney Int.* **2013**, *84*, 198–205. [CrossRef] [PubMed]
29. Chen, H.J.; Bai, C.H.; Yeh, W.T.; Chiu, H.C.; Pan, W.H. Influence of metabolic syndrome and general obesity on the risk of ischemic stroke. *Stroke* **2006**, *37*, 1060–1064. [CrossRef] [PubMed]
30. Go, A.S.; Lee, W.Y.; Yang, J.; Lo, J.C.; Gurwitz, J.H. Statin therapy and risks for death and hospitalization in chronic heart failure. *JAMA* **2006**, *296*, 2105–2111. [CrossRef] [PubMed]
31. Kip, K.E.; Hollabaugh, K.; Marroquin, O.C.; Williams, D.O. The problem with composite end points in cardiovascular studies: The story of major adverse cardiac events and percutaneous coronary intervention. *J. Am. Coll. Cardiol.* **2008**, *51*, 701–707. [CrossRef] [PubMed]
32. Wu, V.C.; Chang, C.H.; Wang, C.Y.; Lin, Y.H.; Kao, T.W.; Lin, P.C.; Chu, T.S.; Chang, Y.S.; Chen, L.; Wu, K.D.; et al. Risk of fracture in primary aldosteronism: A population-based cohort study. *J. Bone Miner. Res.* **2017**, *32*, 743–752. [CrossRef] [PubMed]
33. Wu, V.C.; Chueh, S.J.; Chen, L.; Chang, C.H.; Hu, Y.H.; Lin, Y.H.; Wu, K.D.; Yang, W.S.; Taiwan Primary Aldosteronism Investigation Study Group. Risk of new-onset diabetes mellitus in primary aldosteronism: A population study over 5 years. *J. Hypertens.* **2017**, *35*, 1698–1708. [CrossRef] [PubMed]
34. Soriano, J.B.; Abajobir, A.A.; Abate, K.H.; Abera, S.F.; Agrawal, A.; Ahmed, M.B.; Aichour, A.N.; Aichour, I.; Aichour, M.T.E.; Alam, K.; et al. Global, regional, and national deaths, prevalence, disability-adjusted life years, and years lived with disability for chronic obstructive pulmonary disease and asthma, 1990–2015: A systematic analysis for the global burden of disease study 2015. *Lancet Respi. Med.* **2017**, *5*, 691–706. [CrossRef]
35. Baty, F.; Putora, P.M.; Isenring, B.; Blum, T.; Brutsche, M. Comorbidities and burden of COPD: A population based case-control study. *PLoS ONE* **2013**, *8*, e63285. [CrossRef] [PubMed]
36. Faubel, S.; Edelstein, C.L. Mechanisms and mediators of lung injury after acute kidney injury. *Nat. Rev. Nephrol.* **2016**, *12*, 48–60. [CrossRef] [PubMed]
37. Lie, M.L.; White, L.E.; Santora, R.J.; Park, J.M.; Rabb, H.; Hassoun, H.T. Lung T lymphocyte trafficking and activation during ischemic acute kidney injury. *J. Immunol.* **2012**, *189*, 2843–2851. [CrossRef] [PubMed]
38. Altmann, C.; Andres-Hernando, A.; McMahan, R.H.; Ahuja, N.; He, Z.; Rivard, C.J.; Edelstein, C.L.; Barthel, L.; Janssen, W.J.; Faubel, S. Macrophages mediate lung inflammation in a mouse model of ischemic acute kidney injury. *Am. J. Physiol. Ren. Physiol.* **2012**, *302*, 421–432. [CrossRef] [PubMed]
39. Caramori, G.; Adcock, I.M.; Di Stefano, A.; Chung, K.F. Cytokine inhibition in the treatment of COPD. *Int. J. Chron. Obstruct. Pulmon. Dis.* **2014**, *9*, 397–412. [PubMed]

40. Pandey, K.C.; De, S.; Mishra, P.K. Role of proteases in chronic obstructive pulmonary disease. *Front. Pharmacol.* **2017**, *8*, 512. [CrossRef] [PubMed]
41. Martinez-Aguilar, N.E.; Vargas-Camano, M.E.; Hernandez-Pliego, R.R.; Chaia-Semerena, G.M.; Perez-Chavira, M.R. Immunopathology of chronic obstructive pulmonary disease. *Rev. Alerg. Mex.* **2017**, *64*, 327–346. [PubMed]
42. Polosa, R.; Malerba, M.; Cacciola, R.R.; Morjaria, J.B.; Maugeri, C.; Prosperini, G.; Gullo, R.; Spicuzza, L.; Radaeli, A.; Di Maria, G.U. Effect of acute exacerbations on circulating endothelial, clotting and fibrinolytic markers in COPD patients. *Intern. Emerg. Med.* **2013**, *8*, 567–574. [CrossRef] [PubMed]
43. Muir, K.W.; Tyrrell, P.; Sattar, N.; Warburton, E. Inflammation and ischaemic stroke. *Curr. Opin. Neurol.* **2007**, *20*, 334–342. [CrossRef] [PubMed]
44. Wu, V.C.; Young, G.H.; Huang, P.H.; Lo, S.C.; Wang, K.C.; Sun, C.Y.; Liang, C.J.; Huang, T.M.; Chen, J.H.; Chang, F.C.; et al. In acute kidney injury, indoxyl sulfate impairs human endothelial progenitor cells: Modulation by statin. *Angiogenesis* **2013**, *16*, 609–624. [CrossRef] [PubMed]
45. Bonventre, J.V. Pathophysiology of AKI: Injury and normal and abnormal repair. *Contrib. Nephrol.* **2010**, *165*, 9–17. [PubMed]
46. Hosohata, K. Role of oxidative stress in drug-induced kidney injury. *Int. J. Mol. Sci.* **2016**, *17*, 1826. [CrossRef] [PubMed]
47. Reis, A.H. Acidemia and blood free fatty acids: Analysis of cardiovascular risk factors in a new context. *Discov. Med.* **2017**, *23*, 183–188. [PubMed]
48. Gorter, K.A.; Stehouwer, M.C.; Van Putte, B.P.; Vlot, E.A.; Urbanus, R.T. Acidosis induced by carbon dioxide insufflation decreases heparin potency: A risk factor for thrombus formation. *Perfusion* **2017**, *32*, 214–219. [CrossRef] [PubMed]
49. Checherita, I.A.; David, C.; Ciocalteu, A.; Lascar, I.; Budala, L. Oral treatment of metabolic acidosis in hemodialyzed patients and the implications on the hemodynamic status. *Rom. J. Morphol. Embryol.* **2013**, *54*, 539–543. [PubMed]
50. Hu, M.C.; Shiizaki, K.; Kuro-o, M.; Moe, O.W. Fibroblast growth factor 23 and Klotho: Physiology and pathophysiology of an endocrine network of mineral metabolism. *Annu. Rev. Physiol.* **2013**, *75*, 503–533. [CrossRef] [PubMed]
51. Hu, M.C.; Shi, M.; Cho, H.J.; Adams-Huet, B.; Paek, J.; Hill, K.; Shelton, J.; Amaral, A.P.; Faul, C.; Taniguchi, M.; et al. Klotho and phosphate are modulators of pathologic uremic cardiac remodeling. *J. Am. Soc. Nephrol.* **2015**, *26*, 1290–1302. [CrossRef] [PubMed]
52. Li, L.; Wang, Y.; Gao, W.; Yuan, C.; Zhang, S.; Zhou, H.; Huang, M.; Yao, X. Klotho reduction in alveolar macrophages contributes to cigarette smoke extract-induced inflammation in chronic obstructive pulmonary disease. *J. Biol. Chem.* **2015**, *290*, 27890–27900. [CrossRef] [PubMed]
53. Majumdar, V.; Nagaraja, D.; Christopher, R. Association of the functional kL-VS variant of Klotho gene with early-onset ischemic stroke. *Biochem. Biophys. Res. Commun.* **2010**, *403*, 412–416. [CrossRef] [PubMed]
54. Xie, J.; Yoon, J.; An, S.W.; Kuro-o, M.; Huang, C.L. Soluble Klotho protects against uremic cardiomyopathy independently of fibroblast growth factor 23 and phosphate. *J. Am. Soc. Nephrol.* **2015**, *26*, 1150–1160. [CrossRef] [PubMed]
55. Druml, W. Acute renal failure is not a "cute" renal failure! *Intensive. Care Med.* **2004**, *30*, 1886–1890. [CrossRef] [PubMed]
56. Griffo, R.; Spanevello, A.; Temporelli, P.L.; Faggiano, P.; Carone, M.; Magni, G.; Ambrosino, N.; Tavazzi, L.; Investigators, S. Frequent coexistence of chronic heart failure and chronic obstructive pulmonary disease in respiratory and cardiac outpatients: Evidence from suspirium, a multicentre Italian survey. *Eur. J. Prev. Cardiol.* **2017**, *24*, 567–576. [CrossRef] [PubMed]
57. Macchia, A.; Rodriguez Moncalvo, J.J.; Kleinert, M.; Comignani, P.D.; Gimeno, G.; Arakaki, D.; Laffaye, N.; Fuselli, J.J.; Massolin, H.P.; Gambarte, J.; et al. Unrecognised ventricular dysfunction in COPD. *Eur. Respir. J.* **2012**, *39*, 51–58. [CrossRef] [PubMed]
58. Agarwal, M.; Agrawal, S.; Garg, L.; Garg, A.; Bhatia, N.; Kadaria, D.; Reed, G. Effect of chronic obstructive pulmonary disease on in-hospital mortality and clinical outcomes after ST-segment elevation myocardial infarction. *Am. J. Cardiol.* **2017**, *119*, 1555–1559. [CrossRef] [PubMed]
59. Anand, I.S.; Chandrashekhar, Y.; Rao, S.K.; Malhotra, R.M.; Ferrari, R.; Chandana, J.; Ramesh, B.; Shetty, K.J.; Boparai, M.S. Body fluid compartments, renal blood flow, and hormones at 6000 m in normal subjects.

*J. Appl. Physiol.* **1993**, *74*, 1234–1239. [CrossRef] [PubMed]

60. Walley, K.R.; Lewis, T.H.; Wood, L.D. Acute respiratory acidosis decreases left ventricular contractility but increases cardiac output in dogs. *Circ. Res.* **1990**, *67*, 628–635. [CrossRef] [PubMed]
61. Mishra, J.; Ma, Q.; Prada, A.; Mitsnefes, M.; Zahedi, K.; Yang, J.; Barasch, J.; Devarajan, P. Identification of neutrophil gelatinase-associated lipocalin as a novel early urinary biomarker for ischemic renal injury. *J. Am. Soc. Nephrol.* **2003**, *14*, 2534–2543. [CrossRef] [PubMed]
62. Solak, Y.; Yilmaz, M.I.; Siriopol, D.; Saglam, M.; Unal, H.U.; Yaman, H.; Gok, M.; Cetinkaya, H.; Gaipov, A.; Eyileten, T.; et al. Serum neutrophil gelatinase-associated lipocalin is associated with cardiovascular events in patients with chronic kidney disease. *Int. Urol. Nephrol.* **2015**, *47*, 1993–2001. [CrossRef] [PubMed]
63. Wang, Y.; Jia, M.; Yan, X.; Cao, L.; Barnes, P.J.; Adcock, I.M.; Huang, M.; Yao, X. Increased neutrophil gelatinase-associated lipocalin (NGAL) promotes airway remodelling in chronic obstructive pulmonary disease. *Clin. Sci. (Lond).* **2017**, *131*, 1147–1159. [CrossRef] [PubMed]
64. Hasegawa, M.; Ishii, J.; Kitagawa, F.; Takahashi, H.; Sugiyama, K.; Tada, M.; Kanayama, K.; Takahashi, K.; Hayashi, H.; Koide, S.; et al. Plasma neutrophil gelatinase-associated lipocalin as a predictor of cardiovascular events in patients with chronic kidney disease. *BioMed Res. Int.* **2016**, *2016*, 8761475. [CrossRef] [PubMed]
65. Nymo, S.H.; Ueland, T.; Askevold, E.T.; Flo, T.H.; Kjekshus, J.; Hulthe, J.; Wikstrand, J.; McMurray, J.; Van Veldhuisen, D.J.; Gullestad, L.; et al. The association between neutrophil gelatinase-associated lipocalin and clinical outcome in chronic heart failure: Results from CORONA*. *J. Intern. Med.* **2012**, *271*, 436–443. [CrossRef] [PubMed]
66. Donaldson, G.C.; Hurst, J.R.; Smith, C.J.; Hubbard, R.B.; Wedzicha, J.A. Increased risk of myocardial infarction and stroke following exacerbation of COPD. *Chest* **2010**, *137*, 1091–1097. [CrossRef] [PubMed]
67. Qaseem, A.; Wilt, T.J.; Weinberger, S.E.; Hanania, N.A.; Criner, G.; van der Molen, T.; Marciniuk, D.D.; Denberg, T.; Schunemann, H.; Wedzicha, W.; et al. Diagnosis and management of stable chronic obstructive pulmonary disease: A clinical practice guideline update from the American College of Physicians, American College of Chest Physicians, American Thoracic Society, and European Respiratory Society. *Ann. Int. Med.* **2011**, *155*, 179–191. [CrossRef] [PubMed]
68. Suissa, S.; Dell'Aniello, S.; Ernst, P. Concurrent use of long-acting bronchodilators in COPD and the risk of adverse cardiovascular events. *Eur. Respir. J.* **2017**, *49*. [CrossRef] [PubMed]

6

# Norepinephrine Administration is Associated with Higher Mortality in Dialysis Requiring Acute Kidney Injury Patients with Septic Shock

**Ying-Ying Chen [1,2], Vin-Cent Wu [3], Wei-Chieh Huang [4], Yu-Chang Yeh [5], Mai-Szu Wu [6], Chiu-Ching Huang [7], Kwan-Dun Wu [3], Ji-Tseng Fang [8], Chih-Jen Wu [1,9,10,11,12,*], The NSARF [†] and CAKS Group [‡]**

1 Division of Nephrology, Department of Internal Medicine, MacKay Memorial Hospital, No. 92, Sec. 2, Zhongshan North Road, Taipei 10449, Taiwan; akochen45@hotmail.com
2 Graduate Institute of Clinical Medicine, College of Medicine, National Taiwan University, No.7.Chung San South Road, Taipei 10002, Taiwan
3 Division of Nephrology, Department of Internal Medicine, National Taiwan University Hospital, No.7.Chung San South Road, Taipei 10002, Taiwan; q91421028@ntu.edu.tw (V.-C.W.); kdwu@ntuh.gov.tw (K.-D.W.)
4 Division of Cardiology, Department of Internal Medicine, Taipei Veterans General Hospital, No.201, Sec. 2, Shipai Road, Taipei 11217, Taiwan; hwcc0314@gmail.com
5 Department of Anesthesiology, National Taiwan University Hospital, No.7.Chung San South Road, Taipei 10002, Taiwan; tonyyeh@ntuh.gov.tw
6 Division of Nephrology, Department of Internal Medicine, Taipei Medical University-Shuang Ho Hospital, No.291, Zhongzheng Road, Zhonghe District, New Taipei City 23561, Taiwan; maiszuwu@gmail.com
7 Division of Nephrology, Department of Internal Medicine, China Medical University Hospital, No. 2, Yude Road, North District, Taichung 40447, Taiwan; cch@mail.cmuh.org.tw
8 Chang Gung University College of Medicine, Taoyuan, Taiwan; Kidney Research Center, Department of Nephrology, Chang Gung Memorial Hospital, 5. Fu-Hsing Street. Kuei Shan Hsiang, Taoyuan City 333, Taiwan; fangjits@cgmh.org.tw
9 Department of Medicine, Mackay Medical College, No.46, Sec. 3, Zhongzheng Road, Sanzhi District, New Taipei City 252, Taiwan
10 Graduate Institute of Medical Sciences and Department of Pharmacology, School of Medicine, College of Medicine, Taipei Medical University, 250 Wuxing St., Taipei 11031, Taiwan
11 Department of Medical Research, China Medical University Hospital, China Medical University, No.91, Hsueh-Shih Road, Taichung 40402, Taiwan
12 Mackay Junior College of Medicine, Nursing and Management, No.92, Shengjing Road, Taipei 11260, Taiwan
* Correspondence: yaliwcj@gmail.com
† Membership of the NSARF Group is provided in the Acknowledgments.
‡ Membership of the CAKS Group is provided in the Acknowledgments.

**Abstract:** (1) Background: Norepinephrine (NE) is the first-line vasoactive agent used in septic shock patients; however, the effect of norepinephrine on dialysis-required septic acute kidney injury (AKI-D) patients is uncertain. (2) Methods: To evaluate the impact of NE on 90-day mortality and renal recovery in septic AKI-D patients, we enrolled patients in intensive care units from 30 hospitals in Taiwan. (3) Results: 372 patients were enrolled and were divided into norepinephrine users and non-users. After adjustment by Inverse probability of treatment weighted (IPTW), there was no significant difference of baseline comorbidities between the two groups. NE users had significantly higher 90-day mortality rate and using NE is a strong predictor of 90-day mortality in the multivariate Cox regression (HR = 1.497, $p = 0.027$) after adjustment. The generalized additive model disclosed norepinephrine alone exerted a dose–dependent effect on 90-day mortality, while other vasoactive agents were not. (4) Conclusion: Using norepinephrine in septic AKI-D patients is associated with higher 90-day mortality and the effect is dose-dependent. Further study to explore the potential mechanism is needed.

**Keywords:** critical care; vasoactive agents; norepinephrine; sepsis; acute kidney injury; dialysis

## 1. Introduction

Sepsis is defined as a life-threatening organ dysfunction due to dysregulated host response to infection in accordance to recent Sepsis-3 consensus [1]; it is the leading cause of acute kidney injury (AKI) in critically ill patients in intensive care units (ICU) [2,3]. Using sepsis-3 criteria, analysis of data from a large cohort from 409 hospitals in the USA from 2004–2009 revealed that more than 40% of patients with sepsis also had AKI [4]. Septic AKI is associated with high mortality [3,5,6], extended hospitalization [5], and costly long-term treatment [7].

Septic shock, which is a condition of systemic vasodilatation and arterial hypotension, is now evidenced by a serum lactate level >2 mmol/L and vasopressor requirement to maintain a mean arterial pressure (MAP) of at least 65 mm Hg in the absence of hypovolemia [4]. The use of vasopressors is necessary, especially when fluid resuscitation fails to restore arterial blood pressure; they are still the cornerstone of hypotension management in patients with septic AKI for maintaining adequate organ perfusion [8,9]. Although norepinephrine (NE) is still recommended as the first-line vasoactive agent used in these patients [10], little is known about the impact of NE and other vasoactive agents on the progression of septic AKI.

However, in AKI patients with septic shock, the different effects of NE, and other vasoactive agents has not been surveyed. In this study, we compare the impact of NE and other vasoactive agents on mortality and dialysis dependency in acute kidney injury patients who require dialysis (AKI-D).

## 2. Material and Methods

### 2.1. Study Design and Population

The nephrologists and intensivists in Taiwan have appealed for the development of a consortium to unite strength in the field of critical nephrology in Taiwan. The Consortium for Acute Kidney Injury and Renal Diseases (CAKs) and a division focusing on AKI (CAKs-AKI) were launched in the beginning of 2014. This study group has established a multicenter database since 2002 to improve the quality of care and the prognosis of AKI in critically ill patients and then set up a national registry program of AKI to prospectively enroll a large number of dialysis-requiring AKI (AKI-D) patients. This nationwide epidemiology and prognosis of AKI (NEP-AKI-D) requiring dialysis study is the first flagship study of CAKs-AKI, which aims to explore the epidemiology, risk factors, modality, dose, and frequency of renal replacement therapy (RRT), as well as prognoses of the patients with AKI-D, by using the established anonymous nationwide AKI database launched in the beginning of 2014. Up to January of 2016, 30 hospitals have joined this consortium. These hospitals are distributed widely through the four geographical regions (north, middle, south, and east) of Taiwan, and have a 1:1 ratio of medical centers to regional hospitals in each region [11]. In the included hospitals, adult patients fulfilling the diagnosis of septic shock according to the sepsis-3 criteria [1] at initialized RRT in the ICU were prospectively enrolled in the study and followed until hospital discharge from the six seasonally sampled months (October 2014, along with January, April, July, October 2015, and January 2016). Patients who had ever received dialysis treatment or arteriovenous creation before the index hospitalization were excluded. The use of vasoactive agents was assessed, and septic shock patients were separated into NE (NE) users and other inotropic users (NE nonusers). The outcomes of interest were 90-day mortality and recovery from dialysis-dependency after hospital discharge.

### 2.2. Data Collection and Variable Definitions

Sepsis is defined in Sepsis-3 as life-threatening organ dysfunction, which is known as an acute change in total SOFA score $\geq$2 points, caused by a dysregulated host response to infection. And septic shock is defined by a serum lactate level >2 mmol/L and persistent hypotension after fluid resuscitation; it also requires vasopressors to maintain MAP >65 mmHg [1,4].

Other organ failure is classified as the following [12,13]: (1) respiratory failure: requiring ventilator support; (2) central nervous system failure: Glasgow Coma Score <9; (3) cardiac failure: signs of low cardiac output with a central venous pressure >12 mmHg; and (4) liver dysfunction: total bilirubin >2.0 mg/dL and international normalized ratio (INR) >1.4 [12].

Disease severity was assessed by using the Acute Physiology and Chronic Health Evaluation II (APACHE II) score [14], the Sequential Organ Failure Assessment (SOFA) score [15], and inotropic equivalent (IE) score [16]. We also recorded ICU procedure, infection site, the use of vasoactive agents, and laboratory data at the time of dialysis initiation. We defined "baseline serum creatinine (SCr)" as the latest SCr value during outpatient department (OPD) follow-up for patients who had not visited an OPD within 6 months before index admission. The etiologies of AKI, which included sepsis and other etiologies in the meantime, were documented as well. RRT in this study was performed via a double-lumen catheter. The modality of RRT was chosen according to clinical judgment of the consulting nephrologist and the in-charge intensivist. (Supplemental methods) Because the type and dosage of catecholamines preferred by physicians can vary, this study compared the dosage of catecholamines according to inotropic equivalents (IE, μg/kg/min = dopamine + dobutamine + 100 × epinephrine + 100 × NE + 100 × isoproterenol + 15 × milrinone) in order to compare the severity of heart failure, [16] which was composed of most common used vasoactive agents nowadays. This score had been used in other studies [16,17] for evaluating the severity of cardiovascular dysfunction and it is a valid surrogate outcome measure in pediatric sepsis by testing its association with important short-term outcomes [17–20]. In this study, the vasoactive agents we recorded included dopamine, dobutamine, norepinephrine, epinephrine, isoproterenol, and milrinone. The "other vasoactive agents" were identified as vasoactive agents, except norepinephrine, which was included in the IE score. We evaluated the disease severity before dialysis.

### 2.3. Statistical Analyses

Continuous variables between groups were compared using the Student t test. The chi-square test was applied for categorical variables with Yates' correction where applicable. The inverse probability of treatment weighting (IPTW) using the propensity score was applied to correct the bias of the two groups in basic characteristics and outcomes [21]. Applying these weights has the effect of creating a pseudo-population with a covariate distribution of the individual treatment groups similar to that of the overall study population. Covariate balance was assessed by examining the magnitude of any residual differences between the treatment groups after applying the weight [22]. Accumulated hazard ratio was modeled by Cox regression models and adjusted for the covariates for the outcomes of interest (Table 1). The significance levels for entry (SLE) and for stay (SLS) were set to 0.15 for being conservative. Then, with the aid of substantive knowledge, the best candidate final logistic regression model was identified manually by dropping the covariates with $p$ value > 0.05 one at a time until all regression coefficients were significantly different from 0 [13,23].

**Table 1.** Comparison of baseline characteristic and outcomes of septic shock patients with norepinephrine (NE) or other vasoactive agents at dialysis initiation.

| Variables | Before IPTW | | | After IPTW | | |
|---|---|---|---|---|---|---|
| | NE Non-User ($n$ = 57) | NE User ($n$ = 315) | $p$ * Value | NE Non-User ($n$ = 57) | NE User ($n$ = 315) | $p$ * Value |
| Age (year) | 65.79 ± 15.22 | 64.77 ± 15.72 | 0.637 | 66.56 ± 14.53 | 64.66 ± 15.95 | 0.587 |
| Gender (male) | 36 (63.16%) | 224 (71.11%) | 0.272 | 21 (31.11%) | 91 (29.82%) | 0.797 |
| DM | 29 (50.88%) | 155 (49.21%) | 0.886 | 29 (47.73%) | 155 (50.00%) | 0.772 |
| CAD | 17 (29.82%) | 65 (20.63%) | 0.163 | 17 (22.22%) | 65 (22.59%) | 0.946 |
| CVA | 5 (8.77%) | 33 (10.48%) | 0.816 | 5 (11.11%) | 33 (16.27%) | 0.293 |
| CHF | | | | | | |
| I | 13 (22.81%) | 3 (5.26%) | <0.001 | 13 (31.11%) | 3 (41.99%) | 0.551 |
| II | 12 (21.05%) | 153 (48.57%) | | 12 (28.89%) | 153 (22.66%) | |
| III | 12 (21.05%) | 68 (21.59%) | | 12 (26.67%) | 68 (16.92%) | |
| IV | 17 (29.82%) | 59 (18.73%) | | 17 (11.11%) | 59 (10.57%) | |
| BUN (mg/dL) | 57.59 ± 47.42 | 50.19 ± 40.14 | 0.225 | 51.01 ± 49.62 | 50.19 ± 39.48 | 0.700 |
| Lactate(mmol/L) | 10.65 ± 9.03 | 8.77 ± 6.98 | 0.160 | 9.14 ± 8 | 9.62 ± 7.36 | 0.734 |
| Baseline Cr (mg/dL) | 1.62 ± 1.16 | 1.36 ± 1.02 | 0.074 | 1.65 ± 1.18 | 1.37 ± 1.03 | 0.254 |
| eGFR (mL/min/1.73 m$^2$) | 57.03 ± 35.28 | 69.63 ± 46.76 | 0.048 | 57.34 ± 36.15 | 68.12 ± 44.9 | 0.319 |
| Etiology of AKI | | | | | | |
| Shock | 29 (50.88%) | 242 (76.83%) | <0.001 | 29 (60.00%) | 242 (68.37%) | 0.306 |
| CRS | 34 (59.65%) | 82 (26.03%) | <0.001 | 34 (35.56%) | 82 (33.13%) | 0.663 |
| Drug | 2 (3.51%) | 21 (6.67%) | 0.551 | 2 (8.89%) | 21 (5.72%) | 0.363 |
| Rhabdomyolysis | 4 (7.02%) | 43 (13.65%) | 0.198 | 4 (4.44%) | 43 (13.86%) | 0.054 |
| Pigmentation | 0 (0.00%) | 14 (4.44%) | 0.140 | 0 (0.00%) | 14 (6.02%) | 0.092 |
| Hepatorenal | 4 (7.02%) | 23 (7.30%) | 0.999 | 4 (8.89%) | 23 (6.93%) | 0.648 |
| Contrast | 4 (7.02%) | 24 (7.62%) | 0.999 | 4 (11.11%) | 24 (10.54%) | 0.956 |
| Others | 4 (7.02%) | 33 (10.48%) | 0.630 | 4 (4.44%) | 33 (9.04%) | 0.299 |
| Infection site | | | | | | |
| Respiratory | 22 (38.60%) | 157 (49.84%) | 0.149 | 22 (46.67%) | 157 (46.08%) | 0.999 |
| GU | 19 (33.33%) | 77 (24.44%) | 0.188 | 19 (20.00%) | 77 (22.36%) | 0.738 |
| Bacteremia | 12 (21.05%) | 96 (30.48%) | 0.204 | 12 (26.67%) | 96 (28.61%) | 0.903 |
| Abdomen | 3 (5.26%) | 53 (16.83%) | 0.026 | 3 (6.67%) | 53 (14.16%) | 0.157 |
| Others | 6 (10.53%) | 39 (12.38%) | 0.827 | 6 (8.89%) | 39 (12.95%) | 0.435 |
| Disease severity score | | | | | | |
| Total IE Score | 13.97 ± 14.11 | 31.99 ± 25.36 | <0.001 | 24.23 ± 23.62 | 29.17 ± 24.21 | 0.261 |
| SIRS | 2.7 ± 0.89 | 2.92 ± 0.83 | 0.080 | 2.87 ± 0.95 | 2.87 ± 0.81 | 0.822 |
| SOFA | 14.02 ± 2.66 | 15.6 ± 2.96 | <0.001 | 15.42 ± 2.69 | 15.28 ± 2.99 | 0.663 |
| qSOFA | 2.3 ± 0.46 | 2.37 ± 0.48 | 0.311 | 2.25 ± 0.45 | 2.35 ± 0.48 | 0.300 |
| APACHEII | 25.79 ± 7.57 | 27.27 ± 6.46 | 0.289 | 26.51 ± 6.74 | 27.21 ± 6.49 | 0.851 |
| Outcome | | | | | | |
| ICU day | 28.65 ± 38.07 | 17.22 ± 17.88 | 0.014 | 30.94 ± 37.27 | 17.58 ± 18.32 | 0.204 |
| Length of hospital dialysis | 26.07 ± 36.97 | 12.68 ± 19.19 | <0.001 | 18.67 ± 27.78 | 12.85 ± 19.47 | 0.012 |
| Hospital Mortality | 41 (71.93%) | 252 (80.00%) | 0.217 | 41 (75.56%) | 252 (81.02%) | 0.330 |
| 90-day outcome | | | 0.142 | | | 0.753 |
| Mortality | 42 (73.68%) | 260 (82.54%) | | 42 (76.09%) | 260 (83.13%) | |
| Recovery from dialysis | 13 (22.81%) | 52 (16.51%) | | 13 (21.74%) | 52 (15.66%) | |
| Dialysis-dependent | 2 (3.51%) | 3 (0.95%) | | 2 (2.17%) | 3 (1.20%) | |

Abbreviations: AKI: acute kidney injury; APACHEII: acute physiology and chronic health evaluation; BUN: blood urea nitrogen; CAD: coronary artery disease; CHF: congestive heart failure; Cr: creatinine; CRS: cardiorenal syndrome; CVA: cerebrovascular accident; DM: diabetes mellitus; eGFR: estimated glomerular filtration rate; GU: genitourinary; IABP: intra-aortic balloon pump; ICU: intensive care unit; IE: inotropic equivalent; IHD: intermittent dialysis; IPTW: inverse probability of treatment weighting; qSOFA: quick sequential organ failure assessment; SOFA: sequential organ failure assessment; SIRS: systemic inflammatory response syndrome. * All statistics were two-tailed, and significance was accepted for $p < 0.05$.

Forest plot was constructed for odds ratio of NE use (vs. other vasoactive agents) on 90-day mortality according to prior comorbidities and clinical conditions. The generalized additive model was used to analyze the dose-response relationship between vasoactive agents and the 90-day mortality [24,25]. Because of the high mortality rate in sepsis patients after AKI-D, competing risk regression was also performed to show the risks for dialysis dependence using the Fine and Gray model considering the subdistribution hazard [26,27].

We used R software version 3.2.2 (Free Software Foundation, Inc., Vienna, Austria) for the time-varying Cox model and Stata/MP version 14 (Stata Corporation, College Station, TX, USA) for the competing risk analysis. Two-sided $p$ values < 0.05 were considered statistically significant.

### 2.4. Ethics Approval and Consent to Participate

Approval of this prospective multi-center study follows the regulations of the National Research Program for Biopharmaceuticals (NRPB)-Institutional Review Board (IRB). All clinical trial consortiums have to fill in the application forms on the official website of the NRPB-IRB. Written t informed consent was obtained from all participants before inclusion. (Approval No. NRPB2014050014).

## 3. Results

### 3.1. Baseline Characteristics of the Study Cohort

A total of 372 AKI-D patients fulfilled the criteria of septic shock at initialization of dialysis and 315 patients were NE users. The characteristics of patients are listed in Table 1. The mean SOFA score was 15.42 ± 2.69 in the non-user group and 15.28 ± 2.99 in the user group. The APACHE II score was 26.51 ± 6.74 in the user group and 27.21 ± 6.49 in the non-user group. The mean age was 65.8 ± 15.2 years in the non-NE user group and 64.8 ± 15.7 years in the NE user group. After adjustment by IPTW (Table 1), there was no significant difference of baseline comorbidities between the two groups. The biochemical data and ICU procedure were similar. There was the sum of 263 (70.7%) patients who received surgery during admission. Regarding disease severity, there was no significant difference in APACHEII score (25.79 ± 7.57 in NE non-user and 27.27 ± 6.46 in NE user, $p$ = 0.289) between the two groups initially, and other scoring systems including IE score and SOFA (15.42 ± 2.69 in NE non-user and 15.28 ± 2.99 in NE user, $p$ = 0.663) were similar after adjustment. We record the etiology of acute kidney injury included with/without cardiorenal syndrome, drug, rhabdomyolysis, pigmentation (pigment nephropathy), hepatorenal syndrome, and contrast. And there was no significant difference in the etiologies of AKI between two groups. Besides, no significant difference was noted in major infection site which included respiratory tract, genitourinary tract, blood stream, or abdomen between NE user and non-user. Oliguria (81.9%) is the leading cause for RRT, followed by fluid overloaded (67.8%). The indications for RRT were similar except for oliguria ($p$ = 0.009). Regarding the RRT modality, NE users tended to receive CVVH, and SLEDD ($p$ = 0.034). The detail of these baseline characteristics is in the Supplementary Table S1.

### 3.2. 90-Day Mortality in Septic-Shock-Related AKI-D

A total of 302 (81.2%) patients died within 90 days of hospital discharge (Table 1) and 260 (92.54%) patients were NE users and 42 (73.68%) were NE non-users. The median ICU stay for NE users was similar to that of NE non-users ($p$ = 0.204). The number of dialysis days of the NE non-user groups was larger than that of the NE user group (user vs. non-user = 12.9 ± 19.5 vs. 18.7 ± 27.8 days, $p$ = 0.012).

Table 2 showed the independent risk predictors for 90-day mortality analyzed by multivariate Cox proportional hazards model incorporated with IPTW. After adjustment by age, sex, comorbidities, kidney function, APACHE II score, indication for dialysis, and dialysis modalities, the use of NE was an independent risk for 90-day mortality (hazard ratio = 1.504, $p$ = 0.026).

**Table 2.** Cox regression for 90-day m4.ortality in septic shock patients with NE or other vasoactive agents at dialysis initiation *.

| Variables | HR | Lower 95% CI | 95% CI | *p* |
|---|---|---|---|---|
| NE user (yes) | 1.497 | 1.046 | 2.141 | 0.027 |
| Hepatorenal syndrome (yes) | 1.992 | 1.320 | 3.007 | 0.001 |
| Cr (mg/dL) | 0.840 | 0.776 | 0.910 | <0.001 |
| BUN (mg/dL) | 1.008 | 1.004 | 1.012 | <0.001 |
| APACHEII Score | 1.042 | 1.030 | 1.836 | <0.001 |

Concordance = 0.645; R square = 0.152; APACHEII: acute physiology and chronic health evaluation; BUN: blood urea nitrogen; CHF: congestive heart failure; CI: confidence interval; Cr.: creatinine; HR: hazard ratio; NE: norepinephrine; NYHA: New York heart association; * Cox proportional hazard model adjusted with IPTW.

We further analyzed the outcomes of the use of NE; subgroup analysis using forest plots was performed to calculate IPTW adjusted HRs (HRs) of 90-day mortality. The detrimental effects of NE were consistent across the subgroups stratified by respiratory tract infection, congestive heart failure, diabetes mellitus, BUN with more than 64 mg/dL, and patients who did not have cerebrovascular disease (Figure 1).

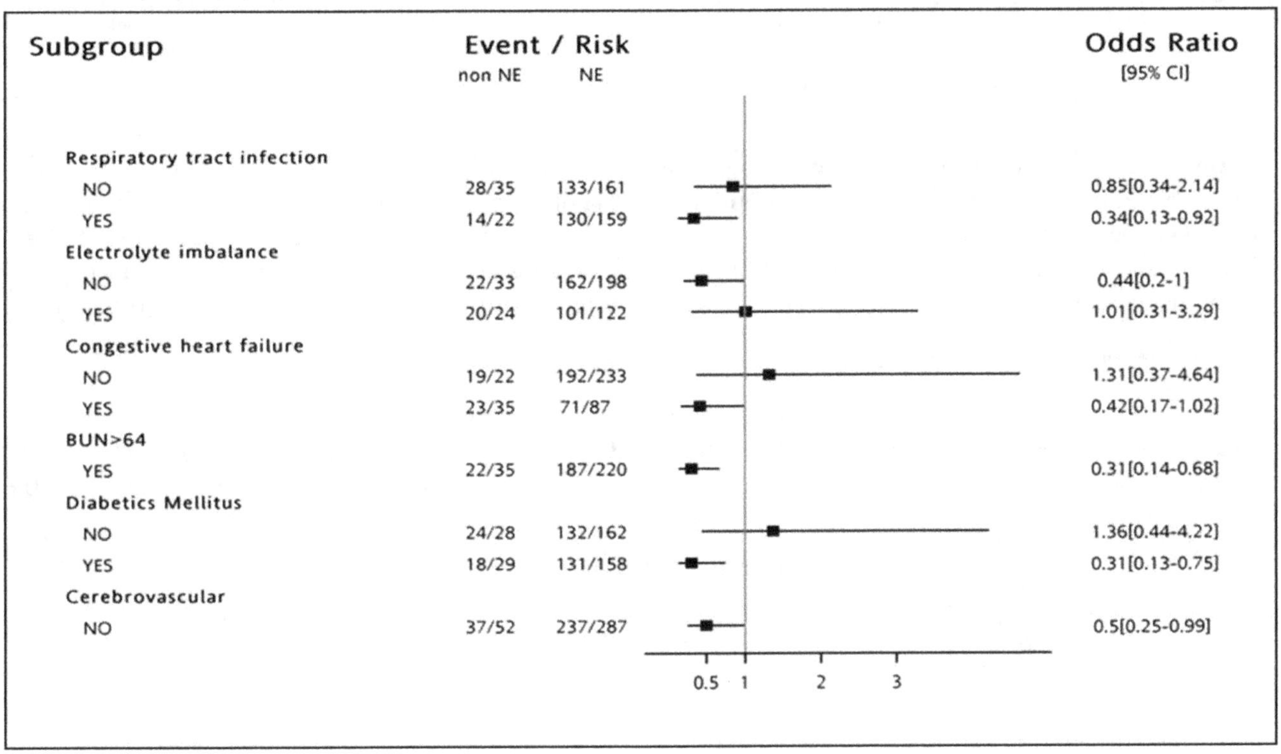


**Figure 1. Odds ratio of Norepinephrine user on the development of 90 days mortality.** Odds ratio of Norepinephrine users (vs. other vasoactive agents) on the development of 90-day mortality, according to demographics in septic shock patients at dialysis initiation. Patients those who had respiratory tract infection, congestive heart failure, diabetes mellitus, BUN with more than 64 mg/dL, and did not have cerebrovascular disease tended to have a higher 90-day mortality while norepinephrine (NE) was prescribed.

### *3.3. The Dose-Response Relationship between NE and 90-Day Mortality*

The quantity of NE was plotted against the log odds of predicting 90-day mortality by using generalized additive mode (GAM) after adjusting the risk factors in the final model (Figure 2). We separated the use of vasoactive agents into 3 groups by measurement of IE score which included vasoactive agents mentioned above (Figure 2A), NE alone (Figure 2B), and vasoactive agents other than NE (Figure 2C). The dose of total vasoactive agents and those without NE did not show a dose-dependent effect relating to 90 day-mortality. However, NE equivalence showed a positive relationship to 90-day mortality. In terms of the risks of 90-day mortality, the GAM plot disclosed with NE alone exerted a significant disadvantage when compared to other vasoactive agents; it was dose-dependent (Figure 2).

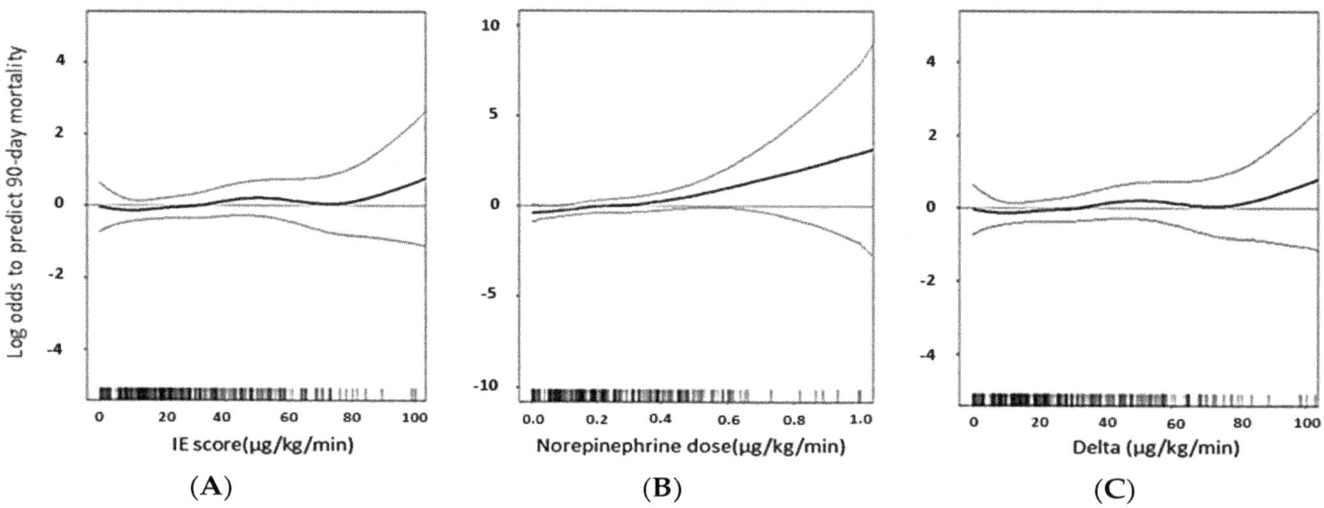


**Figure 2.** Generalized additive mode (GAM) plot of the probability of 90-day mortality regarding the dose equivalent of inotropes. The model incorporates subject-specific (longitudinal) random effects, expressed as the logarithm of the odd (logit). The probability of mortality was constructed with the equivalent dose of (**A**) inotropes (**B**) NE (**C**) inotropic dose deduct NE dose and was centered to have an average of zero over the range of the data as constructed with the GAM. IE: inotropic equivalent.

*3.4. Dialysis Dependency in Septic Shock Patients with or without NE*

In the evaluation of the relation between the use of NE and dialysis dependency, we conducted a competing-risk regression model which took mortality as a competing risk (Figure 3). It revealed that the use of NE was not associated with the cumulative proportions of weaning from dialysis ($p$ = 0.651).

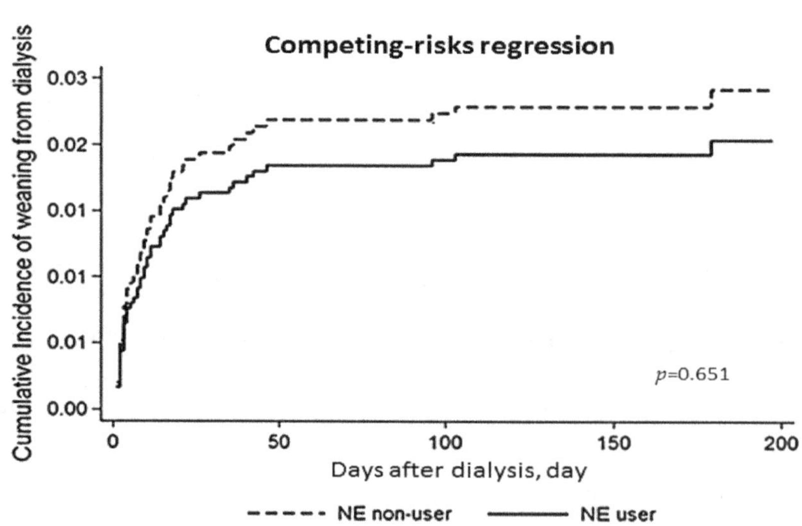


**Figure 3. Cox proportional plot depict cumulative proportions of renal recovery between NE user and non-user groups.** There was no significant difference ($p$ = 0.651) in weaning from dialysis between NE user group and non-user group when taking mortality as a competing risk. BUN: blood urea nitrogen; GAM: generalized additive model; NE: norepinephrine.

## 4. Discussion

### 4.1. Main Finding

In this multi-center, observational study of AKI-D patients with septic shock at initialization of dialysis, we found that 81.2% of patients died within 90 days of hospital discharge. Our report first showed the high mortality of AKI-D patients with septic shock according to Sepsis-3 criteria. The use of NE was associated with a higher 90-day mortality rate than other vasoactive agents and that the detrimental effect is dose-dependence. We applied inverse probability of treatment weighting (IPTW), to minimize the effect of confounding in observational study [28]. And importantly, the risk of NE on 90-day mortality is constant after adjusting for the bias of baseline characteristics by using inverse probability of treatment weighting.

### 4.2. The Use of NE in AKI-D Patients with Septic Shock

In the general population, the use of NE is the first-line choice of vasoactive agents to restore organ perfusion and maintain the blood pressure in septic shock patients [29]. The influence of the use of NE on AKI-D patients with septic shock is still warranted.

Chou et al [30]. conducted a retrospective study which prescribed a high-dose of vasopressor used before the initiation of continuous renal replacement therapy (CRRT). A high dose of NE is associated with higher mortality by way of the catecholamine effect on the cardiovascular system [31]. In a multi-center, double-blind, randomized, controlled trial, vasopressin reduce progression to mortality in early stage AKI patients when compared to NE [32].

Thus, differences between vasopressin and nor epinephrine-treated patient outcomes may be due to the beneficial effects of vasopressin or, alternatively, due to reduction in the detrimental effects of norepinephrine. This result is also consistent with the primary subgroup analysis of the VASST study in which vasopressin treatment was associated with decreased mortality in patients who had less severe shock and not in patients who had more severe shock [33].

In a recent prospective cohort study [34], Passos et al. tried to establish a scoring system to predict 7-day mortality in septic patients requiring CRRT. The use of norepinephrine was recognized as one of the predictors in the study based on the magnitude of regression coefficients in the multivariate analysis. One multi-center, prospective, observational study which enrolled 897 patients with community-acquiring sepsis from seventeen Portuguese ICUs evaluated the impact of vasopressor on mortality. The study reported that the use of NE, either used as single agents or in combination, was associated with worse outcome due to increased cardiovascular events when compared to dopamine in community-acquired sepsis patients during ICU stay [35].

Adequate fluid resuscitation is recommended and it is closely associated with blood pressure maintenance with the ultimate aim of maintaining tissue perfusion and oxygenation [36]. However, insufficiency of fluid resuscitation insufficiency may occur in oliguric septic AKI-D patients because clinician are often anxious to aggressive hydration related fluid overload. One retrospective study enrolled dialysis patients who had sepsis revealed severely under resuscitated and it might contribute to the patients' mortality [37]. To maintain the hemodynamic status, even in dialysis patients, clinicians should add sufficient fluid supplement before adding more vasoactive agents [37]. In addition to fluid resuscitation, antimicrobials therapy should be initiated as soon as possible when the diagnosis of sepsis and septic shock is established [10].

In our study we found worse outcomes when using NE in AKI-D patients with septic shock when compared to other vasoactive agents, even after adjustment for the disease severity. Besides, the disease severity was more severe in our study population in accordance with SOFA score and APACHEII score which might lead to higher mortality rate in our study. In previous study, the highest SOFA scores, higher than 11, were associated with a mortality rate greater than 80% [38]. The mean SOFA score was 15.6–2.96 in the NE user group and 14.02–2.66 in the NE non-user group in our study. Besides, almost 80% patients were from a medical center that assembled very ill patients in our country. Septic shock patients who were not candidates for NE could differ from patients who were candidates, and it will be noted as an indication bias in this observational study. However, the disease severity score, the dose of inotropic equivalent, and even the level of serum lactate, in terms of the severity of septic shock, were similar between the two groups. Therefore, the indication bias, if any, will be trivial in this observational study. NE was known as a more potent vasopressor than dopamine and had favorable outcome on mortality in earlier studies [39]. However, one current large randomized trial—the SOAP II trial, demonstrated that there was no significant difference-in 28-day mortality between the use of NE and dopamine in patients with shock. The result was similar in septic shock and hypovolemic shock, except in cardiogenic shock when the researchers conducted subgroup analysis [40]. Recently, the NE as Initial Therapy in Septic Shock (VANISH) trial [41] reported that AKI occurred in about 45% of patients, and AKI requiring RRT developed in 30% of patients. Although the clinical use of inotropic agents is common in patients with septic AKI requiring dialysis, little was known about which inotropic agent is preferable in these patients. In light of our study, the use of NE in septic AKI requiring dialysis was associated with higher 90-day mortality, and the detrimental effect was dose-dependent. Further study is warranted to reconsider the early use of NE in AKI-D patients with septic shock.

### *4.3. NE and Renal Recovery*

In general, the infusion of NE deceases the renal blood flow [42] and renal vasoconstriction, which may lead to reversible AKI [43]. In light of our study, the vasopressin and septic shock trial (VASST) did not show any difference in the incidence of AKI or need for RRT with the use of vasopressin or NE [33].

However, in acute endotoxemic status, the infusion of NE appears to improve renal blood flow, and had favorable effects on renal function in septic patients. One recent animal study [44] tried to evaluate the NE effects on the kidney in septic AKI ovine, and it found that medullary hypoxia and ischemia were exacerbated after NE infusion. In our study, we showed that the use of NE could not be the crucial factor for recovery from dialysis.

### *4.4. Study Limitation*

This is the first study evaluating NE in critical AKI-D patients with septic shock according to the sepsis-3 criteria from a nationwide cohort. We followed up patients with septic AKI on dialysis to 90 days after hospital discharge, and further evaluated the recovery from AKI promptly. However, our study still had some limitations. First, our study did not evaluate the catecholamine-sparing effect of NE, in addition to the different patient population; and we did not evaluate the vascular response to NE under critical dialysis. Secondly, the indication for the use of NE or other vasoactive agents is not standardized. However, due to the difficulty in the randomness of enrolling patients with septic shock, an observational study could provide valuable information. Third, there could be a selection bias in choosing vasoactive agents due to current guidelines showed that norepinephrine is the first choice for septic shock and low dose dopamine for prophylactic use is no longer recommended. Last but not the least, we did not record pre-dialysis data of hemodynamic status, such as central venous pressure or volume of fluid resuscitation completely. Therefore, we could not evaluate the impact of fluid status when dialysis-required septic AKI developed and the association with the vasoactive agent usage to mortality.

## **5. Conclusions**

The use of NE in septic AKI patients at the initialization of dialysis is associated with a higher 90-day mortality after we adjusted for severity by IPTW compared to other vasoactive agents, and the detrimental effect was dose-dependent. Therefore, consideration of early treatment to block septic AKI vicious cycle to stabilize the hemodynamic status should nonetheless precede increased doses of norepinephrine at dialysis initiation. Further study to explore the potential and possible mechanism is needed.

**Supplementary Materials:**

**Author Contributions:** Writing-Original Draft Preparation: Y.-Y.C.; Conceptualization: V.-C.W., C.-J.W., Y.-C.Y., M.-S.W., C.-C.H., K.-D.W., J.-T.F.; Methodology: V.-C.W. and C.-J.W.; Formal Analysis: W.-C.H.; Resources: the NSARF and CAKS group; All the authors interpreted and had full access to the data, revised the manuscript critically, and approved the final article.

**Acknowledgments:** This work was supported by the Ministry of Science and Technology (MOST) of the Republic of China (Taiwan) (grant number, MOST 106-2321-B-182-002). We also express our sincere gratitude to all the staff of the Taiwan Clinical Trial Consortium, TCTC. This work was carried out with the technical and scientific support of the NSARF: [National Taiwan University Hospital]: Vin-Cent Wu, MD, PhD, Tai-Shuan Lai, MD, PhD, Yu-Feng Lin, MD, I-Jung Tsai, MD, PhD, Chun-Fu Lai, MD, PhD, Tao-Min Huang, MD, Tzong-Shinn Chu, MD, PhD, Yung-Ming Chen, MD, Yu-hsing Chang, MD, Yu-Chang Yeh, MD, PhD, Chien-Heng Lai, RN, Li -Jung Tseng, RN, and Kwan-Dun Wu, MD, PhD. [Chi-Mei Medical Center, Liouying]: Jian-Jhong Wang, MD. [Mackay Memorial Hospital, Hsinchu]: Cheng-Yi Chen, MD. [Saint Mary's Hospital Luodong]: Chih-Chung Shiao, MD. [Taoyuan General Hospital, Ministry of Health and Welfare]: Wei-Jie Wang, MD, PhD, Jui-Hsiang Lin, MD. [Taipei Tzu Chi Hospital, Buddhist Tzu Chi Medical Foundation]: Che-Hsiung Wu, MD. [Mackay Memorial Hospital, Taipei]: Chih-Jen Wu, MD, PhD. The authors appreciate and thank all the members of the CAKS, which are listed in alphabetical order of their affiliation names: [Fu Jen Catholic University Hospital]: Kuo-Cheng Lu, MD. [Chi-Mei Medical Center, Liouying]: Jian-Jhong Wang, MD. [Chi-Mei Medical Center, Yongkang]: Wei-Chih Kan, MD. [China Medical University Hospital]: Chiu-Ching Huang, MD, PhD, Che-Yi Chou, MD, PhD, Ya-Fei Yang, MD. [Dalin Tzu-Chi Hospital]: Jen-Pi Tsai, MD, PhD. [International-Harvard Statistical Consulting Company]: Fu-Chang Hu, Ph.D. [Kaohsiung Chang Gung Memorial Hospital]: Chien-Te Lee, MD, PhD, Jin-Bor Chen, MD, Chih-Hsiung Lee, MD, Wen-Chin Lee, MD, PhD, Lung-Chih Li, MD, PhD, Te-Chuan Chen, MD. [Kaohsiung Municipal Ta-Tung Hospital]: Hugo You-Hsien Lin, MD. [Keelung Chang Gung Memorial Hospital]: Yung-Chang Chen, MD, Chin-Chan Lee, MD, Chiao-Yin Sun, MD, Heng-Chih Pan, MD. [Linkou Chang Gung Memorial Hospital]: Ming-Yang Chang, MD, PhD, Chang-Chyi Jenq, MD, Chan-Yu Lin, MD, PhD, Chih-Hsiang Chang, MD, Tsung-Yu Tsai, MD. [Lin-Shin Hospital]: Cheng-Min Chen, MD. [Lotung Poh-Ai Hospital]: En-Tzu Lin, MD. [Saint Mary's Hospital Luodong]: Chih-Chung Shiao, MD. [Mackay Memorial Hospital]: Chih-Jen Wu, MD, PhD, Cheng-Jua Lin, MD, Pei-Chen Wu, MD. [Mackay Memorial Hospital Taitung Branch]: Feng-Chi Kuo, MD. [Min-Sheng General Hospital]: Chih-Jen Weng, MD. [National Health Research Institutes]: Li-Kwang Chen, PhD. [National Taiwan University Hospital]: Kwan-Dun Wu, MD, PhD, Tzong-Shinn Chu, MD, PhD, Yung-Ming Chen, MD, Shuei-Liong Lin, MD, PhD, Vin-Cent Wu, MD, PhD, Tao-Min Huang, MD, Yu-Feng Lin, MD, Chun-Fu Lai, MD, PhD. Tai-Shuan Lai, MD, PhD: [National Taiwan University Hospital Hsin Chu Branch]: Wei-Shun Yang, MD. [New Taipei City Hospital Sanchong Branch]: Wen-Ding Hsu, MD, MS. [Shin-Kong Wo Ho-Su Memorial Hospital]: Jyh-Gang Leu, MD, PhD, Jui-Ting Chang MD. [Sin-Ren Hospital]: Hung-Hsiang Liou, MD. [Taichung Veteran General Hospital]: Kuo-Hsiung Hsu, MD, Ming-Ju Wu, MD, PhD, Chun-Te Huang, MD. [Taichung Veteran General Hospital Chiayi Branch]: Zi-hong You, MD. [Taipei City Hospital Heping Branch]: Chao-Fu Chang, MD. [Taipei Medical University Hospital]: Tzen-Wen Chen, MD, PhD, Hsi-Hsien Chen, MD, PhD, Fan-Chi Chang, MD, PhD, Yen- Chung Lin, MD, Mai-Szu Wu, MD, Chih-Chin Kao, MD. [Taipei Tzu Chi Hospital]: Szu-Chun Hung, MD, Ko-Lin Kuo, MD, PhD, Che-Hsiung Wu, MD. [Taipei Veterans General Hospital]: Der-Cherng Tarng, MD, PhD, Jinn-Yang Chen, MD, Chih-Yu Yang, MD, PhD, Kuo-Hua Lee, MD. [Taoyuan General Hospital, Ministry of Health and Welfare]: Wei-Jie Wang, MD, PhD, Sheng-Wen Ko, MD, Jui-Hsiang Lin, MD. The authors thank the English editing by Eric B. Chueh of Case Western University, Cleveland, Ohio, USA.

## References

1. Singer, M.; Deutschman, C.S.; Seymour, C.W.; Shankar-Hari, M.; Annane, D.; Bauer, M.; Bellomo, R.; Bernard, G.R.; Chiche, J.D.; Coopersmith, C.M.; et al. The Third International Consensus Definitions for Sepsis and Septic Shock (Sepsis-3). *JAMA* **2016**, *315*, 801–810. [CrossRef] [PubMed]
2. Hoste, E.A.; Bagshaw, S.M.; Bellomo, R.; Cely, C.M.; Colman, R.; Cruz, D.N.; Edipidis, K.; Forni, L.G.; Gomersall, C.D.; Govil, D.; et al. Epidemiology of acute kidney injury in critically ill patients: The multinational AKI-EPI study. *Intensive Care Med.* **2015**, *41*, 1411–1423. [CrossRef] [PubMed]
3. Uchino, S.; Kellum, J.A.; Bellomo, R.; Doig, G.S.; Morimatsu, H.; Morgera, S.; Schetz, M.; Tan, I.; Bouman, C.; Macedo, E.; et al. Acute renal failure in critically ill patients: A multinational, multicenter study. *JAMA* **2005**, *294*, 813–818. [CrossRef] [PubMed]
4. Rhee, C.; Dantes, R.; Epstein, L.; Murphy, D.J.; Seymour, C.W.; Iwashyna, T.J.; Kadri, S.S.; Angus, D.C.; Danner, R.L.; Fiore, A.E.; et al. Incidence and Trends of Sepsis in US Hospitals Using Clinical vs. Claims Data, 2009-2014. *JAMA* **2017**, *318*, 1241–1249. [CrossRef] [PubMed]
5. Bagshaw, S.M.; George, C.; Bellomo, R. Committee ADM: Early acute kidney injury and sepsis: A multicentre evaluation. *Crit. Care* **2008**, *12*, R47. [CrossRef] [PubMed]

6. Thakar, C.V.; Christianson, A.; Freyberg, R.; Almenoff, P.; Render, M.L. Incidence and outcomes of acute kidney injury in intensive care units: A Veterans Administration study. *Crit. Care Med.* **2009**, *37*, 2552–2558. [CrossRef] [PubMed]
7. Bagshaw, S.M.; Uchino, S.; Bellomo, R.; Morimatsu, H.; Morgera, S.; Schetz, M.; Tan, I.; Bouman, C.; Macedo, E.; Gibney, N.; et al. Septic acute kidney injury in critically ill patients: Clinical characteristics and outcomes. *Clin. J. Am. Soc. Nephrol.* **2007**, *2*, 431–439. [CrossRef] [PubMed]
8. Chawla, L.S.; Busse, L.; Brasha-Mitchell, E.; Davison, D.; Honiq, J.; Alotaibi, Z.; Seneff, M.G. Intravenous angiotensin II for the treatment of high-output shock (ATHOS trial): A pilot study. *Crit. Care* **2014**, *18*, 534. [CrossRef] [PubMed]
9. Myburgh, J.A.; Higgins, A.; Jovanovska, A.; Lipman, J.; Ramakrishnan, N.; Santamaria, J. Investigators CATS: A comparison of epinephrine and norepinephrine in critically ill patients. *Intensive Care Med.* **2008**, *34*, 2226–2234. [CrossRef] [PubMed]
10. Rhodes, A.; Evans, L.E.; Alhazzani, W.; Levy, M.M.; Antonelli, M.; Ferrer, R.; Kumar, A.; Sevransky, J.E.; Sprung, C.L.; Nunnally, M.E.; et al. Surviving Sepsis Campaign: International Guidelines for Management of Sepsis and Septic Shock: 2016. *Crit. Care Med.* **2017**, *45*, 486–552. [CrossRef] [PubMed]
11. Shiao, C.C.; Wu, P.C.; Wu, V.C.; Lin, J.H.; Pan, H.C.; Yang, Y.F.; Lai, T.S.; Huang, T.M.; Wu, C.H.; Yang, W.S.; et al. Nationwide epidemiology and prognosis of dialysis-requiring acute kidney injury (NEP-AKI-D) study: Design and methods. *Nephrology (Carlton)* **2016**, *21*, 758–764. [CrossRef] [PubMed]
12. Wu, V.C.; Ko, W.J.; Chang, H.W.; Chen, Y.W.; Lin, Y.F.; Shiao, C.C.; Chen, Y.M.; Chen, Y.S.; Tsai, P.R.; Hu, F.C.; et al. Risk factors of early redialysis after weaning from postoperative acute renal replacement therapy. *Intensive Care Med.* **2008**, *34*, 101–108. [CrossRef] [PubMed]
13. Wu, V.C.; Ko, W.J.; Chang, H.W.; Chen, Y.S.; Chen, Y.W.; Chen, Y.M.; Hu, F.C.; Lin, Y.H.; Tsai, P.R.; Wu, K.D. Early renal replacement therapy in patients with postoperative acute liver failure associated with acute renal failure: Effect on postoperative outcomes. *J. Am. Coll. Surg.* **2007**, *205*, 266–276. [CrossRef] [PubMed]
14. Knaus, W.A.; Draper, E.A.; Wagner, D.P.; Zimmerman, J.E. APACHE II: A severity of disease classification system. *Crit. Care Med.* **1985**, *13*, 818–829. [CrossRef] [PubMed]
15. Vincent, J.L.; Moreno, R.; Takala, J.; Willatts, S.; De Mendonca, A.; Bruining, H.; Reinhart, C.K.; Suter, P.M.; Thijs, L.G. The SOFA (Sepsis-related Organ Failure Assessment) score to describe organ dysfunction/failure. On behalf of the Working Group on Sepsis-Related Problems of the European Society of Intensive Care Medicine. *Intensive Care Med.* **1996**, *22*, 707–710. [CrossRef] [PubMed]
16. Chen, Y.S.; Ko, W.J.; Lin, F.Y.; Huang, S.C.; Chou, T.F.; Chou, N.K.; Hsu, R.B.; Wang, S.S.; Chu, S.H. Preliminary result of an algorithm to select proper ventricular assist devices for high-risk patients with extracorporeal membrane oxygenation support. *J. Heart Lung Transplant.* **2001**, *20*, 850–857. [CrossRef]
17. Gaies, M.G.; Jeffries, H.E.; Niebler, R.A.; Pasquali, S.K.; Donohue, J.E.; Yu, S.; Gall, C.; Rice, T.B.; Thiagarajan, R.R. Vasoactive-inotropic score is associated with outcome after infant cardiac surgery: An analysis from the Pediatric Cardiac Critical Care Consortium and Virtual PICU System Registries. *Pediatr. Crit. Care Med.* **2014**, *15*, 529–537. [CrossRef] [PubMed]
18. Gaies, M.G.; Gurney, J.G.; Yen, A.H.; Napoli, M.L.; Gajarski, R.J.; Ohye, R.G.; Charpie, J.R.; Hirsch, J.C. Vasoactive-inotropic score as a predictor of morbidity and mortality in infants after cardiopulmonary bypass. *Pediatr. Crit. Care Med.* **2010**, *11*, 234–238. [CrossRef] [PubMed]
19. Kumar, M.; Sharma, R.; Sethi, S.K.; Bazaz, S.; Sharma, P.; Bhan, A.; Kher, V. Vasoactive Inotrope Score as a tool for clinical care in children post cardiac surgery. *Indian J. Crit. Care Med.* **2014**, *18*, 653–658. [PubMed]
20. McIntosh, A.M.; Tong, S.; Deakyne, S.J.; Davidson, J.A.; Scott, H.F. Validation of the Vasoactive-Inotropic Score in Pediatric Sepsis. *Pediatr. Crit. Care Med.* **2017**, *18*, 750–757. [CrossRef] [PubMed]
21. Wu, V.C.; Hu, Y.H.; Wu, C.H.; Kao, C.C.; Wang, C.Y.; Yang, W.S.; Lee, H.H.; Chang, Y.S.; Lin, Y.H.; Wang, S.M.; et al. Administrative data on diagnosis and mineralocorticoid receptor antagonist prescription identified patients with primary aldosteronism in Taiwan. *J. Clin. Epidemiol.* **2014**, *67*, 1139–1149. [CrossRef] [PubMed]
22. Roy, J.; Lum, K.J.; Daniels, M.J. A Bayesian nonparametric approach to marginal structural models for point treatments and a continuous or survival outcome. *Biostatistics* **2017**, *18*, 32–47. [CrossRef] [PubMed]
23. Wu, V.C.; Young, G.H.; Huang, P.H.; Lo, S.C.; Wang, K.C.; Sun, C.Y.; Liang, C.J.; Huang, T.M.; Chen, J.H.; Chang, F.C.; et al. In acute kidney injury, indoxyl sulfate impairs human endothelial progenitor cells: Modulation by statin. *Angiogenesis* **2013**, *16*, 609–624. [CrossRef] [PubMed]

24. Wu, V.C.; Huang, T.M.; Shiao, C.C.; Lai, C.F.; Tsai, P.R.; Wang, W.J.; Huang, H.Y.; Wang, K.C.; Ko, W.J.; Wu, K.D.; et al. The hemodynamic effects during sustained low-efficiency dialysis versus continuous veno-venous hemofiltration for uremic patients with brain hemorrhage: A crossover study. *J. Neurosurg.* **2013**, *119*, 1288–1295. [CrossRef] [PubMed]
25. Wu, C.H.; Yang, Y.W.; Hung, S.C.; Tsai, Y.C.; Hu, Y.H.; Lin, Y.H.; Chu, T.S.; Wu, K.D.; Wu, V.C. Effect of Treatment on Body Fluid in Patients with Unilateral Aldosterone Producing Adenoma: Adrenalectomy versus Spironolactone. *Sci. Rep.* **2015**, *5*, 15297. [CrossRef] [PubMed]
26. Wu, V.C.; Chang, C.H.; Wang, C.Y.; Lin, Y.H.; Kao, T.W.; Lin, P.C.; Chu, T.S.; Chang, Y.S.; Chen, L.; Wu, K.D.; et al. Risk of Fracture in Primary Aldosteronism: A Population-Based Cohort Study. *J. Bone Miner. Res.* **2017**, *32*, 743–752. [CrossRef] [PubMed]
27. Wu, V.C.; Chueh, S.J.; Chen, L.; Chang, C.H.; Hu, Y.H.; Lin, Y.H.; Wu, K.D.; Yang, W.S.; Group, T.S. Risk of new-onset diabetes mellitus in primary aldosteronism: A population study over 5 years. *J. Hypertens.* **2017**, *35*, 1698–1708. [CrossRef] [PubMed]
28. Austin, P.C. Variance estimation when using inverse probability of treatment weighting (IPTW) with survival analysis. *Stat. Med.* **2016**, *35*, 5642–5655. [CrossRef] [PubMed]
29. Dellinger, R.P.; Levy, M.M.; Rhodes, A.; Annane, D.; Gerlach, H.; Opal, S.M.; Sevransky, J.E.; Sprung, C.L.; Douglas, I.S.; Jaeschke, R.; et al. Surviving Sepsis Campaign: International guidelines for management of severe sepsis and septic shock, 2012. *Intensive Care Med.* **2013**, *39*, 165–228. [CrossRef] [PubMed]
30. Chou, C.Y.; Yeh, H.C.; Chen, W.; Liu, J.H.; Lin, H.H.; Liu, Y.L.; Yang, Y.F.; Wang, S.M.; Huang, C.C. Norepinephrine and hospital mortality in critically ill patients undergoing continuous renal replacement therapy. *Artif. Organs* **2011**, *35*, E11–E17. [CrossRef] [PubMed]
31. Levy, B.; Dusang, B.; Annane, D.; Gibot, S.; Bollaert, P.E. College Interregional des Reanimateurs du N-E: Cardiovascular response to dopamine and early prediction of outcome in septic shock: A prospective multiple-center study. *Crit. Care Med.* **2005**, *33*, 2172–2177. [CrossRef] [PubMed]
32. Gordon, A.C.; Russell, J.A.; Walley, K.R.; Singer, J.; Ayers, D.; Storms, M.M.; Holmes, C.L.; Hebert, P.C.; Cooper, D.J.; Mehta, S.; et al. The effects of vasopressin on acute kidney injury in septic shock. *Intensive Care Med.* **2010**, *36*, 83–91. [CrossRef] [PubMed]
33. Russell, J.A.; Walley, K.R.; Singer, J.; Gordon, A.C.; Hebert, P.C.; Cooper, D.J.; Holmes, C.L.; Mehta, S.; Granton, J.T.; Storms, M.M.; et al. Vasopressin versus norepinephrine infusion in patients with septic shock. *N. Engl. J. Med.* **2008**, *358*, 877–887. [CrossRef] [PubMed]
34. da Hora Passos, R.; Ramos, J.G.; Mendonca, E.J.; Miranda, E.A.; Dutra, F.R.; Coelho, M.F.; Pedroza, A.C.; Correia, L.C.; Batista, P.B.; Macedo, E.; et al. A clinical score to predict mortality in septic acute kidney injury patients requiring continuous renal replacement therapy: The HELENICC score. *BMC Anesthesiol.* **2017**, *17*, 21. [CrossRef] [PubMed]
35. Povoa, P.R.; Carneiro, A.H.; Ribeiro, O.S.; Pereira, A.C. Portuguese Community-Acquired Sepsis Study G: Influence of vasopressor agent in septic shock mortality. Results from the Portuguese Community-Acquired Sepsis Study (SACiUCI study). *Crit. Care Med.* **2009**, *37*, 410–416. [CrossRef] [PubMed]
36. Vincent, J.L.; Gerlach, H. Fluid resuscitation in severe sepsis and septic shock: An evidence-based review. *Crit. Care Med.* **2004**, *32* (Suppl. 11), S451–S454. [CrossRef] [PubMed]
37. Abou Dagher, G.; Harmouche, E.; Jabbour, E.; Bachir, R.; Zebian, D.; Bou Chebl, R. Sepsis in hemodialysis patients. *BMC Emerg. Med.* **2015**, *15*, 30. [CrossRef] [PubMed]
38. Ferreira, F.L.; Bota, D.P.; Bross, A.; Melot, C.; Vincent, J.L. Serial evaluation of the SOFA score to predict outcome in critically ill patients. *JAMA* **2001**, *286*, 1754–1758. [CrossRef] [PubMed]
39. Martin, C.; Viviand, X.; Leone, M.; Thirion, X. Effect of norepinephrine on the outcome of septic shock. *Crit. Care Med.* **2000**, *28*, 2758–2765. [CrossRef] [PubMed]
40. De Backer, D.; Biston, P.; Devriendt, J.; Madl, C.; Chochrad, D.; Aldecoa, C.; Brasseur, A.; Defrance, P.; Gottignies, P.; Vincent, J.L.; et al. Comparison of dopamine and norepinephrine in the treatment of shock. *N. Engl. J. Med.* **2010**, *362*, 779–789. [CrossRef] [PubMed]
41. Gordon, A.C.; Mason, A.J.; Thirunavukkarasu, N.; Perkins, G.D.; Cecconi, M.; Cepkova, M.; Pogson, D.G.; Aya, H.D.; Anjum, A.; Frazier, G.J.; et al. Effect of Early Vasopressin vs. Norepinephrine on Kidney Failure in Patients With Septic Shock: The VANISH Randomized Clinical Trial. *JAMA* **2016**, *316*, 509–518. [CrossRef] [PubMed]
42. Richer, M.; Robert, S.; Lebel, M. Renal hemodynamics during norepinephrine and low-dose dopamine infusions in man. *Crit. Care Med.* **1996**, *24*, 1150–1156. [CrossRef] [PubMed]

43. Cronin, R.E.; Erickson, A.M.; de Torrente, A.; McDonald, K.M.; Schrier, R.W. Norepinephrine-induced acute renal failure: A reversible ischemic model of acute renal failure. *Kidney Int.* **1978**, *14*, 187–190. [CrossRef] [PubMed]
44. Lankadeva, Y.R.; Kosaka, J.; Evans, R.G.; Bailey, S.R.; Bellomo, R.; May, C.N. Intrarenal and urinary oxygenation during norepinephrine resuscitation in ovine septic acute kidney injury. *Kidney Int.* **2016**, *90*, 100–108. [CrossRef] [PubMed]

# 7

# Proteomic Analysis of Urinary Extracellular Vesicles Reveals a Role for the Complement System in Medullary Sponge Kidney Disease

**Maurizio Bruschi [1,†], Simona Granata [2,†], Giovanni Candiano [1], Antonia Fabris [2], Andrea Petretto [3], Gian Marco Ghiggeri [4], Giovanni Gambaro [2] and Gianluigi Zaza [2,*]**

1 Laboratory of Molecular Nephrology, IRCCS Istituto Giannina Gaslini, 16147 Genova, Italy; mauriziobruschi@gaslini.org (M.B.); giovannicandiano@gaslini.org (G.C.)

2 Renal Unit, Department of Medicine, University/Hospital of Verona, Piazzale A. Stefani 1, 37126 Verona, Italy; simona.granata@univr.it (S.G.); antoniafabris21@gmail.com (A.F.); giovanni.gambaro@univr.it (G.G.)

3 Laboratory of Mass Spectrometry—Core Facilities, IRCCS Istituto Giannina Gaslini, 16147 Genova, Italy; a.petretto@gmail.com

4 Division of Nephrology, Dialysis and Transplantation, IRCCS Istituto Giannina Gaslini, 16147 Genova, Italy; GMarcoGhiggeri@gaslini.org

* Correspondence: gianluigi.zaza@univr.it

† These authors contributed equally to the study.

**Abstract:** Medullary sponge kidney (MSK) disease is a rare and neglected kidney condition often associated with nephrocalcinosis/nephrolithiasis and cystic anomalies in the precalyceal ducts. Little is known about the pathogenesis of this disease, so we addressed the knowledge gap using a proteomics approach. The protein content of microvesicles/exosomes isolated from urine of 15 MSK and 15 idiopathic calcium nephrolithiasis (ICN) patients was investigated by mass spectrometry, followed by weighted gene co-expression network analysis, support vector machine (SVM) learning, and partial least squares discriminant analysis (PLS-DA) to select the most discriminative proteins. Proteomic data were verified by ELISA. We identified 2998 proteins in total, 1764 (58.9%) of which were present in both vesicle types in both diseases. Among the MSK samples, only 65 (2.2%) and 137 (4.6%) proteins were exclusively found in the microvesicles and exosomes, respectively. Similarly, among the ICN samples, only 75 (2.5%) and 94 (3.1%) proteins were exclusively found in the microvesicles and exosomes, respectively. SVM learning and PLS-DA revealed a core panel of 20 proteins that distinguished extracellular vesicles representing each clinical condition with an accuracy of 100%. Among them, three exosome proteins involved in the lectin complement pathway maximized the discrimination between MSK and ICN: Ficolin 1, Mannan-binding lectin serine protease 2, and Complement component 4-binding protein β. ELISA confirmed the proteomic results. Our data show that the complement pathway is involved in the MSK, revealing a new range of potential therapeutic targets and early diagnostic biomarkers.

**Keywords:** medullary sponge kidney; idiopathic calcium nephrolithiasis; complement system; proteomics

## 1. Introduction

In the last decade, great efforts have been undertaken to characterize the biological networking associated with medullary sponge kidney (MSK) disease, a rare clinical condition (prevalence of approximately 5 cases per 100,000 in the general population) often associated with nephrocalcinosis and nephrolithiasis, urinary acidification and concentration defects, and cystic anomalies in the precalyceal ducts [1]. Most of these studies, based on clinical observations, as well as molecular analysis, have provided evidence that supports the genetic transmission of MSK and an association with metabolic disorders (such as hyperparathyroidism) and bone diseases [2–11].

More recently, we used proteomic analysis to catalog the MSK-specific protein profile, as well as the protein content of urinary extracellular vesicles [12]. This revealed the presence of several key regulators of epithelial cell differentiation, kidney development, cell migration/adhesion, and extracellular matrix organization, providing a new insight into the pathophysiology of MSK [12]. The most abundant protein found in MSK urinary extracellular vesicles was laminin subunit α2 (LAMA2, Merosin), a well-characterized member of the laminin family of at least 15 αβɣ heterotrimeric proteins, which contributes to the extracellular matrix and is a major component of the basement membrane [12,13]. This protein is thought to promote cyst formation [14–16]. It also regulates extracellular laminin assembly, and the laminin then determines the orientation of the apical pole [17].

In our most recent publication [18], we compared the protein content of extracellular vesicles (exosomes and microvesicles) from MSK and autosomal dominant polycystic kidney disease (ADPKD) patients by mass spectrometry (MS) and identified a profile including 34 proteins that discriminate between the two clinical conditions. The most abundant protein in MSK vesicles was SPP1, also known as osteopontin, which is implicated in physiological/pathological bone mineralization and kidney stone formation [19]. This protein is synthesized in the kidney and secreted into the urine by epithelial cells, including those lining the loop of Henle, distal convoluted tubule, and papillary duct [20]. SPP1 inhibits the nucleation, growth, and aggregation of calcium oxalate crystals [21] and the binding of these crystals to kidney epithelial cells [22]. Although it has been recently found that osteopontin was up-regulated in the kidney from established rat models for polycystic kidney disease compared with wild-type mice [23,24], no data are available for MSK (no animal model is available for this disease). Therefore, based on our in vivo data, we can assume that in MSK patients, osteopontin could be also more up-regulated than ADPKD. A reason could be that in MSK, this biological element may be implicated not only in cystic development, but also in nephrolithiasis, a major clinical condition associated with medullary sponge kidney.

The diagnostic accuracy for MSK is currently low because it depends on personal experience (MSK is often confused with other causes of nephrocalcinosis or with papillary ductal plugging) and diagnosis requires invasive radiation and/or nephrotoxic contrast agents for medical imaging. Although the studies described above have shed light on the biological mechanisms associated with MSK, the pathogenesis of this disorder is only partially defined and further studies are necessary to identify suitable diagnostic biomarkers. To address this knowledge gap, we carried out a comprehensive comparative proteomic analysis of urinary microvesicles and exosomes to identify biological differences between MSK and idiopathic calcium nephrolithiasis (ICN) as a control group. The analysis of urinary extracellular vesicles is ideal because they can be obtained without invasive procedures and they contain elevated levels of cell-specific proteins from every segment of the nephron, representing diverse cellular processes including metabolic, immunity-related, and coagulation responses [25,26]. These intrinsic characteristics of extracellular vesicles could, therefore, provide a panel of informative marker proteins that not only allow the diagnosis and monitoring of MSK but could also provide insight into the underlying pathophysiological and biochemical processes.

## 2. Results

### *2.1. Characterization of Exosomes and Microvesicles*

The size and purity of the microvesicles and exosomes isolated by ultracentrifugation were confirmed by dynamic light scattering (DLS), revealing a Gaussian distribution profile with peak means at 1000 ± 65 and 90 ± 5 nm, the typical size for microvesicles and exosomes, respectively (Figure S1A). There was no difference in size between the MSK and ICN patients for either type of vesicle. Western blot analysis revealed that the exosomes were positive for CD63 and CD81 but not CD45, whereas the microvesicles showed the opposite antigen profile (Figure S1B).

*2.2. Protein Composition of Exosomes and Microvesicles*

The protein composition of microvesicles and exosomes from the urine of ICN and MSK patients was determined by MS analysis. We identified 2998 proteins in total, 1764 (58.9%) of which were present in all four sample types. Among the ICN samples, only 75 (2.5%) and 94 (3.1%) proteins were exclusively found in the microvesicles and exosomes, respectively. Similarly, among the MSK samples, only 65 (2.2%) and 137 (4.6%) proteins were exclusively found in the microvesicles and exosomes, respectively (Figure 1).

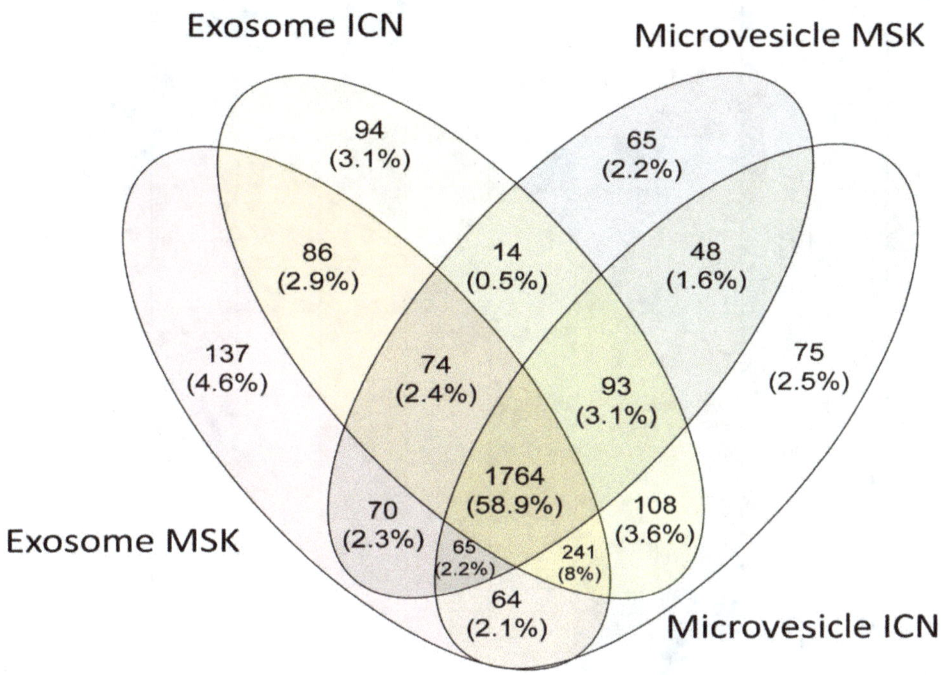


**Figure 1.** Venn diagram showing all the proteins identified in exosomes and microvesicles isolated from the urine of idiopathic calcium nephrolithiasis (ICN) and medullary sponge kidney (MSK) patients. Venn diagram shows common and exclusive proteins in the ICN and MSK groups. The numbers (and percentages) of proteins in the overlapping and non-overlapping areas are indicated.

About 2% of the total proteins found in extracellular vesicles were associated with one or both kidney diseases according to the DisGeNET database [27]. Among these associated proteins, 40% were found in the ICN and 100% in the MSK samples (Figure S2). The cellular origins of the proteins in the microvesicles were very similar in the ICN and MSK disease samples, with 35% of proteins originating from membranes, 25% from the cytoplasm, 7% from the nucleus, and 33% from other organelles. Similar results were observed for the exosome proteins, with 19% originating from membranes, 31% from the cytoplasm, 11% from the nucleus, and 38% from other organelles.

The overlapping protein content of each sample was confirmed by constructing a two-dimensional scatter plot of the multidimensional scaling (MDS) analysis (Figure S3). No samples were excluded during the quality check, performed by non-hierarchical clustering. We used weighted-gene co-expression network analysis (WGCNA) to identify proteins associated with each type of extracellular vesicle and disease, revealing a total of 14 modules comprising proteins with similar expression profiles. To distinguish between modules, we chose an arbitrary color for each module. The number of proteins included in each module ranged from 31 (salmon) to 950 (turquoise). The lime, pink, violet, and tan modules showed closer relationships with the microvesicles or exosomes from the ICN samples, whereas the gray, yellow, and green modules showed closer relationships with the microvesicles from the MSK samples (Figure 2).

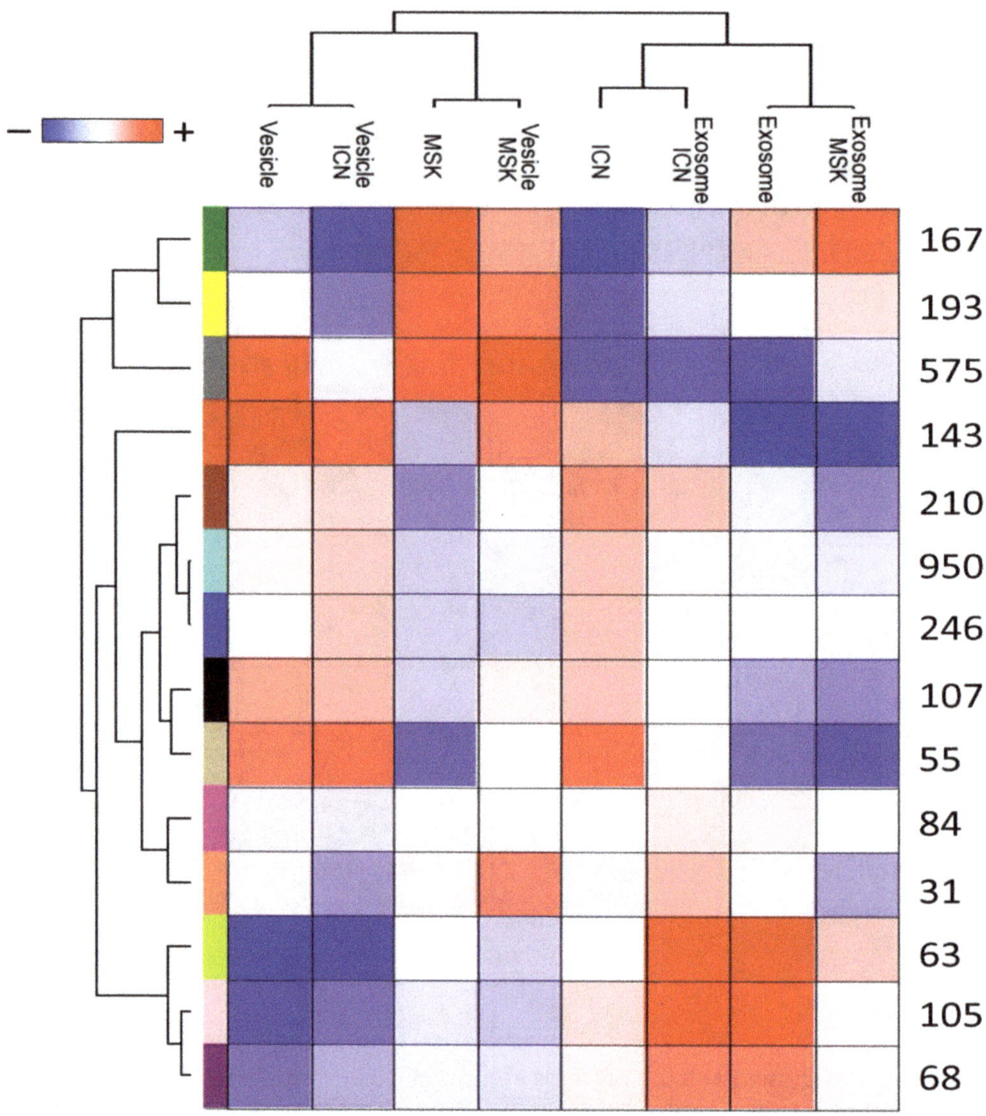


**Figure 2.** Module identification and relationships with clinical traits. Heat map of the relationships between module eigengenes and the trait indicator of each sample. The grade of the relationship ranges from −1 (blue) to 1 (red), where blue represents a perfect negative correlation and red a perfect positive correlation.

Next, we applied the Mann–Whitney *U*-test to identify the proteins that best distinguish the type of disease in the microvesicles or exosomes (Figure 3A,B).

This revealed a total of 142 discriminatory proteins (Tables S1 and S2): 105 distinguished between ICN and MSK microvesicles and 43 distinguished between ICN and MSK exosomes, with six featuring in both vesicle types (Figure S4A). Their expression profiles after Z-score analysis are shown in Figure S4B. support vector machine (SVM) learning and partial least squares discriminant analysis (PLS-DA) were then used to highlight the proteins that maximize the discrimination between different sample types, revealing a core panel of 20 proteins that identified the four sample types with an accuracy of 100% (Figure 4A). Following the Z-score analysis, we built a heat map of the corresponding expression profiles (Figure 4B).

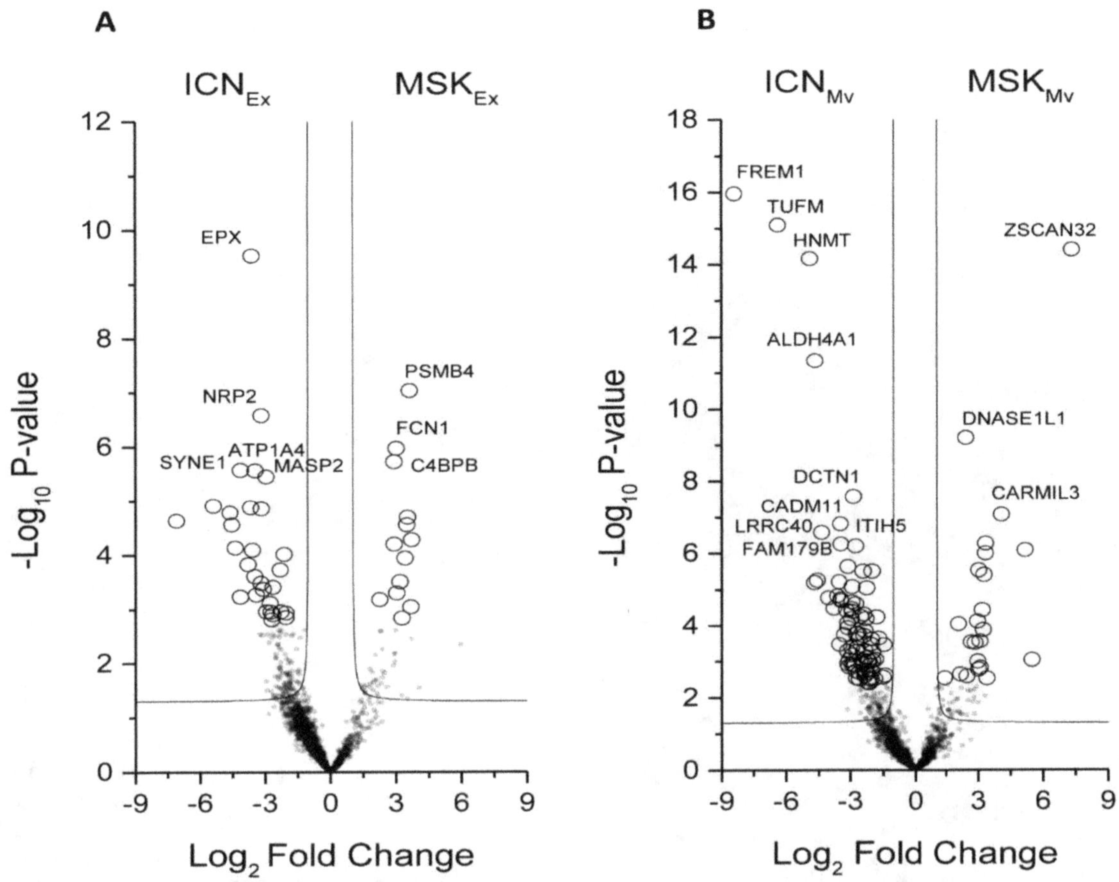


**Figure 3.** Volcano plot showing the univariate statistical analysis of urinary exosome (**A**) and microvesicle (**B**) fractions from ICN and MSK patients. The plot is based on the fold change ($\log_2$) and p-value ($-\log_{10}$) of all proteins identified in all samples. White circles indicate proteins with statistically significant differences in abundance between the two groups of patients.

The diversity of expression profiles among the proteins that showed significant and high levels of sample discrimination indicated an equally diverse range of functions, so we assigned Gene Ontology (GO) functional annotations to build a network of biochemical pathways among the different groups (Figure S5). In this network, circles and lines represent the biochemical pathways and their interconnections, respectively. In addition, the different pathways were clustered into 12 functional groups based on their GO annotations (ellipses): immune system, production of reactive oxygen species, IL-8 regulation, transport, regulation of ERBB signaling, tyrosine phosphorylation, receptor activity, peptidyl serine modification, hydrolase activity, DNA regulation, nucleoside metabolism, and cell and organ development. These 12 clusters were grouped into four macro-areas: regulation of metabolism, signal transduction, inflammation, and regulation of cell development. To generate a more concise picture of the biochemical process associated with the three proteins that maximize the discrimination between the exosomes of ICN and MSK samples [Mannan-binding lectin serine protease 2 (MASP2), Ficolin 1 (FCN1), and Complement component 4-binding protein β (C4BPB)], we explored the enrichment of GO annotations in greater detail. This highlighted the lectin-based complement activation pathway as the perturbed biochemical process most likely associated with all three potential biomarkers (Figure 5). The diagram shows the pathway mapped as a network of proteins (nodes) and their interactions (edges). Node color represents the fold change in protein abundance in the urinary exosome fraction of MSK (red) versus ICN (blue) patients, and the node size represents the corresponding p-values.

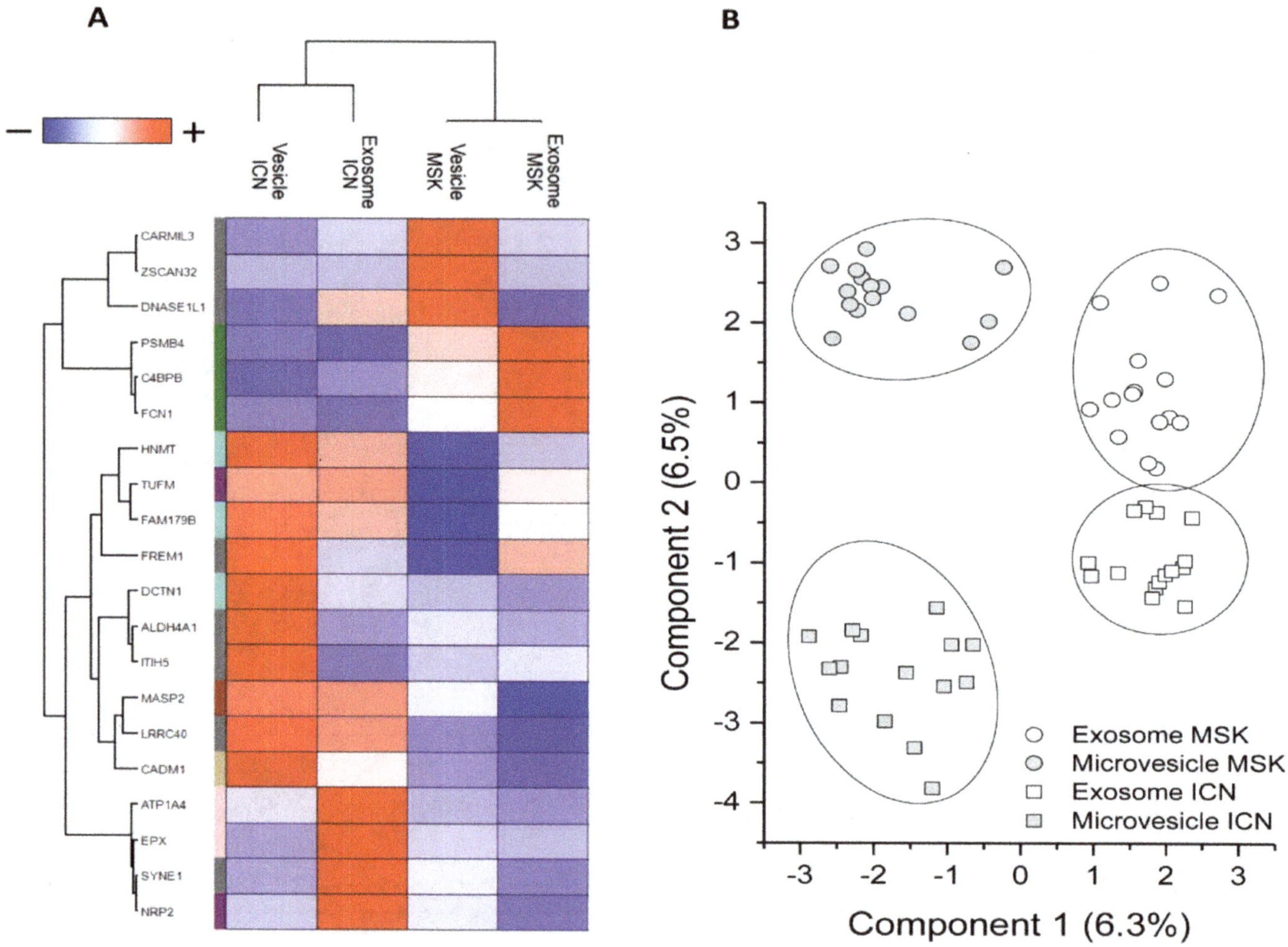


**Figure 4.** Proteins that achieve maximum discrimination between the exosome and microvesicle fractions of ICN and MSK patients. (**A**) Heat map of 20 core proteins identified through the combined use of univariate statistical analysis, machine learning, and partial least squares discriminant analysis. In the heat map, each row represents a protein, and each column corresponds to a sample type (exosome and microvesicle fractions from ICN and MSK patients). Normalized Z-scores of protein abundance are depicted by a pseudocolor scale with red indicating positive expression, white equal expression, and blue negative expression compared to each protein value, whereas the dendrogram displays the outcome of unsupervised hierarchical clustering, placing similar proteome profile values near each other. (**B**) Two-dimensional scatter plot representing the partial least squares discriminant analysis of exosomes (white symbols) and microvesicles (gray symbols) from MSK (circle) and ICN (square) patients, using the 20 core proteins. The ellipsis indicates 95% confidence interval. Visual inspection of the dendrogram, heat map, and scatter plot confirm the ability of these proteins to clearly distinguish among the four different sample types.

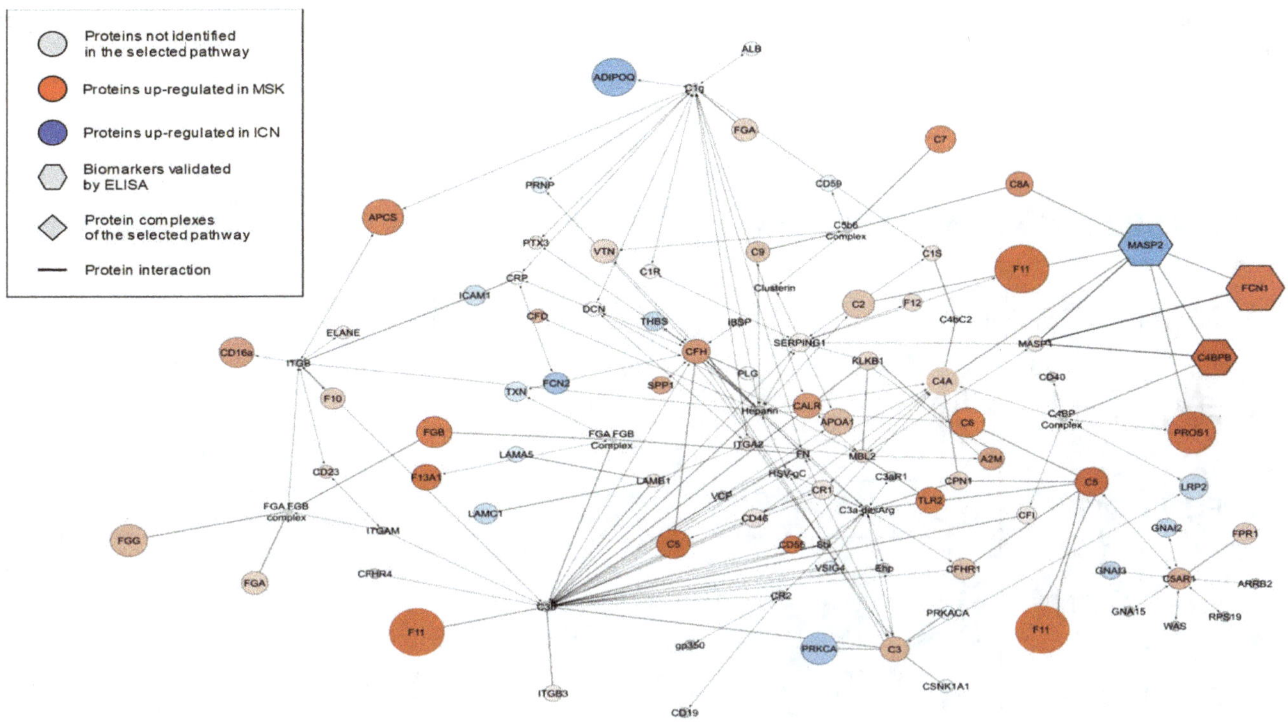


**Figure 5.** Complement lectin pathway activation. The diagram shows the zoom-in of the immune system enrichment results mapped as a network. Nodes and edges represent, respectively, the proteins and their interaction in the pathway of complement lectin activation. The color intensity of each protein (node) indicates the fold change increment in the urinary exosome fraction of MSK (red) versus ICN (blue) patients and the node size is representative of their p-value. The gray nodes represent unidentified proteins (circle) and protein complexes (diamonds) in the lectin pathway. The hexagons indicate the three proteins that maximize the discrimination between ICN and MSK samples as highlighted by the combined use of univariate/multivariate statistical analysis and machine learning algorithms.

### 2.3. *ELISA Analysis of MASP2, FCN1, and C4BPB to Confirm the MS Data*

The mass spectrometry (MS) results were verified by ELISA for all patients enrolled in the study using an in-house assay setup (Figure 6). We found that MASP2 was expressed more strongly in ICN patients compared to MSK patients (Figure 6A, black circle). The median (and interquartile range) values for ICN and MSK were 1.05 (0.41–1.4) and 0.2 (0.1–0.4), respectively ($p < 0.0001$). Received operating characteristic (ROC) analysis revealed that the expression of MASP2 in the urinary exosome can distinguish between ICN and MSK patients (Figure 6B, black line). The area under the curve (AUC), 95% confidence interval (CI), and p-value for the ROC analysis were 0.89, 0.81–0.97, and $p < 0.0001$, respectively. The cutoff, sensitivity, specificity, and likelihood ratio were 0.62, 67%, 97%, and 20, respectively.

In contrast to MASP2, FCN1 (Figure 6A, red circle) and C4BPB (Figure 6A, green circle) were more strongly expressed in MSK patients compared to ICN patients. For FCN1, the median (and interquartile range) values for ICN and MSK were 0.34 (0.28–0.47) and 1.06 (0.59–1.5), respectively ($p < 0.0001$). ROC analysis revealed that the expression of FCN1 in the urinary exosome can distinguish between ICN and MSK patients (Figure 6B, red line). The AUC, 95% CI and p-values for the ROC analysis were 0.9, 0.82–0.98, and $p < 0.0001$, respectively. The cutoff, sensitivity, specificity, and likelihood ratio were 0.55, 77%, 87%, and 5.7, respectively. For C4BPB, the median (and interquartile range) values for ICN and MSK were 0.45 (0.3–0.59) and 1.2 (0.67–1.67), respectively ($p < 0.0001$). ROC analysis revealed that the expression of C4BPB in the urinary exosome can distinguish between ICN and MSK patients (Figure 6B, green line). The AUC, 95% CI, and p-values for the ROC analysis were 0.9, 0.82–0.98, and $p < 0.0001$, respectively. The cutoff, sensitivity, specificity, and likelihood ratio were 0.62, 77%, 87%, and 5.7, respectively.

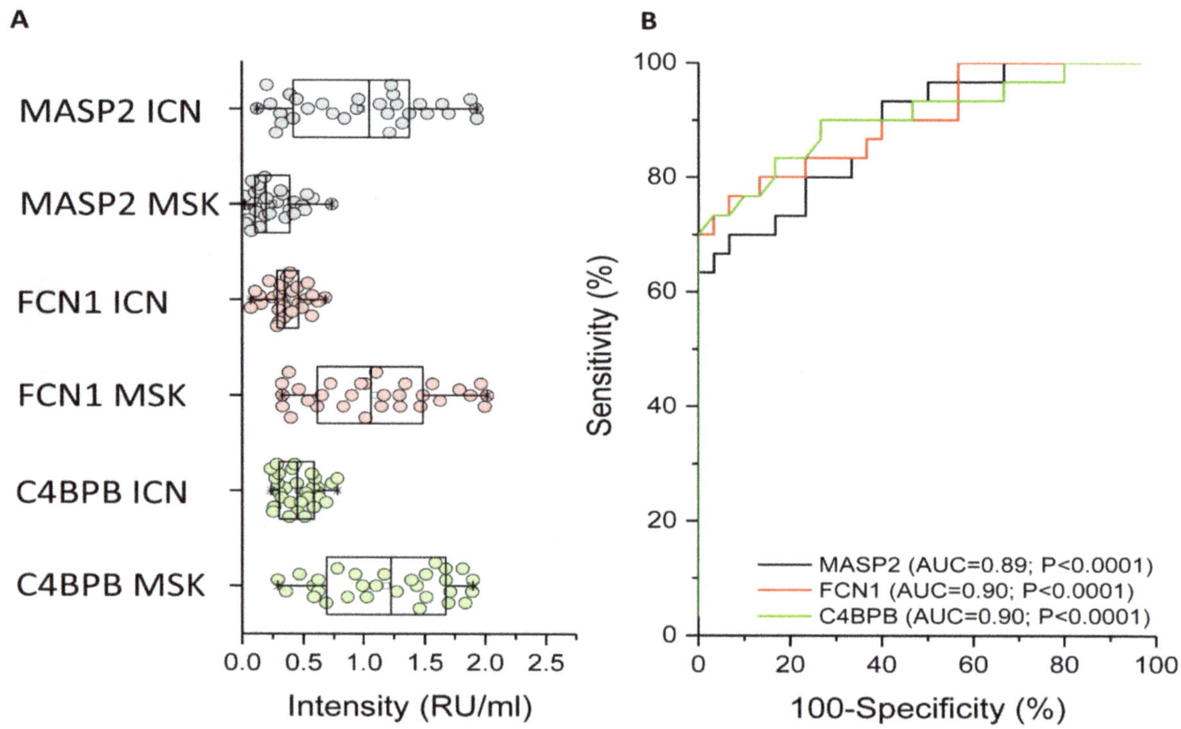


**Figure 6.** ELISA experiments to verify the proteomic data. (**A**) Box plot showing the median and interquartile range values of MASP2 (black), FCN1 (red), and C4BPB (green) in the urinary exosome of all patients. In particular, MASP2 was strongly expressed in the urinary exosome of ICN compared to MSK patients, whereas FCN1 and C4BPB showed the opposite profile. (**B**) Received operating characteristic (ROC) curve analysis confirming that the expression of all three proteins discriminates between ICN and MSK patients.

## 3. Discussion

MSK is a rare kidney disease that is currently difficult to diagnose because the molecular basis of pathogenesis is unclear and robust diagnostic biomarkers are not available in the clinic. We, therefore, carried out a comprehensive comparative proteomic analysis of urinary microvesicles and exosomes from MSK patients and a control group with the distinct kidney disorder ICN. We defined the protein profiles of both vesicles in both diseases and applied innovative statistical methods (including SVM learning and PLS-DA) to identify specific proteins (and the corresponding biological networks) that can accurately discriminate between patients with each disease. These proteins and networks not only represent a source of novel biomarker candidates and potential therapeutic targets but should also shed light on the molecular basis of MSK.

Statistical analysis identified a core panel of 20 highly discriminative proteins, the most promising were FCN1, MASP2, and C4BPB, all of which are major functional or regulatory components of the lectin complement pathway. These three proteins were not associated with either MSK or ICN according to the DisGeNET, a database containing one of the largest publicly available collections of genes and variants associated with human diseases [27]. FCN1 and C4BPB were more abundant in the exosomes of MSK patients compared to ICN controls, whereas MASP2 showed the opposite profile. It is possible that all three proteins, because of their molecular weight and the absence of proteinuria and/or renal impairment in our enrolled patients, did not pass through an intact glomerular membrane but were instead derived from renal epithelial cells [28].

FCN1 (also known as M-ficolin) is an oligomeric pattern-recognition protein consisting of an N-terminal collagen-like domain and a C-terminal globular fibrinogen-like domain [29,30]. It can form complexes with MASP2 to activate the lectin complement pathway [31]. FCN1 may also interact with C-reactive protein (CRP) via a conformational change induced by mild acidosis at the local site of infection [32,33], and with pentraxin 3 (PTX3) in a $Ca^{2+}$-dependent manner [34]. The high level of FCN1 in urinary exosomes isolated from our MSK patients suggests that the lectin complement pathway may be involved in the complex biological process leading to the growth of cysts. This agrees with previous studies based on mouse models deficient in complement factors, which develop fewer kidney cysts and suffer less severe pericystic tissue inflammation, helping to preserve normal renal functions [35]. Further evidence that the complement pathway is involved in cystic disorders has been gathered from patients affected by ADPKD, whose urine and cyst fluids were found to be enriched for complement proteins [36–38].

The downregulation of MASP2 in our MSK patients was accompanied by the upregulation of C4BPB, a multimeric protein that inhibits the activation of the complement cascade by preventing the formation of the classical C3 and C5 convertases [39]. This may reflect the physiological attempt of the kidneys to mitigate the activation of the lectin complement pathway. This could also explain the contra-regulation of FCN1 and MASP2. However, additional studies are necessary to confirm this effect. Indeed, the hyperactivation of complement may induce glomerular and tubulointerstitial injury [40].

Taken together, our data suggest for the first time that the lectin complement pathway may be involved in the complex biological machinery associated with MSK, but it is clearly not associated with nephrolithiasis. Extracellular vesicles may, therefore, be part of the pathological machinery leading to the growth of cysts. Although we cannot exclude that the complement system could be a secondary response to the disease, this might offer a therapeutic option for progression blockade. Additionally, urinary vesicles may provide a source of valuable clinical biomarkers allowing MSK to be distinguished from other cystic disorders (including ADPKD) and types of nephrolithiasis.

However, our results must be validated using a larger cohort of patients, and additional functional studies are required to better define the biological role of the lectin complement cascade in the pathogenesis of MSK.

## 4. Materials and Methods

### 4.1. *Patients*

Having obtained informed written consent, we enrolled 15 adult MSK patients and 15 adult ICN patients matched for age, gender, and geographical origin, followed up at our renal unit. The inclusion criteria for the MSK group were the same as described in our previous study [12]. Particularly, patients had both kidneys involved, nephrocalcinosis and/or cysts in at least 2 papillae in each kidney. For MSK, patients had papillary precalyceal ectasias on films obtained at least 10 min after contrast medium injection in the absence of compression maneuvers and signs of obstruction. The X-ray films were reviewed by an independent radiologist to confirm the diagnosis. For ICN patients the inclusion criteria were calcium stone disease, normal serum creatinine and electrolyte concentrations, and urinary pH $\leq 5.5$ measured in spot morning urine (after overnight fasting) to exclude tubular acidosis. Exclusion criteria for ICN patients were: the presence of endocrine diseases and cystic kidney disorders, nephrocalcinosis, and obstructive nephropathy. In all ICN patients, the MSK disease was ruled out by careful clinical examination.

Clinical data were registered in an electronic database. Informed consent was obtained from all patients in accordance with the Declaration of Helsinki and the ethical board of the University Hospital of Verona approved the study (1312CESC, 24 May 2017).

### 4.2. Isolation of Microvesicles and Exosomes

Second morning urine samples were obtained from all patients. Microvesicles and exosomes were isolated by centrifugation as previously reported [18]. Briefly, 16 ml aliquots of urine were centrifuged at 16,000× *g* for 30 min at 16 °C in order to remove alive and dead cells and organelles. The obtained supernatant was centrifuged for 120 min at 22,000× *g* at 16 °C to obtain the microvesicle fraction. The microvesicle-containing pellet was washed in phosphate-buffered saline (PBS) and repelleted as above for a total of five wash cycles to obtain a clean microvesicle fraction. To obtain the exosome, the supernatant was centrifuged for 120 min at 100,000× *g* at 16 °C. Then one-step sucrose cushion ultracentrifugation for 120 min at 100,000× *g* at 16 °C was performed to further purify exosomes according to their density. The exosome-containing pellet was washed in PBS and repelleted as above for a total of five wash cycles to obtain a clean exosome fraction. This procedure was carried out for each sample and the microvesicle and exosome fractions were stored at –80 °C until use.

### 4.3. Dynamic Light Scattering

The size of the exosomes and microvesicles was determined by dynamic light scattering (DLS) using a Zetasizer nano ZS90 particle sizer (Malvern Instruments, Worcestershire, UK) at a 90° fixed angle. The particle diameter was calculated using the Stokes–Einstein equation. For particle sizing in solution, exosome and microvesicle aliquots were diluted in 10% PBS and analyzed at a constant 25 °C.

### 4.4. Western Blot

Microvesicle and exosome fractions from 16 ml urine samples were separated by SDS-PAGE (8–16% acrylamide gradient) and then transferred to a nitrocellulose membrane. The membrane was blocked with 1% bovine serum albumin (BSA) in PBS plus 0.1% Tween-20 (PBST), rinsed in PBST, and labeled with one of the following primary human antibodies diluted in 1% BSA in PBST: anti-CD63 (Novus Biological, Littleton, CA, USA), anti-CD81 (Novus Biological, Littleton, CA, USA), or anti-CD45 (LifeSpan BioSciences, Seattle, WA, USA) [41]. After rinsing again in PBST, the membrane was incubated with horseradish peroxidase (HRP)-conjugated anti-mouse secondary antibodies (Novus Biological, Littleton, CA, USA). Chemiluminescence was detected and quantified using the ChemiDoc Touch Imaging System and Image Lab software (Bio-Rad, Hercules, CA, USA).

### 4.5. Mass Spectrometry

Samples were processed with in-StageTip (iST) method with two poly (styrene divinylbenzene) reversed-phase sulfonate (SDB-RPS) disks. The microvesicle- and exosome-containing pellets were solubilized with a solution containing 10 mM Tris(2-carboxyethyl)phosphine, 40 mM chloro-acetamide, 100 mM Tris (pH 8.5), and 2% sodium deoxycholate. Lysis, reduction, and alkylation of the samples were performed in a single step and then loaded into the StageTip. The samples were then diluted with a buffer containing 25 mM Tris (pH 8.5) and 1 µg of trypsin. After the acidification step with 1% trifluoroacetic acid (TFA), the samples were washed with 0.2% TFA three times. The proteins were eluted in 60 µl 5% v/v ammonium hydroxide containing 80% v/v acetonitrile. The desalted peptides were dried in a speed vacuum and resuspended in 2% acetonitrile containing 0.2% formic acid (FA). They were then separated on a 50-cm reversed-phase Easy Spray column (75-µm internal diameter × 50 cm; 2 µm/100 Å C18) on an Ultimate 3000 RSLCnano device (Thermo Fisher Scientific, Waltham, MA, USA) with a binary buffer system comprising buffer A (0.1% FA) and buffer B (80% acetonitrile, 5% dimethylsulfoxide, 0.1% FA). The program consisted of a 70-min gradient (2–45% buffer B) at a flow rate of 250 µl/min, with the column temperature maintained at 60 °C. The chromatography system was coupled to an Orbitrap Fusion Tribrid mass spectrometer (Thermo Fisher Scientific, Waltham, MA, USA), acquiring data in Charge Ordered Parallel Ion aNalysis (CHOPIN) mode. The precursors were ionized using an EASY-spray source held at +2.2 kV and the iICNet capillary temperature was held at 300 °C. Single MS survey scans were performed over the mass window 375–1500 *m/z* with an AGC target of 250,000, a maximum injection time of 50 ms, and a resolution of 120,000 at 200 *m/z*. Monoisotopic precursor selection was enabled for peptide isotopic distributions, precursors of z = 2–5 were selected for 2 s of cycle time, and dynamic exclusion was set to 25 s with a ± 10 ppm window set around the precursor. The following CHOPIN conditions were applied: a) if the precursor charge state is 2, then follow with collision-induced dissociation (CID) and scan in the ion trap with an isolation window of 1.8, CID energy of 35%, and a rapid ion trap scan rate; b) if the precursor charge state is 3–5 and precursor intensity >500,000, then follow with higher-energy C-trap dissociation (HCD) and scan in the Orbitrap with an isolation window of 1.8, HCD energy of 28%, and a resolution of 15,000; c) if the precursor charge state is 3–5 and precursor intensity < 500,000, then follow with CID as described for option (a). For all $MS^2$ events, the following options were set: "Injection Ions for All Available Parallelizable Time" with an AGC target value of 4000 and a maximum injection time of 250 ms for CID, or an AGC target value of 10,000 and a maximum injection time of 40 ms for HCD.

### *4.6. MS Data Analysis*

Raw MS files were processed in the MaxQuant v1.6.0.16 environment using the MaxLFQ algorithm for label-free quantification and Andromeda search engine. Peptide and protein false discovery rate (FDRs) were both set at < 0.01. The search contained variable modifications for the oxidation of methionine (M), N-terminal protein acetylation (protein N-terminus), and fixed carbamidomethyl modifications (C). For protease digestion, up to two missed cleavages were allowed. Peptides of length greater than six amino acids have been considered for the identification. The "match between runs" algorithm with a setting of 1 min time window was used for the quantification of MS missed data in each individual measurement. UniProt FASTA Homo sapiens database (access August 2017) was used for the identification of peptides and proteins.

### *4.7. ELISA*

MASP2, FNC1, and C4BPB levels were determined using an in-house ELISA setup. Briefly, polyclonal antibody anti-MASP2, anti-FCN1, or anti-C4BPB (LifeSpan Biosciences) was used to coat overnight at 4 °C 96-well MaxiSorp Nunc plates (Thermo Fisher Scientific, Waltham, MA, USA). The plates were then blocked with 3% BSA in PBS. Exosome fractions were solubilized in 10 µl of mild detergent solution (1% Nonidet P-40, 0.5% Tween-20 in PBS), supplemented with 90 µl 3% BSA in PBST and incubated at 4 °C overnight. After three washes in PBST, the plates were incubated for 4h with the corresponding monoclonal antibody (anti-MASP2, anti-FCN1, or anti-C4BPB, all from LifeSpan Biosciences, Seattle, WA, USA) diluted 1:1000 with 1% BSA in PBST. After three washes with PBST, the plates were incubated with HRP-conjugated anti-mouse IgG diluted 1:5000 in 1% BSA in PBST for 1h. After washing, the peroxidase substrate (TMB, Bio-Rad, Hercules, CA, USA) was added. The reaction was stopped with an $H_2SO_4$ solution. The absorbance at 450 nm was measured using an iMark microplate reader (Bio-Rad, Hercules, CA, USA). To standardize the response of the antibodies, we used a pool of strongly positive controls. The optical density results were expressed as relative units per milliliter (RU/ml).

### *4.8. Statistical Analysis*

After normalization, unsupervised hierarchical clustering and multidimensional scaling (MDS) with Spearman's rank correlation and *k*-means were used to recognize outliers and sample dissimilarity. Weighted-gene co-expression network analysis (WGCNA) package in *R* was used for building the co-expression network with the normalized expression profiles of the identified proteins. A weighted adjacency matrix was constructed using the power function. After choosing the appropriate beta parameter of power (with the value of independence scale set to 0.8), the adjacency matrix was transformed into a topological overlap matrix (TOM), which measures the network connectivity of all the proteins. To classify proteins with co-expression profiles into protein modules, hierarchical clustering analysis was conducted according to the TOM dissimilarity with a minimum size of

30 proteins per module. To identify the relationship between each module and clinical trait, we used module eigengenes (MEs) and calculated the correlation between MEs and each clinical trait and their statistical significance corrected for multiple interactions. A heat map was then used to visualize the degree and significance of each relationship.

A non-parametric Mann–Whitney *U*-test, machine learning methods, such as non-linear support vector machine (SVM) learning, and partial least squares discriminant analysis (PLS-DA) were used to identify the hub proteins of modules that maximize the discrimination between the selected clinical traits. For the Mann–Whitney *U*-test, proteins were considered to be significantly differentially expressed between the two conditions with power of 80% and an adjusted p-value $\leq 0.05$ after correction for multiple interactions (Benjamini–Hochberg) and a fold change of $\geq 2$. In addition, the proteins needed to show at least 70% identity in the samples in one of two conditions. Volcano plots were used to visualize this analysis. In SVM learning, a fourfold cross-validation approach was applied to estimate the prediction and classification accuracy. The whole matrix was also randomly divided into two parts, one for learning (65%) and the other to verify the accuracy of the prediction (35%). Finally, the resulting core panel of hub proteins was uploaded to Cytoscape using the EnrichmentMap, ClusterMaker2, and AutoAnnotate apps to construct a protein–protein interaction network and identify the principal biological processes and pathways involved in each condition. Gene Ontology (GO) annotations were extracted from the Gene Ontology Consortium (http://www.geneontology.org/).

For ELISA data analysis, the Mann–Whitney *U*-test was used to assess differences in MASP2, FCN1, or C4BPB protein levels between the two study groups, and the results were expressed as medians and interquartile ranges. A value of $p < 0.05$ was considered to be statistically significant. Received operating characteristic (ROC) curves were generated to assess the diagnostic efficiency of each assay. Youden's index and likelihood ratio were used, to identify the cutoff and the diagnostic performance of the tests, respectively. All statistical tests were performed using the latest version of the software package *R* available at the time of the experiments.

**Supplementary Materials:**
Figure S1. Characterization of exosome and microvesicle fractions purified from the urine samples of ICN and MSK patients. Figure S2. Venn diagram of all proteins identified in exosomes and microvesicles isolated from the urine of ICN and MSK patients, and proteins associated with ICN and MSK. Figure S3. Multidimensional scaling analysis of extracellular vesicles from the urine of ICN and MSK patients. Figure S4. Exosome and microvesicle proteins that show significant differences in abundance between ICN and MSK patients. Figure S5. Enrichment network map of the significant proteins found in urinary microvesicles and exosomes from MSK and ICN patients. Table S1. List of identification values for all significant proteins between MSK and ICN in exosome and microvesicle fraction. Table S2. List of all significant proteins between MSK and ICN in exosome and microvesicle fraction.

**Author Contributions:** Conceptualization: S.G. and G.Z.; data curation: M.B., S.G., and G.Z.; formal analysis: M.B., G.M.G., G.G., and G.Z.; methodology: M.B., S.G., G.C., A.F., and A.P.; supervision: G.Z.; validation: M.B. and G.C.; writing—original draft preparation: M.B., S.G., and G.Z.; writing—review and editing: G.M.G. and G.G.

**Acknowledgments:** This study was performed (in part) in the LURM (Laboratorio Universitario di Ricerca Medica) Research Center, University of Verona.

## Abbreviations

| | |
|---|---|
| MSK | medullary sponge kidney |
| ICN | idiopathic calcium nephrolithiasis |
| LAMA2 | laminin subunit $\alpha 2$ |
| SVM | support vector machine |
| PLS-DA | partial least squares discriminant analysis |
| ADPKD | autosomal dominant polycystic kidney disease |
| MS | mass spectrometry |

| | |
|---|---|
| SPP1 | osteopontin |
| PBS | phosphate-buffered saline |
| DLS | dynamic light scattering |
| iST | in-StageTip |
| SDB-RPS | poly (styrene divinylbenzene) reversed-phase sulfonate |
| TFA | trifluoroacetic acid |
| BSA | bovine serum albumin |
| PBST | PBS plus 0.1% Tween-20 |
| HRP | horseradish peroxidase |
| ROC | Received operating characteristic |
| AUC | area under the curve |
| CI | confidence interval |
| FCN1 | Ficolin 1 |
| MASP2 | Mannan-binding lectin serine protease 2 |
| C4BPB | Complement component 4-binding protein β |
| PTX3 | pentraxin 3 |
| CRP | C-reactive protein |

## References


1. Fabris, A.; Anglani, F.; Lupo, A.; Gambaro, G. Medullary sponge kidney: State of the art. *Nephrol. Dial. Transplant.* **2013**, *28*, 1111–1119. [CrossRef] [PubMed]
2. Indridason, O.S.; Thomas, L.; Berkoben, M. Medullary sponge kidney associated with congenital hemihypertrophy. *J. Am. Soc. Nephrol.* **1996**, *7*, 1123–1130. [PubMed]
3. El-Sawi, M.; Shahein, A.R. Medullary sponge kidney presenting in a neonate with distal renal tubular acidosis and failure to thrive: A case report. *J. Med. Case Rep.* **2009**, *3*, 6656. [CrossRef] [PubMed]
4. Patriquin, H.B.; O'Regan, S. Medullary sponge kidney in childhood. *AJR Am. J. Roentgenol.* **1985**, *145*, 315–319. [CrossRef] [PubMed]
5. Lambrianides, A.L.; John, D.R. Medullary sponge disease in horseshoe kidney. *Urology* **1987**, *29*, 426–427. [CrossRef]
6. Gambaro, G.; Fabris, A.; Citron, L.; Tosetto, E.; Anglani, F.; Bellan, F.; Conte, M.; Bonfante, L.; Lupo, A.; D'Angelo, A. An unusual association of contralateral congenital small kidney reduced renal function and hyperparathyroidism in sponge kidney patients: On the track of the molecular basis. *Nephrol. Dial. Transplant.* **2005**, *20*, 1042–1047. [CrossRef] [PubMed]
7. Janjua, M.U.; Long, X.D.; Mo, Z.H.; Dong, C.S.; Jin, P. Association of medullary sponge kidney and hyperparathyroidism with RET G691S/S904S polymorphism: A case report. *J. Med. Case Rep.* **2018**, *12*, 197. [CrossRef]
8. Ria, P.; Fabris, A.; Dalla Gassa, A.; Zaza, G.; Lupo, A.; Gambaro, G. New non-renal congenital disorders associated with medullary sponge kidney (MSK) support the pathogenic role of GDNF and point to the diagnosis of MSK in recurrent stone formers. *Urolithiasis* **2017**, *45*, 359–362. [CrossRef]
9. Osther, P.J.; Hansen, A.B.; Røhl, H.F. Renal acidification defects in medullary sponge kidney. *Br. J. Urol.* **1988**, *61*, 392–394. [CrossRef]
10. Fabris, A.; Bernich, P.; Abaterusso, C.; Marchionna, N.; Canciani, C.; Nouvenne, A.; Zamboni, M.; Lupo, A.; Gambaro, G. Bone disease in medullary sponge kidney and effect of potassium citrate treatment. *Clin. J. Am. Soc. Nephrol.* **2009**, *4*, 1974–1979. [CrossRef]
11. McPhail, E.F.; Gettman, M.T.; Patterson, D.E.; Rangel, L.J.; Krambeck, A.E. Nephrolithiasis in medullary sponge kidney: Evaluation of clinical and metabolic features. *Urology* **2012**, *79*, 277–281. [CrossRef] [PubMed]
12. Fabris, A.; Bruschi, M.; Santucci, L.; Candiano, G.; Granata, S.; Dalla Gassa, A.; Antonucci, N.; Petretto, A.; Ghiggeri, G.M.; Gambaro, G.; et al. Proteomic-based research strategy identified laminin subunit alpha 2 as a potential urinary-specific biomarker for the medullary sponge kidney disease. *Kidney Int.* **2017**, *91*, 459–468. [CrossRef] [PubMed]
13. Colognato, H.; Yurchenco, P.D. Form and function: The laminin family of heterotrimers. *Dev. Dyn.* **2000**, *218*, 213–234. [CrossRef]

14. Vijayakumar, S.; Dang, S.; Marinkovich, M.P.; Lazarova, Z.; Yoder, B.; Torres, V.E.; Wallace, D.P. Aberrant expression of laminin-332 promotes cell proliferation and cyst growth in ARPKD. *Am. J. Physiol. Renal. Physiol.* **2014**, *306*, F640–F654. [CrossRef] [PubMed]
15. Joly, D.; Berissi, S.; Bertrand, A.; Strehl, L.; Patey, N.; Knebelmann, B. Laminin 5 regulates polycystic kidney cell proliferation and cyst formation. *J. Biol. Chem.* **2006**, *281*, 29181–29189. [CrossRef]
16. Shannon, M.B.; Patton, B.L.; Harvey, S.J.; Miner, J.H. A hypomorphic mutation in the mouse laminin alpha5 gene causes polycystic kidney disease. *J. Am. Soc. Nephrol.* **2006**, *17*, 1913–1922. [CrossRef]
17. Weir, M.L.; Oppizzi, M.L.; Henry, M.D.; Onishi, A.; Campbell, K.P.; Bissell, M.J.; Muschler, J.L. Dystroglycan loss disrupts polarity and beta-casein induction in mammary epithelial cells by perturbing laminin anchoring. *J. Cell Sci.* **2006**, *119 (Pt 19)*, 4047–4058. [CrossRef]
18. Bruschi, M.; Granata, S.; Santucci, L.; Candiano, G.; Fabris, A.; Antonucci, N.; Petretto, A.; Bartolucci, M.; Del Zotto, G.; Antonini, F.; et al. Proteomic Analysis of Urinary Microvesicles and Exosomes in Medullary Sponge Kidney Disease and Autosomal Dominant Polycystic Kidney Disease. *Clin. J. Am. Soc. Nephrol.* **2019**, *14*, 834–843. [CrossRef]
19. Kleinman, J.G.; Wesson, J.A.; Hughes, J. Osteopontin and calcium stone formation. *Nephron Physiol.* **2004**, *98*, 43–47. [CrossRef]
20. Verhulst, A.; Persy, V.P.; Van Rompay, A.R.; Verstrepen, W.A.; Helbert, M.F.; De Broe, M.E. Osteopontin synthesis and localization along the human Nephron. *J. Am. Soc. Nephrol.* **2002**, *13*, 1210–1218.
21. Worcester, E.M.; Beshensky, A.M. Osteopontin inhibits nucleation of calcium oxalate crystals. *Ann. N. Y. Acad. Sci.* **1995**, *760*, 375–387. [CrossRef] [PubMed]
22. Wesson, J.A.; Worcester, E. Formation of hydrated calcium oxalates in the presence of poly-L-aspartic acid. *Scan. Microsc.* **1996**, *10*, 415–424.
23. Cowley, B.D., Jr.; Ricardo, S.D.; Nagao, S.; Diamond, J.R. Increased renal expression of monocyte chemoattractant protein-1 and osteopontin in ADPKD in rats. *Kidney Int.* **2001**, *60*, 2087–2096. [CrossRef] [PubMed]
24. Gauer, S.; Urbschat, A.; Gretz, N.; Hoffmann, S.C.; Kränzlin, B.; Geiger, H.; Obermüller, N. Kidney Injury Molecule-1 Is Specifically Expressed in Cystically-Transformed Proximal Tubules of the PKD/Mhm (cy/+) Rat Model of Polycystic Kidney Disease. *Int. J. Mol. Sci.* **2016**, *17*, 802. [CrossRef] [PubMed]
25. Pisitkun, T.; Shen, R.F.; Knepper, M.A. Identification and proteomic profiling of exosomes in human urine. *Proc. Natl. Acad. Sci. USA* **2004**, *101*, 13368–13373. [CrossRef]
26. Moon, P.G.; You, S.; Lee, J.E.; Hwang, D.; Baek, M.C. Urinary exosomes and proteomics. *Mass Spectrom. Rev.* **2011**, *30*, 1185–1202. [CrossRef]
27. Piñero, J.; Bravo, À.; Queralt-Rosinach, N.; Gutiérrez-Sacristán, A.; Deu-Pons, J.; Centeno, E.; García-García, J.; Sanz, F.; Furlong, L.I. DisGeNET: A comprehensive platform integrating information on human disease-associated genes and variants. *Nucleic Acids Res.* **2017**, *45*, D833–D839. [CrossRef]
28. Salih, M.; Demmers, J.A.; Bezstarosti, K.; Leonhard, W.N.; Losekoot, M.; van Kooten, C.; Gansevoort, R.T.; Peters, D.J.; Zietse, R.; Hoorn, E.J.; et al. Proteomics of Urinary Vesicles Links Plakins and Complement to Polycystic Kidney Disease. *J. Am. Soc. Nephrol.* **2016**, *27*, 3079–3092. [CrossRef]
29. Runza, V.L.; Schwaeble, W.; Männel, D.N. Ficolins: Novel pattern recognition molecules of the innate immune response. *Immunobiology* **2008**, *213*, 297–306. [CrossRef]
30. Kjaer, T.R.; Hansen, A.G.; Sørensen, U.B.; Nielsen, O.; Thiel, S.; Jensenius, J.C. Investigations on the pattern recognition molecule M-ficolin: Quantitative aspects of bacterial binding and leukocyte association. *J. Leukoc. Biol.* **2011**, *90*, 425–437. [CrossRef]
31. Thiel, S. Complement activating soluble pattern recognition molecules with collagen-like regions, mannan-binding lectin, ficolins and associated proteins. *Mol. Immunol.* **2007**, *44*, 3875–3888. [CrossRef] [PubMed]
32. Zhang, J.; Yang, L.; Ang, Z.; Yoong, S.L.; Tran, T.T.; Anand, G.S.; Tan, N.S.; Ho, B.; Ding, J.L. Secreted M-ficolin anchors onto monocyte transmembrane G protein-coupled receptor 43 and cross talks with plasma C-reactive protein to mediate immune signaling and regulate host defense. *J. Immunol.* **2010**, *185*, 6899–6910. [CrossRef] [PubMed]
33. Tanio, M.; Wakamatsu, K.; Kohno, T. Binding site of C-reactive protein on M-ficolin. *Mol. Immunol.* **2009**, *47*, 215–221. [CrossRef] [PubMed]

34. Gout, E.; Moriscot, C.; Doni, A.; Dumestre-Pérard, C.; Lacroix, M.; Pérard, J.; Schoehn, G.; Mantovani, A.; Arlaud, G.J.; Thielens, N.M. M-ficolin interacts with the long pentraxin PTX3: A novel case of cross-talk between soluble pattern-recognition molecules. *J. Immunol.* **2011**, *186*, 5815–5822. [CrossRef]
35. Zhou, J.; Ouyang, X.; Schoeb, T.R.; Bolisetty, S.; Cui, X.; Mrug, S.; Yoder, B.K.; Johnson, M.R.; Szalai, A.J.; Mrug, M. Kidney injury accelerates cystogenesis via pathways modulated by heme oxygenase and complement. *J. Am. Soc. Nephrol.* **2012**, *23*, 1161–1171. [CrossRef] [PubMed]
36. Su, Z.; Wang, X.; Gao, X.; Liu, Y.; Pan, C.; Hu, H.; Beyer, R.P.; Shi, M.; Zhou, J.; Zhang, J.; et al. Excessive activation of the alternative complement pathway in autosomal dominant polycystic kidney disease. *J. Intern. Med.* **2014**, *276*, 470–485. [CrossRef]
37. Lai, X.; Bacallao, R.L.; Blazer-Yost, B.L.; Hong, D.; Mason, S.B.; Witzmann, F.A. Characterization of the renal cyst fluid proteome in autosomal dominant polycystic kidney disease (ADPKD) patients. *Proteom. Clin. Appl.* **2008**, *2*, 1140–1152. [CrossRef]
38. Bakun, M.; Niemczyk, M.; Domanski, D.; Jazwiec, R.; Perzanowska, A.; Niemczyk, S.; Kistowski, M.; Fabijanska, A.; Borowiec, A.; Paczek, L.; et al. Urine proteome of autosomal dominant polycystic kidney disease patients. *Clin. Proteom.* **2012**, *9*, 13. [CrossRef]
39. Rawal, N.; Rajagopalan, R.; Salvi, V.P. Stringent regulation of complement lectin pathway C3/C5 convertase by C4b-binding protein (C4BP). *Mol. Immunol.* **2009**, *46*, 2902–2910. [CrossRef]
40. Salvadori, M.; Rosso, G.; Bertoni, E. Complement involvement in kidney diseases: From physiopathology to therapeutical targeting. *World J. Nephrol.* **2015**, *4*, 169–184. [CrossRef]
41. Nolan, J.P.; Duggan, E. Analysis of Individual Extracellular Vesicles by Flow Cytometry. *Methods Mol. Biol.* **2018**, *1678*, 79–92. [PubMed]

# 8

# Risk of Incident Non-Valvular Atrial Fibrillation after Dialysis-Requiring Acute Kidney Injury

**Chih-Chung Shiao [1,2], Wei-Chih Kan [3,4], Jian-Jhong Wang [5], Yu-Feng Lin [6,7,8], Likwang Chen [9], Eric Chueh [10], Ya-Ting Huang [11], Wen-Po Chiang [12], Li-Jung Tseng [12], Chih-Hsien Wang [12] and Vin-Cent Wu [7,13,*]**

1. Division of Nephrology, Department of Internal Medicine, Saint Mary's Hospital Luodong, Loudong 265, Yilan, Taiwan; chungyy2001@yahoo.com.tw
2. Saint Mary's Junior College of Medicine, Nursing and Management, Sanxing Township, Yilan County 266, Taiwan
3. Division of Nephrology, Department of Internal medicine, Chi Mei Medical Center, Yongkang District, Tainan City 710, Taiwan; rockiekan@ntu.edu.tw
4. Department of Biological Science and Technology, Chung Hwa University of Medical Technology, Rende District, Tainan City 717, Taiwan
5. Division of Nephrology, Department of Internal Medicine, Chi Mei Medical Center, Liouying, Tainan City 736, Taiwan; win7a@yahoo.com.tw
6. Graduate Institute of Clinical Medicine, National Taiwan University College of Medicine, Taipei 106, Taiwan; dr.yufenglin@gmail.com
7. Division of Nephrology, Department of Internal Medicine, National Taiwan University Hospital, Taipei 100, Taiwan
8. Division of Hospital Medicine, Department of Internal Medicine, National Taiwan University Hospital, Taipei 100, Taiwan
9. Institute of Population Health Sciences, National Health Research Institutes, Zhunan, Miaoli County 350, Taiwan; likwang@nhri.org.tw
10. Case Western Reserve University, No. 10900 Euclid Ave., Cleveland, OH 44106, USA; ericc0109@gmail.com
11. Department of Nursing, Saint Mary's Hospital Luodong, Loudong 265, Yilan, Taiwan; frankie7451@gmail.com
12. Department of Surgery, National Taiwan University Hospital, Taipei 100, Taiwan; aillen1111@yahoo.com.tw (W.-P.C.); ntuhtlj@gmail.com (L.-J.T.); wchemail@gmail.com (C.-H.W.)
13. NSARF, National Taiwan University Study Group on Acute Renal Failure

* Correspondence: q91421028@ntu.edu.tw

**Abstract:** The influence of acute kidney injury (AKI) on subsequent incident atrial fibrillation (AF) has not yet been fully addressed. This retrospective nationwide cohort study was conducted using Taiwan's National Health Insurance Research Database from 1 January 2000 to 31 December 2010. A total of 41,463 patients without a previous AF, mitral valve disease, and hyperthyroidism who developed de novo dialysis-requiring AKI (AKI-D) during their index hospitalization were enrolled. After propensity score matching, "non-recovery group" ($n$ = 2895), "AKI-recovery group" ($n$ = 2895) and "non-AKI group" (control group, $n$ = 5790) were categorized. Within a follow-up period of 6.52 $\pm$ 3.88 years (median, 6.87 years), we found that the adjusted risks for subsequent incident AF were increased in both AKI-recovery group (adjusted hazard ratio (aHR) = 1.30; 95% confidence intervals (CI), 1.07–1.58; $p \leq 0.01$) and non-recovery group (aHR = 1.62; 95% CI, 1.36–1.94) compared to the non-AKI group. Furthermore, the development of AF carried elevated risks for major adverse cardiac events (aHR = 2.11; 95% CI, 1.83–2.43), ischemic stroke (aHR = 1.33; 95% CI, 1.19–1.49), and all stroke (aHR = 1.28; 95% CI, 1.15–1.43). (all $p \leq 0.001$, except otherwise expressed) The authors concluded that AKI-D, even in those who withdrew from temporary dialysis, independently increases the subsequent risk of de novo AF.

**Keywords:** acute kidney injury; adverse cardiovascular events; atrial fibrillation; dialysis

## 1. Introduction

Atrial fibrillation (AF) is the most common sustained cardiac arrhythmia with an increasing trend of prevalence following widespread population aging [1]. It is estimated that AF currently affects around 2.3 million adults in the United States, and the number of affected people is projected to increase to 5.6–15.9 million by 2050 [1]. AF has a significant effect on cardiovascular events including stroke, peripheral embolization, and associated morbidities and mortalities [1]. The existence of AF is independently associated with the risk of the development and severity of acute kidney injury (AKI) in both surgical and medical settings [2].

Recent studies suggest that AKI episodes are associated with a higher risk of developing cardiovascular events and overall mortality [3–5]. Nevertheless, the influence of AKI on subsequent incident AF has not been fully addressed in previous research. Most investigations only evaluate the concurrent occurrence of AKI and AF in a limited number of patients undergoing cardiac surgeries within a relatively short follow-up period [6,7]. In these studies, the development of postoperative AKI was found as an independent factor associated with the new-onset postoperative AF [6,7]. In line with these interpretations, new-onset AF after AKI in a nationwide survey for an extended followed-up period is necessary [7–10]. In particular, the National Institute for Health and Clinical Excellence (NICE) guideline raises an ultimate critical point: if the development of AF occurs, the assessment to evaluate the risk of having a stroke is necessary. However, little information is available regarding cardiovascular events and outcomes after new-onset AF in this subset.

A proper understanding of the risk factors associated with kidney disease and AF development may allow primary care physicians to initiate preventive strategies and thereby potentially decrease the risk of AF. Thus, we conducted this study aiming to test the hypothesis that the occurrence of dialysis-requiring AKI (AKI-D), as well as the "recovery pattern" of the AKI, would increase the subsequent risk of subsequent AF and result in worse cardiovascular injury.

## 2. Materials and Methods

### *2.1. Data Source*

This retrospective population-based cohort study was conducted using the data of Taiwan's National Health Insurance Research Database (NHIRD) in the period from 1 January 2000 to 3 December 2010. The NHIRD is an encrypted database released by the National Health Research Institutes (NHRI) for research purposes. The NHIRD includes all information on outpatient visits, hospital admissions, prescriptions, interventional procedures, disease profiles, and vital status of the National Health Insurance (NHI) program which provides comprehensive medical care covering more than 99% of the country's population of 23 million people. The baseline comorbidities were identified from at least three outpatient visits or one inpatient claim within one year preceding the index hospitalization with the first dialysis. This identification method has been well validated with adequate predictive power [3]. The Charlson Comorbidity Index (CCI) was calculated by weighting baseline comorbidities.

For confidentiality purposes, identification numbers were encrypted before being released for research, but the uniqueness of the encrypted identification is retained to ensure valid internal linkage. The study protocol conformed to the ethical guidelines of the 1975 Declaration of Helsinki. The study was approved by the institutional review board of the National Taiwan University Hospital (201212021RINC), and informed consent was waived since all personal data were de-identified in the database to protect privacy.

### *2.2. Study Cohort and Design*

This study included patients aged 18 to 100 years without a history of AF, mitral valve disease, and hyperthyroidism for at least one year preceding study enrollment, and who developed de novo AKI-D during their index hospitalization and survived to at least 30 days after discharge.

Disease diagnoses were classified according to the International Classification of Diseases, Ninth Revision, Clinical Modification (ICD-9-CM). AKI-D was defined by ICD-9 codes for AKI (584.3, 634.3, 635.3, 636.3, 637.3, 638.3, 639.3, 669.3, or 958.5) along with procedure codes for acute dialysis. CKD was defined by ICD-9 codes for CKD (580, 580.x, 584.x, 586, 399.5). Advanced CKD was defined as CKD patients with concomitant erythropoiesis-stimulating agents [3]. The diagnosis accuracy of AKI and chronic kidney disease (CKD) by ICD-9-CM, as well as the definition of advanced CKD, were detailed in Supplementary File 1.

Renal function recovery was defined by withdrawal from dialysis before the 31st day after discharge. The patients who had successfully withdrawn from dialysis within hospitalization or within the 30-day period after hospital discharge were categorized into "AKI-recovery" group, while those had not withdrawn from dialysis within the 30-day period were categorized in "non-recovery" group. In an attempt to make a less biased comparison, we further constructed a control group which contained patients without AKI and who survived to discharge from the remaining hospitalized patients (non-AKI group).

### 2.3. Research Variables

The demographic data including age, gender, monthly income, hospital levels, baseline comorbidities, CHA2DS2-VASc scores before discharge, the frequency of outpatient visits and medications within one year following discharge, and the patients' outcomes were identified and analyzed.

### 2.4. Outcome Variables

Our primary outcome was de novo AF development (ICD-9-CM code 427.31) after hospital discharge. To ensure the accuracy of the AF identification, the diagnosis of AF needed to be confirmed by a doctor, or doctors, and recorded in the diagnosis list of the chart more than twice in outpatient visits, or recorded in the discharge diagnosis list more than once in an inpatient setting. The diagnostic accuracy of AF based on the ICD-9-CM codes has been previously validated [11–13]. The secondary outcomes included major adverse cardiac event (MACE), ischemic stroke (ICD-9-CM code 433.x, 434.x, or 436), and hemorrhage stroke (ICD-9-CM code 431 or 432). MACE was defined as coronary artery disease-related death, nonfatal myocardial infarction, angina, and revascularizations.

We evaluated the influences of AKI-D on the risk of subsequent incident AF in the whole study population as well as in different subgroups. Furthermore, besides testing the association between AKI-D and these outcomes, we also evaluated the association between AF and the above-mentioned secondary outcomes. All enrolled patients were followed from the date of index hospital discharge to the first diagnosed outcomes and were censored at death unrelated to coronary artery disease, or at the end of the study (31 December 2010).

### 2.5. Statistical Analysis

Statistical analyses were performed using SAS 9.4 (SAS Institute, Cary, NC, USA). A two-sided $p$-value of $\leq 0.05$ was considered statistically significant. Continuous variables were presented as the mean $\pm$ standard deviation (SD), and categorical variables were described as counts (percentages). The propensity scores were determined by multivariate logistic regression analysis. The Cox proportional hazard model was applied to examine the effect of non-recovery and AKI-recovery groups on subsequent AF development, as well as the influence of AF on other major adverse events. Because withdrawal from dialysis is likely to adhere to the condition of acute kidney disease, advanced CKD was identified to be a time-varying covariate [3,14].

By using the propensity score matching method, we proposed three matched groups (non-recovery group: AKI-recovery group: non-AKI group) on a 1:1:2 ratio. The propensity scores, containing the baseline characteristics and risk factors listed in Table 1, were calculated by multivariate logistic regression.

**Table 1.** Comparisons of the baseline characteristics among the three groups.

| | Before Matching $n = 20{,}540$ | | | | After Matching $n = 11{,}680$ | | | |
|---|---|---|---|---|---|---|---|---|
| **Variables** | **Non-Recovery** $n = 4807$ | **AKI-Recovery** $n = 5283$ | **Non-AKI** $n = 10{,}450$ | $p$ | **Non-Recovery** $n = 2895$ | **AKI-Recovery** $n = 2895$ | **Non-AKI** $n = 5790$ | $p$ |
| Age, years | 59.7 ± 15.2 | 60.3 ± 17.7 | 59.8 ± 16.1 | <0.001 | 59.6 ± 15.7 | 60.2 ± 17.2 | 60.6 ± 15.7 | 0.01 |
| Gender, men | 2390 (49.7%) | 3172 (60.0%) | 5540 (53.0%) | <0.001 | 1542 (53.3%) | 1535 (53.0%) | 3178 (54.9%) | 0.68 |
| **Monthly income, NTD** | | | | <0.001 | | | | 0.21 |
| <19,100 | 1700 (35.4%) | 2103 (39.8%) | 3649 (34.9%) | | 1064 (36.8%) | 1099 (38.0%) | 2203 (38.1%) | |
| 19,100–41,999 | 2449 (51.0%) | 2434 (46.1%) | 5285 (50.6%) | | 1443 (49.8%) | 1378 (47.6%) | 2925 (50.5%) | |
| ≥42,000 | 658 (13.7%) | 746 (14.1%) | 1516 (14.5%) | | 388 (13.4%) | 418 (14.4%) | 762 (13.2%) | |
| **Hospital level** * | | | | <0.001 | | | | <0.001 |
| Level 1 | 1916 (39.9%) | 2648 (50.1%) | 4046 (38.7%) | | 1218 (42.1%) | 1184 (40.9%) | 2641 (45.6%) | |
| Level 2 | 2092 (43.5%) | 2158 (40.84%) | 3972 (38.0%) | | 1249 (43.1%) | 1340 (46.3%) | 2282 (39.4%) | |
| Levels 3 + 4 | 799 (16.6%) | 477 (9.0%) | 2,432 (23.3%) | | 428 (14.8%) | 371 (12.8%) | 967 (16.7%) | |
| **Baseline Comorbidities** | | | | | | | | |
| CCI | 2.8 ± 1.6 | 2.1 ± 1.5 | 2.4 ± 1.6 | <0.001 | 2.4 ± 1.6 | 2.4 ± 1.6 | 2.4 ± 1.6 | 0.29 |
| Myocardial infarction | 22 (0.5%) | 27 (0.5%) | 37 (0.4%) | 0.31 | 12 (0.4%) | 10 (0.4%) | 22 (0.4%) | 0.91 |
| Congestive heart failure | 287 (6.0%) | 215 (4.1%) | 457 (4.4%) | <0.001 | 131 (4.5%) | 136 (4.7%) | 279 (4.8%) | 0.91 |
| Peripheral vascular disease | 26 (0.5%) | 34 (0.6%) | 54 (0.5%) | 0.59 | 13 (0.5%) | 17 (0.6%) | 39 (0.7%) | 0.47 |
| Cerebrovascular disease | 284 (5.9%) | 335 (6.3%) | 629 (6.0%) | 0.62 | 175 (6.0%) | 173 (6.0%) | 345 (6.0%) | 0.94 |
| Dementia | 24 (0.5%) | 74 (1.4%) | 68 (0.7%) | <0.001 | 20 (0.7%) | 19 (0.7%) | 35 (0.6%) | 0.85 |
| COPD | 333 (6.9%) | 362 (6.9%) | 640 (6.1%) | 0.08 | 179 (6.2%) | 209 (7.2%) | 414 (7.2%) | 0.23 |
| Rheumatologic disease | 47 (1.0%) | 61 (1.2%) | 103 (1.0%) | 0.57 | 30 (1.0%) | 28 (1.0%) | 69 (1.2%) | 0.66 |
| Peptic ulcer disease | 403 (8.4%) | 350 (6.6%) | 691 (6.6%) | <0.001 | 205 (7.1%) | 207 (7.2%) | 450 (7.8%) | 0.55 |
| Hemiplegia or paraplegia | 10 (0.2%) | 20 (0.4%) | 25 (0.2%) | 0.18 | 8 (0.3%) | 9 (0.3%) | 13 (0.2%) | 0.71 |
| CKD | 2396 (49.8%) | 1063 (20.1%) | 3225 (30.9%) | <0.001 | 1005 (34.7%) | 932 (32.2%) | 1910 (33.0%) | 0.06 |
| Liver disease [a] | 178 (3.7%) | 204 (3.9%) | 355 (3.4%) | 0.30 | 96 (3.3%) | 99 (3.4%) | 192 (3.3%) | 0.93 |
| Tumor | 86 (1.8%) | 137 (2.6%) | 195 (1.9%) | 0.004 | 62 (2.1%) | 56 (1.9%) | 113 (2.0%) | 0.77 |
| Diabetes | 1254 (26.1%) | 1186 (22.5%) | 2653 (25.4%) | <0.001 | 687 (23.7%) | 708 (24.5%) | 1504 (26.0%) | 0.16 |

**Table 1.** *Cont.*

| Variables | Before Matching $n = 20{,}540$ | | | | After Matching $n = 11{,}680$ | | | |
|---|---|---|---|---|---|---|---|---|
| | Non-Recovery $n = 4807$ | AKI-Recovery $n = 5283$ | Non-AKI $n = 10{,}450$ | $p$ | Non-Recovery $n = 2895$ | AKI-Recovery $n = 2895$ | Non-AKI $n = 5790$ | $p$ |
| **CHA2DS2-VASc †** | | | | <0.001 | | | | <0.001 |
| 0 | 211 (4.4%) | 706 (13.4%) | 1018 (9.7%) | | 204 (7.1%) | 200 (6.9%) | 400 (6.9%) | |
| 1 | 890 (18.5%) | 996 (18.9%) | 1979 (18.9%) | | 636 (22.0%) | 631 (21.8%) | 1125 (19.4%) | |
| 2 | 1268 (26.4%) | 976 (18.5%) | 1908 (18.3%) | | 834 (28.8%) | 613 (21.2%) | 1144 (19.8%) | |
| 3 | 885 (18.4%) | 858 (16.2%) | 1896 (18.1%) | | 534 (18.5%) | 505 (17.4%) | 1124 (19.4%) | |
| 4 | 706 (14.7%) | 683 (12.9%) | 1462 (14.0%) | | 438 (15.1%) | 410 (14.2%) | 894 (15.4%) | |
| 5 | 456 (9.5%) | 483 (9.1%) | 1123 (10.8%) | | 279 (9.6%) | 307 (10.6%) | 691 (11.9%) | |
| 6 | 245 (5.1%) | 350 (6.6%) | 660 (6.3%) | | 194 (6.7%) | 158 (5.5%) | 306 (5.3%) | |
| 7 | 120 (2.5%) | 174 (3.3%) | 296 (2.8%) | | 98 (3.4%) | 91 (3.1%) | 155 (2.7%) | |
| 8 | 24 (0.5%) | 50 (1.0%) | 99 (1.0%) | | 23 (0.8%) | 27 (0.9%) | 45 (0.8%) | |
| 9 | 2 (0.04%) | 7 (0.1%) | 9 (0.1%) | | 2 (0.1%) | 3 (0.1%) | 6 (0.1%) | |

Note: Continuous variables were presented as a mean ± standard deviation, and statistically analyzed using one-way analysis of variance, while categorical variables were described as counts (percentages) and analyzed using Chi-squared tests. † denotes "before discharge"; [a] moderate or severe liver disease. * Level 1, 2, 3 and 4 denote medical center, regional hospital, district hospital and local medical clinic, respectively; Abbreviations: ACEI, angiotensin-converting enzyme inhibitor; ARB, angiotensin receptor blocker; CCI, Charlson Comorbidity Index; CKD, chronic kidney disease; COPD, chronic obstructive pulmonary disease; ESRD, end-stage renal disease; Gr, group; MACE, major adverse cardiac event; NSAID, non-steroid anti-inflammatory drug; NTD, new Taiwan Dollar.

Several demographic factors were adjusted in the hazard models to evaluate the impact of AKI on AF, as well as the influence of incident AF to other adverse events. Variable selection was performed using stepwise multiple regression methods, with both $p$-to-enter and $p$-to-leave equal to 0.15. Final results of multivariate analyses were presented by hazard ratio (HR) and adjusted HR (aHR) with 95% confidence interval (CI). To exclude the confounding effect of subsequent impaired renal function and the influence of chronic dialysis, we additionally took "advanced CKD" as a "time-varying covariate" in the Cox proportional hazard model determining the adjusted risk for subsequent AF.

## 3. Results

### 3.1. Characteristics of the Three Groups

From the period of 1 January 2000, to 31 December 2010, a total of 10,091 AKI-D patients were eligible for inclusion. Among them, 5284 patients withdrew from dialysis for at least 30 days, but 4807 patients did not. After the exclusion and sampling processes, a total of 10,450 patients without AKI and who survived to hospital discharge were enrolled as control group. After propensity score matching on a 1:1:2 ratio, we categorized these patients into non-recovery ($n$ = 2895), AKI-recovery ($n$ = 2895) and non-AKI ($n$ = 5790) groups (Figure 1).

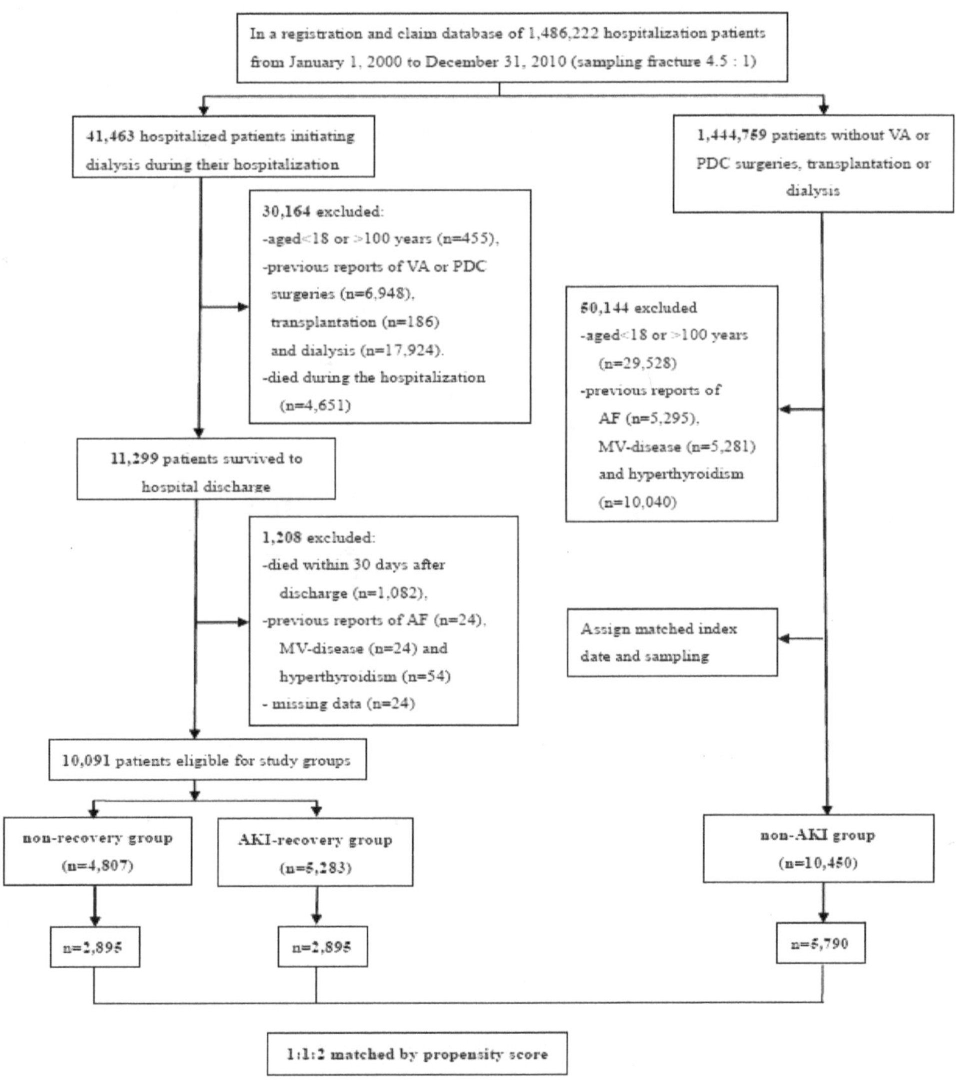


**Figure 1.** Study flow diagram. Abbreviations: AF, atrial fibrillation; MV, mitral valve; PDC, peritoneal dialysis catheter; VA, vascular access.

The follow-up period of the whole post-matching cohort was 6.38 $\pm$ 3.83 years (median, 6.68 years; range, 0.02–10.99 years). Among the three groups, the non-AKI group was the oldest. While the gender, socioeconomic status, baseline comorbidities, as well as outpatient follow-up visits and medication status were not statistically different among the three groups (Table 1). All primary outcome (AF, $p = 0.002$) and secondary outcomes (MACE, ischemic stroke, hemorrhage stroke and all stroke, all $p \leq 0.001$) were of statistical significance among the three groups (Table 2).

### 3.2. Risk of Incident Atrial Fibrillation

The occurrence time of AF since discharge was 3.24 $\pm$ 2.94 years (median, 0.24 years; range, 0.02–10.94 years). The incidence rates of AF were 0.94%, 1.14%, and 1.34% before propensity score matching in "non-AKI group", "AKI-recovery group", and "non-recovery group", respectively.

After propensity score matching, the adjusted risks for subsequent de novo AF development were significantly higher in both the "non-recovery group" (aHR = 1.62; 95% CI, 1.36–1.94; $p \leq 0.001$) and the "AKI-recovery group" (aHR = 1.30; 95% CI, 1.07–1.58; $p \leq 0.01$) compared to the "Non-AKI group" (Table 3 and Figure 2). When compared with "non-recovery group", the "AKI-recovery group" had a significantly lower risk of subsequent AF (aHR = 0.80; 95% CI, 0.616–0.933; $p \leq 0.01$).

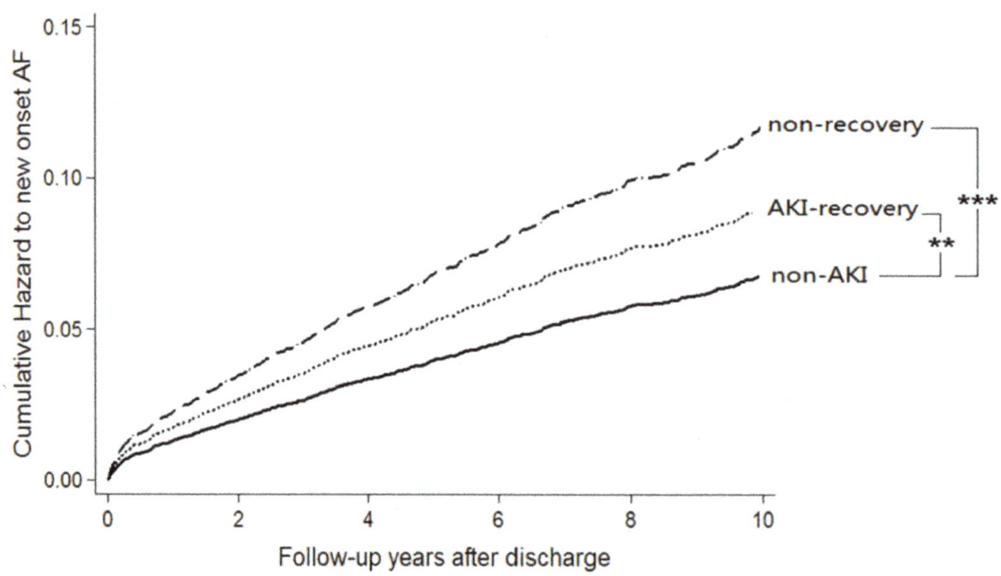


**Figure 2.** Cumulative incidences of atrial fibrillation among the three groups. Note: The analysis was performed using the Cox proportional hazard method with adjustment to the Charlson Comorbidity Index, age, gender and advanced chronic kidney disease (time-varying covariate). *** denotes $p < 0.001$, ** denotes $p < 0.01$. Abbreviations: AF, atrial fibrillation; AKI, acute kidney injury.

**Table 2.** Comparisons of the variables within one year following hospital discharge and outcomes among the three groups.

| | Before Matching $n$ = 20,540 | | | | After Matching $n$ = 11,680 | | | |
|---|---|---|---|---|---|---|---|---|
| **Variables** | **Non-Recovery** $n$ = 4807 | **AKI-Recovery** $n$ = 5283 | **Non-AKI** $n$ = 10,450 | $p$ | **Non-Recovery** $n$ = 2895 | **AKI-Recovery** $n$ = 2895 | **Non-AKI** $n$ = 5790 | $p$ |
| **Outpatient visits, times ‡** | | | | < 0.001 | | | | 0.09 |
| 0–5 visits | 4596 (95.6%) | 4932 (93.3%) | 9297 (89.0%) | | 2763 (95.4%) | 2747 (94.9%) | 5530 (95.5%) | |
| 6–10 visits | 121 (2.5%) | 151 (2.9%) | 450 (4.3%) | | 67 (2.3%) | 74 (2.6%) | 190 (3.3%) | |
| 11–15 visits | 66 (1.4%) | 123 (2.3%) | 479 (4.6%) | | 47 (1.6%) | 50 (1.7%) | 123 (2.1%) | |
| >15 visits | 24 (0.5%) | 77 (1.5%) | 224 (2.1%) | | 18 (0.6%) | 24 (0.8%) | 47 (0.8%) | |
| **Medication for hypertension ‡** | | | | | | | | |
| Alpha-Blocker | 571 (11.9%) | 629 (11.9%) | 1000 (9.6%) | <0.001 | 358 (12.4%) | 341 (11.8%) | 698 (12.1%) | 0.74 |
| Beta-Blocker | 2000 (41.6%) | 1898 (35.9%) | 3904 (37.4%) | <0.001 | 1129 (39.0%) | 1143 (39.5%) | 2369 (40.9%) | 0.52 |
| Calcium-Channel Blocker | 3006 (62.5%) | 2610 (49.4%) | 4986 (47.7%) | <0.001 | 1614 (55.8%) | 1630 (56.3%) | 3360 (58.0%) | 0.49 |
| Diuretic | 1707 (35.5%) | 2485 (47.0%) | 4168 (39.9%) | <0.001 | 1193 (41.2%) | 1231 (42.5%) | 2522 (43.6%) | 0.35 |
| ACEI/ARB | 1725 (35.9%) | 1791 (33.9%) | 4176 (40.0%) | <0.001 | 1057 (36.5%) | 1073 (37.1%) | 2231 (38.5%) | 0.44 |
| **Other Medication ‡** | | | | | | | | |
| Anti-diabetic drugs | 1468 (30.5%) | 1595 (30.2%) | 3230 (30.9%) | 0.57 | 849 (29.3%) | 887 (30.6%) | 1846 (31.9%) | 0.16 |
| Aspirin | 411 (8.6%) | 396 (7.5%) | 1259 (12.1%) | <0.001 | 246 (8.5%) | 247 (8.5%) | 517 (8.9%) | 0.88 |
| Clopidogrel | 143 (3.0%) | 291 (5.5%) | 443 (4.2%) | <0.001 | 104 (3.6%) | 114 (3.9%) | 212 (3.7%) | 0.70 |
| Ticlopidine | 208 (4.33%) | 117 (2.2%) | 370 (3.5%) | <0.001 | 85 (2.9%) | 86 (3.0%) | 194 (3.4%) | 0.57 |
| Dipyridamole | 1059 (22.0%) | 792 (15.0%) | 2224 (21.3%) | <0.001 | 538 (18.6%) | 555 (19.2%) | 1147 (19.8%) | 0.61 |
| Nitrate | 868 (18.1%) | 1050 (19.9%) | 1262 (12.1%) | <0.001 | 501 (17.3%) | 524 (18.1%) | 1053 (18.2%) | 0.71 |
| Statin | 519 (10.8%) | 628 (11.9%) | 1524 (15.6%) | <0.001 | 334 (11.5%) | 355 (12.3%) | 743 (12.8%) | 0.35 |
| Proton pump inhibitor | 26 (0.5%) | 57 (1.1%) | 64 (0.6%) | 0.001 | 24 (0.8%) | 22 (0.8%) | 42 (0.7%) | 0.84 |
| NSAID | 3062 (63.7%) | 2832 (53.6%) | 7863 (75.2%) | <0.001 | 1811 (65.6%) | 1833 (63.3%) | 3707 (64.0%) | 0.84 |
| H2-blocker | 1173 (24.4%) | 1232 (23.3%) | 2718 (26.0%) | <0.001 | 692 (23.9%) | 739 (25.5%) | 1535 (26.5%) | 0.09 |

**Table 2.** *Cont.*

| Variables | Before Matching $n = 20{,}540$ | | | | After Matching $n = 11{,}680$ | | | |
|---|---|---|---|---|---|---|---|---|
| | Non-Recovery $n = 4807$ | AKI-Recovery $n = 5283$ | Non-AKI $n = 10{,}450$ | $p$ | Non-Recovery $n = 2895$ | AKI-Recovery $n = 2895$ | Non-AKI $n = 5790$ | $p$ |
| **Outcome** ‡‡ | | | | | | | | |
| Atrial fibrillation | 384 (8.0%) | 274 (5.2%) | 759 (7.3%) | <0.001 | 214 (7.4%) | 149 (5.2%) | 383 (6.6%) | 0.002 |
| MACE | 830 (17.3%) | 617 (11.7%) | 1449 (13.9%) | <0.001 | 467 (16.1%) | 333 (11.5%) | 772 (13.3%) | <0.001 |
| Ischemia Stroke | 1226 (25.5%) | 824 (15.6%) | 4195 (40.1%) | <0.001 | 696 (24.0%) | 481 (16.6%) | 2286 (39.5%) | <0.001 |
| Hemorrhage Stroke | 367 (7.6%) | 229 (4.3%) | 1176 (11.3%) | <0.001 | 222 (7.7%) | 140 (4.8%) | 719 (13.7%) | <0.001 |
| All stroke | 1399 (29.1%) | 944 (17.9%) | 4748 (45.4%) | <0.001 | 802 (27.7%) | 555 (19.2%) | 2617 (45.2%) | <0.001 |
| Advanced CKD | 988 (20.6%) | 723 (13.7%) | 702 (6.8%) | <0.001 | 822 (28.4%) | 482 (16.6%) | 423 (7.3%) | <0.001 |
| Mortality | 2486 (51.7%) | 2204 (41.7%) | 3025 (29.0%) | <0.001 | 1482 (51.2%) | 1188 (41.0 %) | 1890 (32.6%) | <0.001 |

Note: Continuous variables were presented as a mean ± standard deviation, and statistically analyzed using one-way analysis of variance, while categorical variables were described as counts (percentages) and analyzed using Chi-squared tests. † denotes "before discharge"; ‡ denotes "within one year following hospital discharge"; ‡‡ denotes "follow-up until death or the end of the study (31 December 2010)"; Abbreviations: ACEI, angiotensin-converting enzyme inhibitor; ARB, angiotensin receptor blocker; CKD, chronic kidney disease; COPD, chronic obstructive pulmonary disease; Gr, group; MACE, major adverse cardiac event; NSAID, non-steroid anti-inflammatory drug; NTD, new Taiwan dollar.

**Table 3.** Incidences and risks of atrial fibrillation development among the three groups.

| | Atrial Fibrillation | | | Crude Risk | Adjusted Risk ‡ | Adjusted Risk ‡‡ |
|---|---|---|---|---|---|---|
| | Events | Person-Years | Incidence Rate § | HR (95% CI) | aHR (95% CI) | aHR (95% CI) |
| | | | Before propensity score-matching | | | |
| non-AKI | 759 | 81,186.67 | 0.94 | ref | ref | ref |
| AKI-recovery | 274 | 24,007.06 | 1.14 | 1.08 (0.94–1.24) | 1.16 (1.00–1.33) | 1.15 (1.10–1.32) |
| non-recovery | 384 | 28,726.82 | 1.34 | 1.36 *** (1.20–1.54) | 1.62 *** (1.43–1.83) | 1.58 *** (1.39–1.80) |
| | | | After propensity score-matching | | | |
| non-AKI | 383 | 45,562.79 | 0.84 | ref | ref | ref |
| AKI-recovery | 149 | 13,462.42 | 1.11 | 1.18 (0.98–1.43) | 1.33 ** (1.10–1.61) | 1.30 ** (1.07–1.58) |
| non-recovery | 214 | 17,088.48 | 1.25 | 1.42 *** (1.20–1.68) | 1.72 *** (1.45–2.03) | 1.62 *** (1.36–1.94) |

Note: Cox proportional hazard model was applied to exam the effect of dialysis-requiring AKI on subsequent atrial fibrillation development. § presented as "100 person-year". ‡ Adjusted for Charlson Comorbidity Index, age, and gender. ‡‡ Adjusted for Charlson Comorbidity Index, age, gender, and advanced chronic kidney disease (time-varying covariate). ** denotes $p$-value ≤ 0.01; *** denotes $p$-value ≤ 0.001. Abbreviations: aHR, adjusted hazard ratio; CI, confidence interval; Gr, group; HR, hazard ratio.

### 3.3. *Risk of Incident Atrial Fibrillation in Subgroups*

In the subgroup comparison, we found that "AKI-recovery group" has a significantly higher risk of incident AF than the "non-AKI group" in some subgroups. These subgroups included the patients without congestive heart failure (CHF) (aHR = 1.23; 95% CI, 1.06–1.42) and chronic obstructive pulmonary disease (aHR = 1.18; 95% CI, 1.01–1.36), those with CKD (aHR = 1.37; 95% CI, 1.05–1.80) and diabetes mellitus (aHR = 1.37; 95% CI, 1.05–1.79), as well as those receiving angiotensin-converting-enzyme inhibitor (ACEI)/angiotensin receptor blocker (ARB) (aHR = 1.27; 95% CI, 1.04–1.54) and beta-blocker (aHR = 1.49; 95% CI, 1.24–1.80). Additionally, the subgroups who received anticoagulants (aHR = 1.23; 95% CI, 1.00–1.51) had marginally significant increased risks of AF (Figure 3).

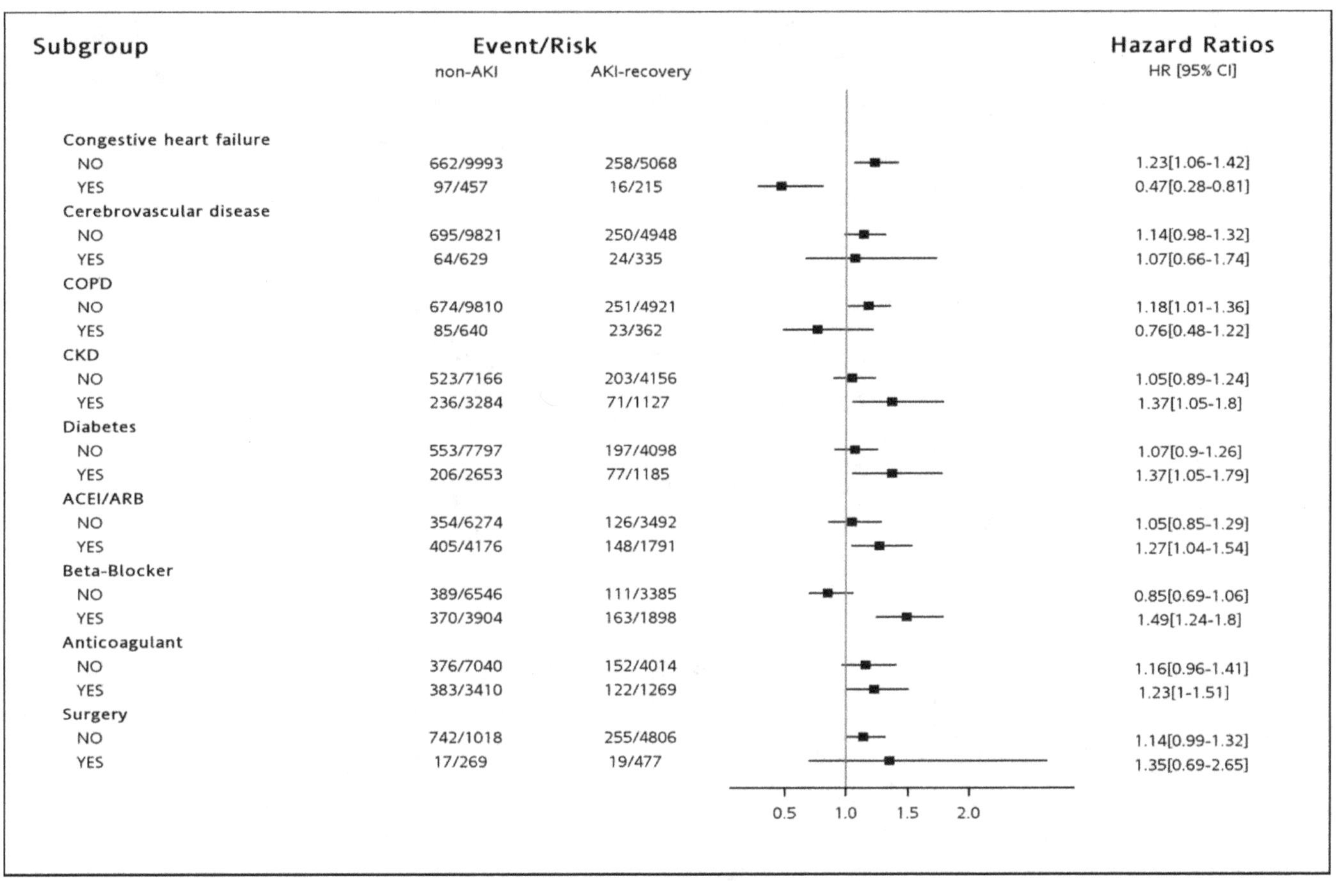


**Figure 3.** Subgroup comparisons for the risk of atrial fibrillation. Note: The forest plot for the comparison of AKI-recovery group versus non-AKI group was drawn using the before-matching population with adjustment to the Charlson Comorbidity Index, age, and gender. Abbreviations: ACEI, angiotensin-converting enzyme inhibitor; ARB, angiotensin receptor blocker; AF, atrial fibrillation; AKI, acute kidney injury; CKD, chronic kidney disease; COPD, chronic obstructive pulmonary disease.

### 3.4. *Risk of Major Adverse Events between Patients with and without Incident Atrial Fibrillation*

After propensity score matching, the patients with de novo AF augmented risks for MACE (aHR = 2.11; 95% CI, 1.83–2.43), ischemic stroke (aHR = 1.33; 95% CI, 1.19–1.49) and all stroke (aHR = 1.28; 95% CI, 1.15–1.43) (all $p \leq 0.001$) (Table 4).

**Table 4.** Incidences and risks of major adverse events between patients with and without atrial fibrillation.

| | AF | | | Non-AF | | | Crude Risk | Adjusted Risk ‡ |
|---|---|---|---|---|---|---|---|---|
| | Event | Person-Year | Incidence Rate § | Event | Person-Year | Incidence Rate § | HR (95% CI) | HR (95% CI) |
| Before propensity score-matching | | | | | | | | |
| MACE | 987 | 9230.59 | 10.69 | 2466 | 117,959.62 | 2.09 | 2.25 ** (2.03–2.49) | 1.88 ** (1.70–2.09) |
| Hemorrhagic stroke | 161 | 10,381.48 | 1.55 | 1611 | 121,543.88 | 1.33 | 1.20 * (1.02–1.41) | 1.24 * (1.05–1.46) |
| Ischemic stroke | 667 | 7077.34 | 9.42 | 5578 | 96,917.20 | 5.76 | 1.62 ** (1.49–1.75) | 1.31 ** (1.21–1.42) |
| Total stroke | 714 | 6867.78 | 10.40 | 6377 | 93,540.77 | 6.82 | 1.50 ** (1.39–1.62) | 1.26 ** (1.17–1.36) |
| After propensity score-matching | | | | | | | | |
| MACE | 511 | 4729.33 | 10.80 | 1337 | 67,595.80 | 1.98 | 2.49 ** (2.17–2.86) | 2.11 ** (1.83–2.43) |
| Hemorrhagic stroke | 89 | 5321.74 | 1.67 | 992 | 68,827.18 | 1.44 | 1.20 (0.97–1.49) | 1.23 (0.99–1.53) |
| Ischemic stroke | 333 | 3766.11 | 8.84 | 3130 | 55,361.13 | 5.65 | 1.57 ** (1.40–1.75) | 1.33 ** (1.19–1.49) |
| All Stroke | 362 | 3654.72 | 9.90 | 3612 | 53,357.19 | 6.77 | 1.46 ** (1.31–1.63) | 1.28 ** (1.15–1.43) |

Note: Cox proportional hazard model was applied to exam the effect of dialysis-requiring AKI on subsequent atrial fibrillation development. § presented as "100 person-year". ‡ Adjusted to Charlson Comorbidity Index, age, and gender. * denotes $p$-value $\leq 0.05$; ** denotes $p$-value $\leq 0.001$; Abbreviations: aHR, adjusted hazard ratio; CI, confidence interval; ESRD, end-stage renal disease; HR, hazard ratio; MACE, major adverse cardiac event.

## 4. Discussion

This study is the first to demonstrate a long-term association between AKI and the subsequent incident AF in critically ill patients using a large nationwide cohort. We found that the experience of severe AKI necessitating dialysis, even in the patients who only required temporary dialysis, was associated with increased risk of subsequent incident AF. Moreover, the experience of incident AF further carried a higher risk of MACE, and ischemic stroke in these patients. Since AKI carries an increased risk of coronary events [3], the increased AF following AKI could at least partially explain the elevated probability of MACE after AKI. Since the current study was designed using a selected population set from a nationwide database to evaluate the influence of AKI-D on the incident AF, the incidence rate of AF in this study was not comparable to other investigations [15,16] for an epidemiological purpose.

Most of the previous studies evaluating the association between AF and AKI were designed with a relatively short study period using patients who underwent cardiac surgeries [6,7]. One such study enrolled 446 cardiac surgical patients and found that the development of postoperative AKI was an independent factor associated with new-onset AF [6]. Another prospective study including 2572 cardiac surgical patients disclosed that the occurrence of postoperative AKI carried the 1.7-fold increased risk of developing postoperative AF [7]. In the subgroup comparison of the current study, although insufficient case numbers made the results not statistically significant, we also observed a tendency that patients receiving cardiac surgeries had a higher risk of incident AF than those without (aHR, 1.35 versus 1.14) (Figure 3). Nevertheless, the results from post-cardiac surgical patients probably could not be extensively applied to other patient settings, because the cardiac surgical patient is a special population with a higher risk of AF due to the relevant involvement of heart structurally and electrically [8,17]. Furthermore, the temporal association between AKI and AF was difficult to be clarified by these studies because of a short period of observation [7,9,10]. Compared to the previous studies, the clarified temporal association between in-hospital AKI and new-onset AF after hospital discharge, along with the long-term follow-up period in the current study, provides more strengthened evidence in this field.

In particular, we provide an important outcome estimate: that is, even after being adjusted with progression to subsequent advanced CKD or ESRD, in the worst of circumstances, AKI still independently contributes to subsequent incident AF or all-cause mortality. Therefore, the risk factors of the kidney injury that had engendered an AKI event may persist and eventually lead to future AF without direct causal association to the subsequent CKD.

### 4.1. *Acute Kidney Injury and Atrial Fibrillation*

An increasing body of evidence has shown that AKI is independently associated with the occurrence of AF [18]. AKI causes "remote organ injury" in the heart by the "classical" acute uremic effect, the inflammatory state and the modulating effect of the underlying morbidities associated with the injured kidneys, as well as the health care dilemma [5].

Several mechanisms are proposed for explaining the association between AKI and the elevated risk of AF: (1) The increased preload because of the AKI-induced salt and water retention at the acute stage could increase the cardiac structural change [19–22]. (2) The myocardial damage and impaired left ventricular function secondary to the enhanced neutrophil trafficking, endothelial dysfunction, myocyte apoptosis, as well as an increased level of inflammatory cytokines [19–22]. Additionally, fibroblast growth factor 23 (FGF-23), a biomarker for predicting early AKI presentation and cardiovascular morbidity and mortality [23], is disclosed to have markedly elevated serum level in patients with AKI. Higher FGF-23 levels were also found to be associated with elevated risk of AF development in both patients with and without clinical cardiovascular disease [24]. Thus, the enhanced AF incidence might be attributed to the atrial remodeling related to increased FGF-23 levels [25]. Taken together, these results provide a new perspective on the pathogenesis of sinoatrial dysfunction after AKI and open new avenues for treatment of the disease. (3) The activation of the sympathetic nervous system: previous studies have demonstrated that ischemia-reperfusion injury related AKI would activate a sympathetic reflex [26]. The activating sympathetic activation of the atrium would subsequently cause remodeling of the cardiac autonomic neural tissue and promote further persistence and recurrence of AF [27].

Of note, in the subgroup of "patients without CHF", the finding that "recovery AKI-D patients had a higher risk of subsequent AF than non-AKI patients" was consistent with the results from our whole study population. This was reasonable when we considered this finding as a result without the confounding the effect of CHF. Nevertheless, diverse observations were disclosed in patients with CHF. In these patients, the indication of dialysis could more likely be "fluid overload", which was associated with a more favorable prognosis than other indications. On the contrary, the mortality risk might be higher in patients with more severe AKI-D and CHF than those who only had AKI-D. Owing to the lack of the etiology and severity of congestive heart failure, and the indication of dialysis in the database for further analysis, the observation among patients with CHF should be inconclusive (Figure 3).

Additionally, the results among the subgroups of "hypertensive patients taking beta-blocker and ACEI/ARB" were also consistent with the findings from the whole population. These findings could be interpreted as the beneficial effects of the aforementioned anti-hypertensive medications minimizing the other confounding effects of the underlying cardiovascular disease. In contrast, the influences of AKI-D on AF were blunted in the patients not taking beta-blockers and ACEI/ARB. In fact, this subgroup contains two patient groups (patients without hypertension, and hypertensive patients not taking beta-blocker or ACEI/ARB for treatment) with different prognostic characteristics. Without doing further analysis, we could not draw any conclusions regarding this issue (Figure 3).

### *4.2. Major Adverse Events Associated with Atrial Fibrillation*

In the current study, incident AF was associated with several major adverse events (Table 4). Similar findings were also demonstrated that the development of AKI-D was associated with increased risk of in-hospital mortality and adverse events among patients with AF [2]. Following our results, patients who have AF and AKI will have a high incidence of cardiovascular events, especially coronary events and ischemic stroke. Distant organ injury, a direct consequence of deleterious systemic effects following AKI, is an important issue for clinical care [5].

The association between AF and abnormal renal function is also an interesting and essential issue to be discussed. Among stable anticoagulated patients with AF, the presence of impaired baseline renal function was reported as an independent risk factor of the occurrence of thrombotic/vascular events, stroke, bleeding, and mortality [28,29]. During the two-year follow-up period, about 21% to 32% of patients had a rapid renal function deterioration (decline of estimated Glomerular filtration rate (eGFR) > 5–10 mL/min/1.73 $m^2$) [28,30]. More renal function deterioration in absolute levels (decreases of eGFR $\geq$ 15–25 mL/min/1.73 $m^2$ within two years) or relative percentage (decline of $\geq$25% eGFR) within 2 years was independently associated with the occurrence of stroke or death in these patients [29]. The independent risk factors for the development of severe kidney disease include diabetes, CHF, coronary artery disease and impaired baseline renal function [28]. However, normal or near-normal baseline renal function did not exclude the subsequent development of severe renal impairment over time [28].

Regarding the therapeutic strategy for AF, the old drug "Warfarin" is thought to be associated with higher risk for AKI, which is probably due to a higher risk of glomerular hemorrhage known as anticoagulation-related nephropathy [31]. In a randomized study enrolling 18,113 patients, Bohm et al. [32] found that patients receiving warfarin, as opposed to those receiving direct oral anticoagulants (DOAC), have more rapid eGFR decline after an average follow-up period of 30 months. Patients with poor international normalized ratio control (i.e., time in the therapeutic range <65%) tend to have a faster decline in eGFR. Similarly, Chan et al. [33] found that DOAC users had an overall 21%

lower risk of AKI compared with warfarin users among Asians with nonvalvular AF. The beneficial effect was especially disclosed in among patients with eGFR > 60 mL/min/1.73 m$^2$.

As to the association between AF and MACE, some information should be addressed. In a prospective cohort of 23,928 participants without coronary artery disease conducted by Soliman et al. [34], AF was associated with around two-fold elevated the risk of myocardial infarction within a 6.9 year (median 4.5 years) follow-up. Consistent findings were found in the study enrolling 4,608 participants by O'Neal et al. [35]. Within the median follow-up period of 12.2 years, 17.3% participants developed myocardial infarction, and AF independently carried 1.7 folds increase the risk of myocardial infarction. The increased cardiovascular risk of AF was further confirmed by a systemic review and meta-analysis including 15 cohort studies. Another work also found that AF is associated with an elevated risk of CHF and all-cause mortality in patients regardless of having coronary artery disease, and additionally with an elevated risk of subsequent myocardial infarction in those without coronary artery disease [36]. Of note, the influences of AF on increasing risk of cardiovascular events were more prominent in women than men and African-Americans than Caucasians [34,35,37].

Despite receiving oral warfarin treatment, patients with AF still have a high rate of cardiovascular events, including fatal/nonfatal myocardial infarction, cardiac revascularization, and cardiovascular death. The independent predictors of cardiovascular events included age, smoking, history of cerebrovascular and cardiac events, metabolic syndrome, CHF, and male gender [38].

The cardiovascular safety of oral anticoagulants has long been debated. By using a systemic review and meta-analysis, Tornyos et al., [39] disclosed that most of the DOACs were of safer than warfarin regarding the risk of subsequent myocardial infarction. A very recent work by Lee et al. [40] further exhibited a favorable effect of DOACs as compared to warfarin in reducing cardiac complications in AF. In the analysis using 31,739 patients, all DOACs were associated with lower risk of myocardial infarction than warfarin.

AKI is now considered a growing global health alert [41]. These findings are noteworthy from the perspective of a clinician caring for an individual with dialysis-requiring AKI. Considerable growth in AKI epidemiology and improvements in post-hospitalization resource utilization [42] allowed us to examine the impact of AKI on AF and identify a large vulnerable population with increased risk of cardiovascular events and all-cause mortality [3,4].

### 4.3. Limitations

Several limitations are worth mentioning. First, the nature of the observational study is subject to bias. Second, the study using administrative data is potentially limited by unmeasured confounding. The epidemiological data, the etiology, and severity of AKI, the indication of dialysis initiation, as well as some known risk factors including alcohol abuse and body mass index, which may further provide meaningful information regarding the association with subsequent AF, are not available in such a nationwide insurance research database. Third, the primary outcome of the current study is "non-valvular AF". The observations accrued here might not be extrapolated to patients with "valvular AF". Fourth, the precision of the disease diagnoses based on ICD-9-CM may be a concern. Fifth, although we have taken "advanced CKD" as a covariate in the Cox model when evaluating the adjusted risk for subsequent AF, the confounding effect of subsequent impaired renal function and chronic dialysis could not be completely excluded. Sixth, the start point of the follow-up period is indeed arguable. Some confounding effect from acute dialysis may exist, which probably increases the risk of AF in "AKI-recovery group", if immediate period after discharge is included in the observation period. Nevertheless, changing the start point from "after discharge" to "the 31st day after discharge" decreases 11% AF events without changing the results of the current study.

However, despite widespread interest and extensive research on AF, our understanding of the etiology and pathogenesis of this disease process is still incomplete. As a result, there are no set primary preventive strategies in a place apart from general cardiac risk factor prevention goals. Our result seems intuitive that a better understanding of acute dialysis as the risk factors for AF would better prepare medical professionals to initially prevent or subsequently treat these patients and follow up with groups who could not wean from acute dialysis.

## 5. Conclusions

In this current nationwide cohort study, we found that the experience of severe AKI necessitating dialysis carries an increased risk of subsequent AF, even in those weaned from acute dialysis. Further study is needed to determine the mechanisms which link AKI and subsequent AF and to identify potentially modifiable risk factors to decrease the burden of AF and subsequent risk of major adverse events.

**Author Contributions:** Formal analysis: C.-C.S., Y.-T.H., and V.-C.W.; Investigation: V.-C.W.; supervision: V.-C.W.; validation: C.-C.S., J.-J.W., Y.-F.L., L.C., E.C., W.-P.C., L.-J.T., C.-H.W., and Y.-T.H.; writing—original draft: C.-C.S., W.C.K., and Y.-T.H.; writing—review and editing: C.-C.S., J.-J.W., Y.-F.L., L.C., E.C., W.-P.C., L.-J.T., C.-H.W., and V.-C.W.

**Acknowledgments:** The study was partly based on data provided by the National Health Insurance Administration, Ministry of Health and Welfare, Taiwan. The interpretation and conclusions shown in this paper do not represent those of National Health Insurance Administration, Ministry of Health and Welfare, National Health Research Institutes, or the National Taiwan University Hospital. We also express our sincere gratitude to all staff of the Taiwan Clinical Trial Consortium, TCTC.

## References

1. Rahman, F.; Kwan, G.F.; Benjamin, E.J. Global epidemiology of atrial fibrillation. *Nat. Rev. Cardiol.* **2014**, *11*, 639–654. [CrossRef] [PubMed]
2. Chan, L.; Mehta, S.; Chauhan, K.; Poojary, P.; Patel, S.; Pawar, S.; Patel, A.; Correa, A.; Patel, S.; Garimella, P.S.; et al. National trends and impact of acute kidney injury requiring hemodialysis in hospitalizations with atrial fibrillation. *J. Am. Hear. Assoc.* **2016**, *5*, e004509. [CrossRef] [PubMed]
3. Wu, V.C.; Wu, C.H.; Huang, T.M.; Wang, C.Y.; Lai, C.F.; Shiao, C.C.; Chang, C.H.; Lin, S.L.; Chen, Y.Y.; Chen, Y.M.; et al. Long-term risk of coronary events after AKI. *J. Am. Soc. Nephrol.* **2014**, *25*, 595–605. [CrossRef] [PubMed]
4. Wu, V.C.; Wu, P.C.; Wu, C.H.; Huang, T.M.; Chang, C.H.; Tsai, P.R.; Ko, W.J.; Chen, L.; Wang, C.Y.; Chu, T.S.; et al. The impact of acute kidney injury on the long-term risk of stroke. *J. Am. Heart Assoc.* **2014**, *3*, e000933. [CrossRef] [PubMed]
5. Shiao, C.C.; Wu, P.C.; Huang, T.M.; Lai, T.S.; Yang, W.S.; Wu, C.H.; Lai, C.F.; Wu, V.C.; Chu, T.S.; Wu, K.D.; et al. Long-term remote organ consequences following acute kidney injury. *Crit. Care* **2015**, *19*, 438. [CrossRef] [PubMed]
6. Diplaris, K.; Ampatzidou, F.; Karagounnis, L.; Drossos, G.; Vlahou, A. The role of blood transfusion in the development of atrial fibrillation after coronary artery bypass grafting. *Thorac. Cardiovasc. Surg.* **2016**, *64*, 688–692. [CrossRef] [PubMed]
7. Ng, R.R.G.; Tan, G.H.J.; Liu, W.; Ti, L.K.; Chew, S.T.H. The association of acute kidney injury and atrial fibrillation after cardiac surgery in an asian prospective cohort study. *Medicine* **2016**, *95*, e3005. [CrossRef] [PubMed]
8. Maesen, B.; Nijs, J.; Maessen, J.; Allessie, M.; Schotten, U. Post-operative atrial fibrillation: A maze of mechanisms. *Europace* **2011**, *14*, 159–174. [CrossRef] [PubMed]
9. Ommen, S.R.; Odell, J.A.; Stanton, M.S. Atrial arrhythmias after cardiothoracic surgery. *New Engl. J. Med.* **1997**, *336*, 1429–1434. [CrossRef] [PubMed]
10. Auer, J.; Lamm, G.; Weber, T.; Berent, R.; Ng, C.-K.; Porodko, M.; Eber, B. Renal function is associated with risk of atrial fibrillation after cardiac surgery. *Can. J. Cardiol.* **2007**, *23*, 859–863. [CrossRef]
11. Lin, L.-J.; Cheng, M.-H.; Lee, C.-H.; Wung, D.-C.; Cheng, C.-L.; Kao Yang, Y.-H. Compliance with antithrombotic prescribing guidelines for patients with atrial fibrillation—A nationwide descriptive study in taiwan. *Clin. Ther.* **2008**, *30*, 1726–1736. [CrossRef] [PubMed]
12. Chao, T.-F.; Huang, Y.-C.; Liu, C.-J.; Chen, S.-J.; Wang, K.-L.; Lin, Y.-J.; Chang, S.-L.; Lo, L.-W.; Hu, Y.-F.; Tuan, T.-C.; et al. Acute myocardial infarction in patients with atrial fibrillation with a cha2ds2-vasc score of 0 or 1: A nationwide cohort study. *Hear. Rhythm.* **2014** *11*, 1941–1947. [CrossRef] [PubMed]

13. Jensen, P.N.; Johnson, K.; Floyd, J.; Heckbert, S.R.; Carnahan, R.; Dublin, S. A systematic review of validated methods for identifying atrial fibrillation using administrative data. *Pharmacoepidemiol. Drug Saf.* **2012**, *21*, 141–147. [CrossRef] [PubMed]
14. Wang, W.J.; Chao, C.T.; Huang, Y.C.; Wang, C.Y.; Chang, C.H.; Huang, T.M.; Lai, C.F.; Huang, H.Y.; Shiao, C.C.; Chu, T.S.; et al. The impact of acute kidney injury with temporary dialysis on the risk of fracture. *J. Bone Miner. Res.* **2013**, *29*, 676–684. [CrossRef] [PubMed]
15. Chao, T.-F.; Liu, C.-J.; Tuan, T.-C.; Chen, T.-J.; Hsieh, M.-H.; Lip, G.Y.H.; Chen, S.-A. Lifetime Risks, Projected Numbers, and Adverse Outcomes in Asian Patients With Atrial Fibrillation: A Report From the Taiwan Nationwide AF Cohort Study. *Chest* **2018**, *153*, 453–466. [CrossRef] [PubMed]
16. Chien, K.-L.; Su, T.-C.; Hsu, H.-C.; Chang, W.-T.; Chen, P.-C.; Chen, M.-F.; Lee, Y.-T. Atrial fibrillation prevalence, incidence and risk of stroke and all-cause death among Chinese. *Int. J. Cardiol.* **2010**, *139*, 173–180. [CrossRef] [PubMed]
17. January, C.T.; Wann, L.S.; Alpert, J.S.; Calkins, H.; Cigarroa, J.E.; Cleveland, J.C., Jr.; Conti, J.B.; Ellinor, P.T.; Ezekowitz, M.D.; Field, M.E.; et al. 2014 AHA/ACC/HRS guideline for the management of patients with atrial fibrillation: A report of the American College of Cardiology/American Heart Association Task Force on Practice Guidelines and the Heart Rhythm Society. *J. Am. Coll. Cardiol.* **2014**, *64*, e1–e76. [CrossRef] [PubMed]
18. Ologunde, R.; Zhao, H.; Lu, K.; Ma, D. Organ cross talk and remote organ damage following acute kidney injury. *Int. Urol. Nephrol.* **2014**, *46*, 2337–2345. [CrossRef] [PubMed]
19. Grams, M.E.; Rabb, H. The distant organ effects of acute kidney injury. *Kidney Int.* **2012**, *81*, 942–948. [CrossRef] [PubMed]
20. Kelly, K.J. Distant effects of experimental renal ischemia/reperfusion injury. *J. Am. Soc. Nephrol.* **2003**, *14*, 1549–1558. [CrossRef] [PubMed]
21. Bhalodia, Y.S.; Sheth, N.R.; Vaghasiya, J.D.; Jivani, N.P. Homocysteine-dependent endothelial dysfunction induced by renal ischemia/reperfusion injury. *J. Nephrol.* **2011**, *24*, 631–635. [CrossRef] [PubMed]
22. Kelly, K.J.; Meehan, S.M.; Colvin, R.B.; Williams, W.W.; Bonventre, J.V. Protection from toxicant-mediated renal injury in the rat with anti-cd54 antibody. *Kidney Int.* **1999**, *56*, 922–931. [CrossRef] [PubMed]
23. Leaf, D.E.; Christov, M.; Jüppner, H.; Siew, E.; Ikizler, T.A.; Bian, A.; Chen, G.; Sabbisetti, V.S.; Bonventre, J.V.; Cai, X.; et al. Fibroblast growth factor 23 levels are elevated and associated with severe acute kidney injury and death following cardiac surgery. *Kidney Int.* **2016**, *89*, 939–948. [CrossRef] [PubMed]
24. Mathew, J.S.; Sachs, M.C.; Katz, R.; Patton, K.K.; Heckbert, S.R.; Hoofnagle, A.N.; Alonso, A.; Chonchol, M.; Deo, R.; Ix, J.H.; et al. Fibroblast growth factor-23 and incident atrial fibrillation: the multi-ethnic study of atherosclerosis (mesa) and the cardiovascular health study (chs). *Circulation* **2014**, *130*, 298–307. [CrossRef] [PubMed]
25. Sciacqua, A.; Perticone, M.; Tripepi, G.; Miceli, S.; Tassone, E.J.; Grillo, N.; Carullo, G.; Sesti, G.; Perticone, F. Renal disease and left atrial remodeling predict atrial fibrillation in patients with cardiovascular risk factors. *Int. J. Cardiol.* **2014**, *175*, 90–95. [CrossRef] [PubMed]
26. Cao, W.; Li, A.; Li, J.; Wu, C.; Cui, S.; Zhou, Z.; Liu, Y.; Wilcox, C.S.; Hou, F.F. Reno-cerebral reflex activates the renin-angiotensin system, promoting oxidative stress and renal damage after ischemia-reperfusion injury. *Antioxid. Redox Signal* **2017**, *27*, 415–432. [CrossRef] [PubMed]
27. Lane, K.; Dixon, J.J.; MacPhee, I.A.M.; Philips, B.J. Renohepatic crosstalk: Does acute kidney injury cause liver dysfunction? *Nephrol. Dial. Transplant.* **2013**, *28*, 1634–1647. [CrossRef] [PubMed]
28. Roldan, V.; Marin, F.; Fernandez, H.; Manzano-Fernandez, S.; Gallego, P.; Valdes, M.; Vicente, V.; Lip, G.Y. Renal impairment in a "real-life" cohort of anticoagulated patients with atrial fibrillation (implications for thromboembolism and bleeding). *Am. J. Cardiol.* **2013**, *111*, 1159–1164. [CrossRef] [PubMed]
29. Peng, X.S.; Meng, G.W.; Zhang, J.; Wang, X.F.; Zhao, L.X.; Wang, Y.W.; Zhang, L.D. Electrochemical fabrication of ordered Ag2S nanowire arrays. *Mater. Res. Bull.* **2002**, *37*, 1369–1375. [CrossRef]
30. Violi, F.; Pastori, D.; Perticone, F.; Hiatt, W.R.; Sciacqua, A.; Basili, S.; Proietti, M.; Corazza, G.R.; Lip, G.Y.H.; Pignatelli, P. Relationship between low ankle-brachial index and rapid renal function decline in patients with atrial fibrillation: A prospective multicentre cohort study. *BMJ Open* **2015**, *5*, e008026. [CrossRef] [PubMed]
31. Brodsky, S.V.; Hebert, L.A. Anticoagulant-Related Nephropathy: Is an AKI Elephant Hiding in Plain View? *J. Am. Coll. Cardiol.* **2016** *68*, 2284–2286. [CrossRef] [PubMed]

32. Bohm, M.; Ezekowitz, M.D.; Connolly, S.J.; Eikelboom, J.W.; Hohnloser, S.H.; Reilly, P.A.; Schumacher, H.; Brueckmann, M.; Schirmer, S.H.; Kratz, M.T.; et al. Changes in renal function in patients with Atrial Fibrillation: An analysis from the RE-LY Trial. *J. Am. Coll. Cardiol.* **2015**, *65*, 2481–2493. [CrossRef] [PubMed]
33. Chan, Y.H.; Yeh, Y.H.; See, L.C.; Wang, C.L.; Chang, S.H.; Lee, H.F.; Wu, L.S.; Tu, H.T.; Kuo, C.T. Acute kidney injury in Asians with atrial fibrillation treated with dabigatran or warfarin. *J. Am. Coll. Cardiol.* **2016**, *68*, 2272–2283. [CrossRef] [PubMed]
34. Soliman, E.Z.; Safford, M.M.; Muntner, P.; Khodneva, Y.; Dawood, F.Z.; Zakai, N.A.; Thacker, E.L.; Judd, S.; Howard, V.J.; Howard, G.; et al. Atrial fibrillation and the risk of myocardial infarction. *JAMA Intern. Med.* **2014**, *174*, 107–114. [CrossRef] [PubMed]
35. O'Neal, W.T.; Sangal, K.; Zhang, Z.-M.; Soliman, E.Z. Atrial fibrillation and incident myocardial infarction in the elderly. *Clin. Cardiol.* **2014**, *37*, 750–755. [CrossRef] [PubMed]
36. Ruddox, V.; Sandven, I.; Munkhaugen, J.; Skattebu, J.; Edvardsen, T.; Otterstad, J.E. Atrial fibrillation and the risk for myocardial infarction, all-cause mortality and heart failure: A systematic review and meta-analysis. *Eur. J. Prev. Cardiol.* **2017**, *24*, 1555–1566. [CrossRef] [PubMed]
37. Emdin, C.A.; Wong, C.X.; Hsiao, A.J.; Altman, D.G.; Peters, S.A.; Woodward, M.; Odutayo, A.A. Atrial fibrillation as risk factor for cardiovascular disease and death in women compared with men: Systematic review and meta-analysis of cohort studies. *BMJ* **2016**, *352*, h7013. [CrossRef] [PubMed]
38. Pastori, D.; Pignatelli, P.; Angelico, F.; Farcomeni, A.; Del Ben, M.; Vicario, T.; Bucci, T.; Raparelli, V.; Cangemi, R.; Tanzilli, G.; Lip, G.Y.H.; Violi, F. Incidence of myocardial infarction and vascular death in elderly patients with atrial fibrillation taking anticoagulants. *Chest* **2015**, *147*, 1644–1650. [CrossRef] [PubMed]
39. Tornyos, A.; Kehl, D.; D'Ascenzo, F.; Komócsi, A. Risk of myocardial infarction in patients with long-term non-vitamin k antagonist oral anticoagulant treatment. *Prog. Cardiovasc. Dis.* **2016**, *58*, 483–494. [CrossRef] [PubMed]
40. Lee, C.J.; Gerds, T.A.; Carlson, N.; Bonde, A.N.; Gislason, G.H.; Lamberts, M.; Olesen, J.B.; Pallisgaard, J.L.; Hansen, M.L.; Torp-Pedersen, C. Risk of myocardial infarction in anticoagulated patients with atrial fibrillation. *J. Am. Coll. Cardiol.* **2018**, *72*, 17–26. [CrossRef] [PubMed]
41. Li, P.K.T.; Burdmann, E.A.; Mehta, R.L. World kidney day 2013: Acute kidney injury—global health alert. *Am. J. Kidney Dis.* **2013**, *61*, 359–363. [CrossRef] [PubMed]
42. Liangos, O.; Wald, R.; O'Bell, J.W.; Price, L.; Pereira, B.J.; Jaber, B.L. Epidemiology and outcomes of acute renal failure in hospitalized patients: A national survey. *Clin. J. Am. Soc. Nephrol.* **2006**, *1*, 43–51. [CrossRef] [PubMed]

9

# Intraoperative Oliguria with Decreased SvO2 Predicts Acute Kidney Injury after Living Donor Liver Transplantation

**Won Ho Kim [1,2,*], Hyung-Chul Lee [1], Leerang Lim [1], Ho-Geol Ryu [1,2] and Chul-Woo Jung [1,2]**

1 Department of Anesthesiology and Pain Medicine, Seoul National University Hospital, Seoul 03080, Korea; azong@hanmail.net (H.-C.L.); erange@snu.ac.kr (L.L.); hogeol@gmail.com (H.-G.R.); jungcwoo@gmail.com (C.-W.J.)

2 Department of Anesthesiology and Pain Medicine, Seoul National University College of Medicine, Seoul 03080, Korea

* Correspondence: wonhokim@snu.ac.kr

**Abstract:** Acute kidney injury (AKI) is a frequent complication after living donor liver transplantation (LDLT), and is associated with increased mortality. However, the association between intraoperative oliguria and the risk of AKI remains uncertain for LDLT. We sought to determine the association between intraoperative oliguria alone and oliguria coupled with hemodynamic derangement and the risk of AKI after LDLT. We evaluated the hemodynamic variables, including mean arterial pressure, cardiac index, and mixed venous oxygen saturation ($SvO_2$). We reviewed 583 adult patients without baseline renal dysfunction and who did not receive hydroxyethyl starch during surgery. AKI was defined using the Kidney Disease Improving Global Outcomes criteria according to the serum creatinine criteria. Multivariable logistic regression analysis was performed with and without oliguria and oliguria coupled with a decrease in $SvO_2$. The performance was compared with respect to the area under the receiver operating characteristic curve (AUC). Intraoperative oliguria <0.5 and <0.3 mL/kg/h were significantly associated with the risk of AKI; however, their performance in predicting AKI was poor. The AUC of single predictors increased significantly when oliguria was combined with decreased $SvO_2$ (AUC 0.72; 95% confidence interval (CI) 0.68–0.75 vs. AUC of oliguria alone 0.61; 95% CI 0.56–0.61; $p < 0.0001$; vs. AUC of $SvO_2$ alone 0.66; 95% CI 0.61–0.70; $p < 0.0001$). Addition of oliguria coupled with $SvO_2$ reduction also increased the AUC of multivariable prediction (AUC 0.87; 95% CI 0.84–0.90 vs. AUC with oliguria 0.73; 95% CI 0.69–0.77; $p < 0.0001$; vs. AUC with neither oliguria nor $SvO_2$ reduction 0.68; 95% CI 0.64–0.72; $p < 0.0001$). Intraoperative oliguria coupled with a decrease in $SvO_2$ may suggest the risk of AKI after LDLT more reliably than oliguria alone or decrease in $SvO_2$ alone. Intraoperative oliguria should be interpreted in conjunction with $SvO_2$ to predict AKI in patients with normal preoperative renal function and who did not receive hydroxyethyl starch during surgery.

**Keywords:** acute kidney injury; urine output; hemodynamics; living-donor liver transplantation

## 1. Introduction

The incidence of acute kidney injury (AKI) after orthotopic liver transplantation has been reported to be as high as 64% [1–4]. AKI is an important complication associated with poor graft survival and increased mortality [1,2,5–8]. Furthermore, post-transplant AKI is associated with the development of chronic kidney disease [3,9,10].

Diagnosis of AKI is based on elevation of serum creatinine and/or decrease in urine output in the currently available KDIGO (Kidney Disease Improving Global Outcomes) criteria [7,11].

However, serum creatinine and urine output criteria have been criticized due to inaccurate reflection of glomerular filtration rate, insensitivity to detect acute change in renal function, [12,13] and being influenced by many factors including use of diuretics and volume status. In this regard, biomarkers to detect the development of AKI early after surgery have been investigated and showed promising performance for early detection [14]. However, the accuracy of the biomarkers are still controversial and there is still no biomarker with performance as good as that of troponin for detecting myocardial infarction [14].

The current urine output criteria of AKI suggest that a urine flow rate of <0.5 mL/kg/h lasting for more than 6 h indicates stage 1 AKI [7,11]. A rate of 0.3 mL/kg/h indicates stage 3 AKI. These criteria are widely regarded as the cutoff values to determine AKI in critically ill patients [15,16]. However, urine output criteria are regarded as unreliable in predicting AKI after surgery, because oliguria may develop during surgery due to decreased preload or nephrotoxic drug in addition to intrarenal oliguria [17]. AKI may develop in the absence of oliguria and oliguria may develop due to external obstruction of urinary tract [18,19]. Furthermore, during living donor liver transplantation (LDLT), urine output is influenced by many other factors, including baseline hepatorenal syndrome, cardiac preload condition, hemodynamics, sympathetic tone, and endocrine factors such as anti-diuretic hormones and aldosterone. Therefore, clinical significance of oliguria that is associated with postoperative AKI may be different from the currently available diagnostic criteria.

The etiology of acute kidney injury during surgery includes hemodynamic instability that may result in decreased renal perfusion. During LDLT, intraoperative hemodynamic variables including continuous arterial pressure, cardiac index, and mixed venous oxygen saturation ($SvO_2$) from pulmonary artery catheter are frequently monitored, although less invasive monitoring is increasingly used. Oliguria coupled with the deterioration in these hemodynamic variables may predict AKI better than oliguria alone because the other causes of oliguria that are not associated with AKI could be excluded. Oliguria developed from poor renal perfusion and oxygen delivery may be more strongly associated with AKI after LDLT.

Therefore, in the present study, we aimed to investigate the specific impact of intraoperative oliguria on the risk of AKI after LDLT determined by KDIGO criteria. We also hypothesized that oliguria coupled with low mean arterial blood pressure, low cardiac index, or low $SvO_2$ may predict AKI after LDLT better than oliguria alone. The objective of this retrospective study was to compare the association of intraoperative oliguria alone with oliguria observed with hemodynamic deterioration on the risk of AKI after LDLT.

## 2. Materials and Methods

### 2.1. Study Design

This retrospective observational study was approved by the institutional review board of Seoul National University Hospital (1608-073-784). We reviewed the electronic medical records of 1211 consecutive adult patients who had undergone liver transplantation at our institution between 2004 and 2015. The need for informed consent was waived because the study had a retrospective design. Patients who received deceased donor liver transplantation ($n$ = 367), those who had baseline renal dysfunction with an estimated glomerular filtration rate of <60 mL/min/1.73m$^2$ and/or with hepatorenal syndrome ($n$ = 73), and those who received hydroxyethyl starch during surgery ($n$ = 188) were excluded from the analysis. The remaining 583 patients who had undergone LDLT were analyzed.

### 2.2. Anesthesia, Surgical Technique and Immunosuppression

During the study period, the anesthesia protocol of our institution was as follows. Anesthesia was induced and maintained using propofol, rocuronium, and sevoflurane. Volume-controlled ventilation was maintained, with a tidal volume of 6–8 mL kg$^{-1}$ and a $FiO_2$ of 0.5. Arterial-line catheters were inserted into the radial and femoral arteries. A Swan-Ganz catheter was inserted through a 9-Fr Advanced Venous Access catheter (Edward Lifesciences, Irvine, CA, USA) that was placed in the right internal jugular vein. Continuous cardiac index and right ventricle-associated variables were monitored using the Vigilance II monitor (Edward Lifesciences, Irvine, CA, USA). The cause of hypotension was determined on the basis of cardiac index, stroke volume variation, $SvO_2$ and systemic vascular resistance and was treated using either (1) ephedrine and continuous dopamine, (2) phenylephrine and norepinephrine, and/or (3) epinephrine. Donor grafts were prepared using a histidine-tryptophan-ketoglutarate solution. The piggyback technique was used to anastomose the graft and donor vessels. End-to-end anastomosis of the hepatic artery and duct-to-duct anastomosis of the bile duct were carried out in succession. During surgery, immunosuppression was induced using 500 mg of methylprednisolone (Solumedrol, Pfizer, Ballerup, Denmark) and 20 mg of intravenous basiliximab (Simulect, Novartis Pharma B.V., Arnhem, The Netherlands). During the postoperative period, immunosuppression was induced using calcineurin inhibitors of either tacrolimus or cyclosporine with mycophenolate mofetil.

When intraoperative oliguria occurred during the study period, we administered crystalloid solutions to increase preload when surgical bleeding is evident or preload indices including central venous pressure, pulmonary artery occlusion pressure, and/or right ventricular end-diastolic volume indicated intravascular hypovolemia. Vasopressor was used to increase renal perfusion pressure when urine output decreased with euvolemia. Diuretics were used only when intravascular volume overload was suspected with elevated central venous pressure, pulmonary artery occlusion pressure, and/or right ventricular end-diastolic volume. Diuretics were not used to treat intraoperative oliguria.

The following crystalloid fluids were used to optimize the preload during LDLT before 2010: lactated Ringer's solution, normal saline, and plasmalyte, and hydroxyethyl starch (Voluven, Fresenius Kabi, Germany). The administration rate of crystalloid during LDLT was adjusted according to the hemodynamic preload index of central venous pressure, pulmonary artery occlusion pressure, and stroke volume variation. The hematocrit threshold for red blood cell transfusion was 20% during LDLT throughout the study period. Intraoperative diuretics (furosemide; 10–20 mg) were used in patients with persistent positive fluid balance and when volume overload was suspected due to a pulmonary artery wedge pressure greater 18 mmHg.

### 2.3. Data Collection

Based on previous literature, demographic and perioperative variables known to be related to postoperative renal dysfunction or AKI were collected [1,4,5,20–22]. Preoperatively, the Model for End-stage Liver Disease (MELD) score, the Child-Turcotte-Pugh (CTP) score, and the Child classification were determined for all recipients [23]. The following variables were also collected: history of hypertension, diabetes mellitus, ABO blood type incompatibility, preoperative serum albumin, preoperative diuretic medication, graft macrosteatosis, graft ischemic time, postoperative platelet count, intraoperative blood loss, intraoperative transfusion volume, intraoperative diuretics use, and mean tacrolimus trough concentration during the first week after surgery [20,24]. The mean urine output during surgery was calculated by averaging the intraoperative data obtained from the electronic medical records. Urine output was measured hourly in a urine bag connected to a Foley catheter.

The resting arterial blood pressure before anesthesia induction was used as baseline blood pressure. The initially measured cardiac index and $SvO_2$ by pulmonary artery catheter and the Vigilance II monitor were used as a baseline. Sudden decrease in mean arterial pressure, cardiac index, and $SvO_2$ lower than 20% from baseline for at least one measurement was identified and recorded as a categorized variable.

The primary outcome variable was postoperative AKI, as defined using the KDIGO criteria, which have been validated in patients undergoing LDLT [10]. We determined postoperative AKI based on the maximal change in serum creatinine level during the first seven postoperative days [25]. No urine output criteria were used due to the purpose of our study. Although the oliguria criteria of

KDIGO requires that oliguria last more than 6 h, oliguria was determined based on the average urine out during surgery, regardless of its duration, in our study.

### 2.4. Statistical Analysis

SPSS software version 23.0 (IBM Corp., Armonk, NY, USA) and STATA/MP version 15.1 (StataCorp, College Station, TX, USA) were used to analyze the data. In all analyses, $p$-values $< 0.05$ were considered statistically significant. The Kolmogorov-Smirnov test was used to determine the normality of the data. All the continuous covariates listed in Table 1 followed non-parametric distribution. To compare all continuous variables in Table 1 and the urine output between those with and without AKI, the Mann-Whitney U test was used. Data were missing in fewer than 5% of records. We imputed the missing values according to the incidence of missing data. If the incidence of missing was < 1%, the missing data were substituted by the mean for continuous variables and by the mode for incidence variables. Missing values of variables with a ratio of missing data >1% and <5% were replaced by hot-deck imputation.

**Table 1.** Patient characteristics and perioperative parameters.

| Characteristic | No AKI Group ($n$ = 378) | AKI Group ($n$ = 205) | $p$-Values |
|---|---|---|---|
| **Demographic data** | | | |
| Age, years | 53 (47–58) | 53 (49–58) | 0.405 |
| Female, n | 85 (22.5) | 63 (30.7) | 0.029 |
| Body-mass index, kg/m$^2$ | 22.9 (21.0–24.8) | 23.3 (21.6–26.1) | 0.008 |
| **Background medical status** | | | |
| Hypertension, $n$ | 39 (10.3) | 12 (5.9) | 0.069 |
| Diabetes mellitus, $n$ | 47 (12.4) | 22 (10.7) | 0.544 |
| Alcoholic liver cirrhosis, $n$ | 44 (11.6) | 25 (12.2) | 0.843 |
| HBV hepatitis, $n$ | 159 (42.1) | 71 (34.6) | 0.080 |
| HCV hepatitis, $n$ | 25 (6.6) | 12 (5.9) | 0.719 |
| Hepatocellular carcinoma, $n$ | 209 (55.3) | 113 (55.1) | 0.969 |
| Cholestatic disease, $n$ | 7 (1.9) | 6 (2.9) | 0.401 |
| Preoperative hemoglobin, g/dL | 11.5 (9.7–13.2) | 10.2 (8.9–11.9) | <0.001 |
| Preoperative serum albumin level, g/dL | 3.0 (2.5–3.6) | 2.8 (2.5–3.2) | 0.002 |
| Preoperative serum creatinine, mg/dL | 0.90 (0.75–1.10) | 0.85 (0.68–1.04) | 0.014 |
| Preoperative estimated glomerular filtration rate, mL/min | 88 (70–109) | 94 (75–122) | 0.021 |
| MELD score | 13 (9–21) | 17 (11–21) | 0.001 |
| Child-Turcotte-Pugh score | 8 (6–11) | 9 (7–11) | <0.001 |
| Child class, n (A/ B/ C) | 109 (33.5)/96 (29.5)/120 (36.9) | 28 (16.2)/61 (35.3)/84 (48.6) | <0.001 |
| Preoperative LVEF. % | 65 (61–68) | 65 (62–68) | 0.254 |
| Preoperative beta-blocker, $n$ | 29 (7.7) | 13 (6.3) | 0.645 |
| Preoperative diuretics, $n$ | 16 (4.2) | 12 (5.9) | 0.382 |
| **Donor/ graft factors** | | | |
| Age, years | 31 (23–41) | 30 (23–38) | 0.302 |
| Estimated GRWR | 1.17 (1.01–1.46) | 1.16 (1.00–1.41 | 0.396 |
| ABO incompatible, $n$ | 19 (5.0) | 10 (4.9) | 0.937 |
| **Operation and anesthesia details** | | | |
| Operation time, h | 7.0 (6.1–8.2) | 7.6 (6.5–8.6) | 0.001 |
| Cold ischemic time, min | 71 (58–83) | 78 (65–95) | <0.001 |
| Warm ischemic time, min | 31 (23–40) | 32 (26–41) | 0.142 |
| Intraoperative furosemide use, $n$ | 71 (18.8) | 52 (25.4) | 0.063 |
| Intraoperative furosemide dose, mg | 0 (0–0) | 0 (0–5) | 0.040 |
| Intraoperative use of epinephrine, $n$ | 148 (39.2) | 81 (39.5) | 0.933 |
| Intraoperative dose of epinephrine, mcg | 0 (0–10) | 0 (0–5) | 0.603 |
| Intraoperative mean blood glucose, mg/dL | 163 (144–178) | 164 (145–183) | 0.216 |
| Intraoperative highest blood glucose, mg/dL | 211 (194–230) | 218 (200–238) | 0.012 |
| Mean trough level of tacrolimus during posmiddleerative first week (ng/mL) | 6.2 (3.2–8.5) | 6.5 (3.4–9.1) | 0.098 |

**Table 1.** *Cont.*

| Characteristic | No AKI Group ($n$ = 378) | AKI Group ($n$ = 205) | $p$-Values |
|---|---|---|---|
| **Bleeding and transfusion amount** | | | |
| pRBC transfusion, units | 4 (0–10) | 6 (3–12) | <0.001 |
| FFP transfusion, units | 4 (0–8) | 6 (2–12) | <0.001 |
| Blood loss per body weight, mL/kg | 33 (18–64) | 47 (23–91) | <0.001 |
| **Input and output during surgery** | | | |
| Intraoperative average urine flow rate, mL/kg/h | 1.36 (0.89–2.08) | 1.15 (0.76–1.72) | 0.007 |
| Crystalloid administration, mL/kg | 53 (37–73) | 57 (40–85) | 0.007 |
| Net fluid balance during surgery, mL/kg | 31 (13–52) | 36 (18–59) | 0.072 |

The values are expressed as the mean (standard deviation) or median [interquartile range] or number (%). AKI = acute kidney injury; MELD score = model for end-stage liver disease score; GRWR = graft to recipient body weight ratio; pRBC = packed red blood cell; FFP = fresh frozen plasma. Net fluid balance was calculated by total input subtracted by total output.

The following is a summary of our statistical analysis. First, we determined the cutoff of intraoperative mean urine output by multivariable logistic regression analysis. Second, according to oliguria using the cutoff, we compared the predictive ability of the oliguria alone with that of oliguria coupled with a decrease in mean arterial pressure, cardiac index, and $SvO_2$. Third, we evaluated whether the oliguria coupled with hemodynamic derangement could enhance the AUC of the multivariable prediction model for AKI after LDLT.

Multivariable logistic regression analysis was performed (1) to find an optimal cutoff of oliguria, and (2) to evaluate the association between perioperative variables and postoperative AKI. The following variables were considered potential risk factors of AKI after LDLT in addition to oliguria and hemodynamic variables: age, sex, body-mass index, year of operation, MELD score, CTP score, hypertension, diabetes mellitus, preoperative hemoglobin level, preoperative serum albumin, preoperative serum creatinine, ABO blood type incompatibility, operation time, graft ischemic time, preoperative diuretics use, intraoperative blood loss, intraoperative crystalloid and colloid administration, transfusion amount and total dose of diuretics administered during surgery. We did not perform any univariable screening before the multivariable analysis. A $p$-value < 0.20 was used to select for significant predictors in the multivariable analysis, with the backward stepwise variable selection. We also performed multivariable logistic regression analysis without stepwise variable selection.

Three different cutoffs of intraoperative mean intraoperative urine flow rate including 1.0, 0.5, and 0.3 mL/kg/h were evaluated, because oliguria less than these cutoffs was significantly associated with postoperative AKI in our preliminary multivariable logistic regression analysis using perioperative baseline variables with mean urine output with different cutoffs (Supplemental Table S1).

To compare the predictive ability of oliguria using these cutoffs with that of oliguria coupled with three hemodynamic variables, the area under the receiver operating characteristic curve (AUC) was calculated for every single potential predictor. Also, performance measurements including sensitivity, specificity, positive predictive value (PPV), and negative predictive value (NPV) were compared.

Multivariable logistic regression analysis was performed again by adding the predictors of oliguria coupled with hemodynamic variables. Then, the AUCs of a multivariable prediction model with and without these oliguria coupled with hemodynamic variables were compared to evaluate whether these combined predictors could increase the predictive ability of multivariable prediction model. The comparison between AUCs was performed using De Long' s method [26].

## 3. Results

During the first postoperative week, AKI, as determined using the KDIGO criteria, occurred in 205 patients (35.2%), and stage $\geq$2 AKI occurred in 43 patients (7.4%). Patient demographics and perioperative variables were compared between the patients with and without AKI in Table 1. The distribution of mean intraoperative mean urine flow rate is shown in Supplemental Figure S1.

The median (interquartile ranges) of mean urine output were 1.15 (0.76–1.71) for those with AKI and 1.36 (0.89–2.08) for those without AKI. The mean intraoperative urine output was significantly lower in patients with AKI than in those without AKI ($p = 0.007$).

The odds ratios, 95% CI and their $p$-values according to oliguria with different cutoffs are shown in Supplemental Table S1. Multivariable logistic regression analysis showed that oliguria <0.5 and <0.3 mL/kg/h were significantly associated with AKI.

The performances to predict postoperative AKI of a single variable of oliguria, a single variable of 20% decrease in hemodynamic variables, and their combined variables were compared in terms of AUC, sensitivity, specificity, PPV, and NPV (Table 2). Three different cutoffs of 0.3, 0.5, and 1.0 mL/kg/h were used, and hemodynamic variables included mean arterial pressure, cardiac index, and $SvO_2$. AUC was largest for oliguria <0.5 mL/kg/h with $SvO_2$ reduction (AUC = 0.72, 95% CI 0.68–0.75).

**Table 2.** Comparisons of performance of risk factors between the oliguria with different cutoffs alone, 20% decreased hemodynamic variables alone, and their combined variables.

| Oliguria | Coupled Hemodynamic Variable | AUC (95% CI) | $p$-Value | Sensitivity | Specificity | PPV | NPV |
|---|---|---|---|---|---|---|---|
| <0.3 | None | 0.55 (0.50–0.60) | 0.031 | 16.1 | 94.7 | 62.3 | 60.5 |
| <0.5 | None | 0.60 (0.56–0.64) | <0.001 | 49.8 | 56.6 | 50.1 | 64.7 |
| <1.0 | None | 0.55 (0.50–0.60) | 0.040 | 53.7 | 48.7 | 38.3 | 69.8 |
| No | $SvO_2$ | 0.66 (0.61–0.70) | <0.001 | 57.1 | 79.1 | 59.7 | 77.3 |
| No | Cardiac index | 0.56 (0.52–0.61) | 0.011 | 62.0 | 50.8 | 40.6 | 71.1 |
| No | Mean arterial pressure | 0.53 (0.48–0.58) | 0.219 | 52.2 | 54.0 | 38.1 | 67.5 |
| <0.3 | $SvO_2$ | 0.61 (0.56–0.66) | <0.001 | 11.3 | 97.4 | 82.5 | 50.0 |
| <0.3 | Cardiac index | 0.55 (0.50–0.60) | 0.046 | 16.1 | 93.9 | 58.9 | 67.4 |
| <0.3 | Mean arterial pressure | 0.53 (0.48–0.58) | 0.191 | 13.2 | 91.4 | 51.9 | 66.5 |
| <0.5 | $SvO_2$ | 0.72 (0.68–0.75) | <0.001 | 59.1 | 86.5 | 69.6 | 78.8 |
| <0.5 | Cardiac index | 0.56 (0.52–0.60) | 0.011 | 37.6 | 75.1 | 45.0 | 68.9 |
| <0.5 | Mean arterial pressure | 0.53 (0.49–0.57) | 0.276 | 29.3 | 73.2 | 40.0 | 65.5 |
| <1.0 | $SvO_2$ | 0.58 (0.53–0.63) | 0.001 | 37.1 | 79.1 | 49.0 | 69.9 |
| <1.0 | Cardiac index | 0.52 (0.47–0.57) | 0.418 | 39.5 | 64.6 | 37.7 | 66.3 |
| <1.0 | Mean arterial pressure | 0.50 (0.45–0.55) | 0.929 | 30.2 | 69.3 | 34.8 | 64.7 |

AUC = area under the receiver operating characteristic curve, CI = confidence interval, $SvO_2$ = mixed venous oxygen saturation, PPV = positive predictive value, NPV = negative predictive value. Coupled hemodynamic variables mean 20% decrease of the hemodynamic variables compared to baseline. AUC of the univariable analysis was reported. $P$-value are the results of testing the null hypothesis of AUC is 0.50.

The AUCs of four single predictors of oliguria <0.5 mL/kg/h alone, oliguria coupled with mean arterial pressure reduction, oliguria with cardiac index reduction, and oliguria with $SvO_2$ reduction were compared in Figure 1. AUC of oliguria ≤0.5 mL/kg/h with $SvO_2$ 20% reduction was significantly greater than all other variables (oliguria with $SvO_2$ reduction: AUC 0.72, 95% CI 0.68–0.75 vs. oliguria alone: 0.60, 95% CI 0.56–0.64, $p < 0.001$; vs. oliguria with mean arterial pressure reduction: 0.53, 95% CI 0.49–0.57, $p < 0.001$; vs. oliguria with cardiac index reduction: 0.56, 95% CI 0.52–0.60, $p < 0.001$).

The results of multivariable logistic regression analysis to predict postoperative AKI with and without including oliguria <0.5 mL/kg/h coupled with $SvO_2$ reduction are shown in Table 3. The Nagelkerke's $R^2$ of the model with and without oliguria with $SvO_2$ reduction were 0.16 and 0.39, respectively. Both models showed good calibration (Hosmer-Lemeshow goodness of fit: chi-square = 2.33, 8.76 and $p = 0.264$, 0.567, respectively). The results of multivariable logistic regression analysis without stepwise variable selection are shown in Supplemental Table S1.

The AUCs of (1) the multivariable prediction without oliguria or $SvO_2$, (2) multivariable prediction with oliguria <0.5 mL/kg/h, and (3) multivariable prediction with oliguria <0.5 mL/kg/h coupled with $SvO_2$ reduction are compared in Figure 2 (AUC of oliguria coupled with $SvO_2$ reduction: 0.87, 95% CI 0.84–0.90 vs. AUC without oliguria or $SvO_2$ reduction: 0.68, 95% CI 0.64–0.72, $p < 0.0001$; vs. AUC with oliguria: 0.73, 95% CI 0.69–0.77, $p < 0.0001$).

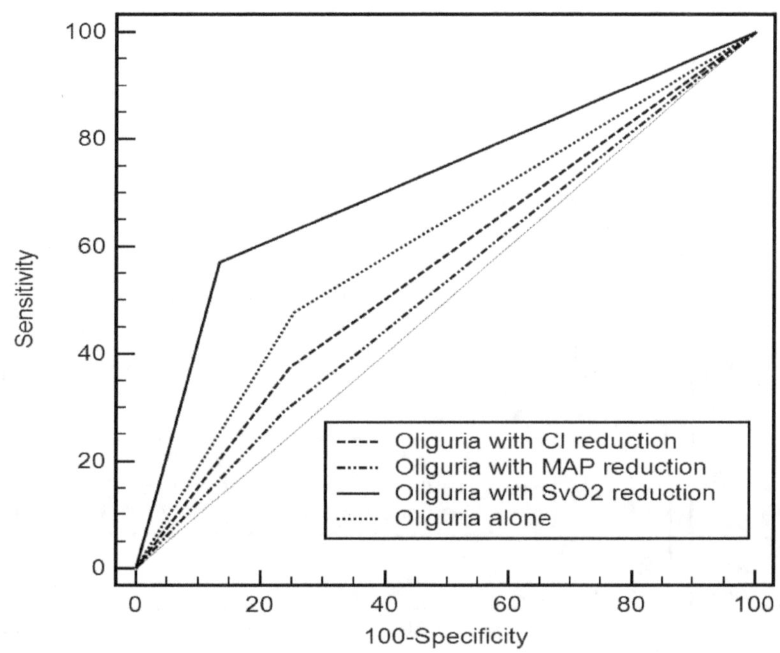


**Figure 1.** Comparison of area under the receiver operating characteristic curve between the four predictors of oliguria alone and oliguria coupled with hemodynamic variables including mean arterial pressure (MAP), cardiac index (CI), and mixed venous oxygen saturation ($SvO_2$). Oliguria used a cutoff of 0.5 mL/kg/h and hemodynamic variables used 20% reduction from their baseline values. AUC of oliguria $\leq$ 0.5 mL/kg/h with $SvO_2$ 20% reduction was significantly greater than all other variables (oliguria coupled with $SvO_2$ reduction: AUC 0.72, 95% CI 0.68–0.75 vs. oliguria alone: 0.60, 95% CI 0.56–0.64, $p < 0.001$; vs. oliguria coupled with mean arterial pressure reduction: 0.53, 95% CI 0.49–0.57, $p < 0.001$; vs. oliguria coupled with cardiac index reduction: 0.56, 95% CI 0.52–0.60, $p < 0.001$).

**Table 3.** Multivariable logistic regression analysis to predict acute kidney injury after liver transplantation with and without oliguria or hemodynamic variables.

| Variable | Odds Ratio | 95% CI | *p*-Value |
|---|---|---|---|
| **Without urine output or hemodynamic variables** | | | |
| Body-mass index, kg/m$^2$ | 1.09 | 1.03–1.16 | 0.004 |
| Preoperative hemoglobin, g/dL | 0.86 | 0.77–0.95 | 0.004 |
| Preoperative albumin, g/dL | 0.88 | 0.68–1.15 | 0.158 |
| Operation time, h | 1.07 | 0.94–1.22 | 0.123 |
| Cold ischemic time, min | 1.02 | 1.01–1.03 | <0.001 |
| Red blood cell transfusion, unit | 1.10 | 1.05–1.12 | 0.010 |
| Crystalloid administration, per 10 mL/kg | 1.07 | 1.00–1.15 | 0.068 |
| **Including urine output coupled with hemodynamic variables** | | | |
| Body-mass index, kg/m$^2$ | 1.12 | 1.05–1.20 | 0.001 |
| Preoperative hemoglobin, g/dL | 0.89 | 0.79–0.99 | 0.041 |
| Preoperative diuretics | 1.68 | 0.58–4.89 | 0.139 |
| Operation time, h | 1.12 | 0.91–1.34 | 0.236 |
| Cold ischemic time, min | 1.02 | 1.01–1.03 | 0.003 |
| Crystalloid administration, per 10 mL/kg | 1.08 | 1.02–1.15 | 0.011 |
| $SvO_2$ reduction with oliguria <0.5 mL/kg/h | 7.64 | 4.82–12.11 | <0.001 |

Two separate logistic regression analysis was performed with and without intraoperative mean urine flow rate and intraoperative hemodynamic variables. CI = confidence interval. Stepwise backward variable selection was used and cutoff of $p < 0.20$ was used to select the variables.

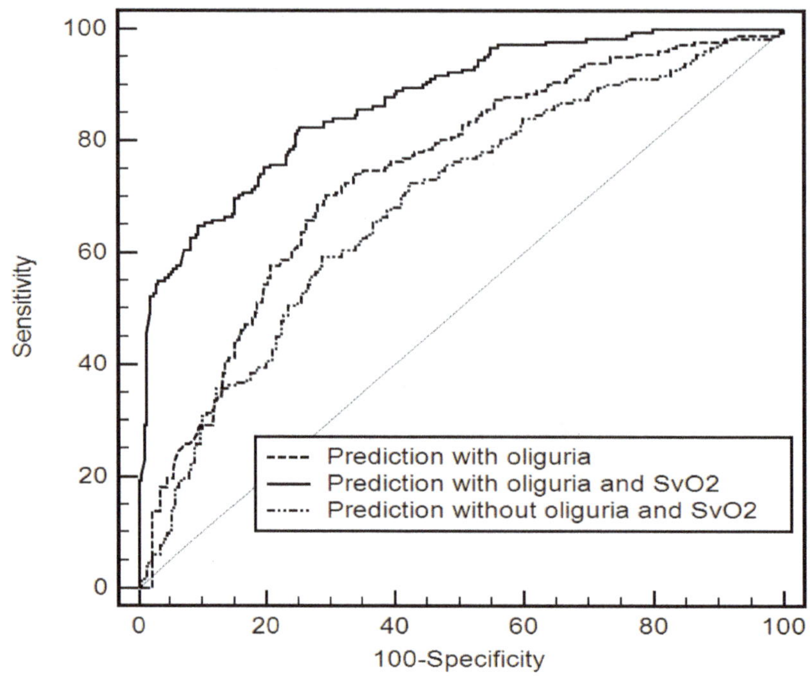


**Figure 2.** Comparison of area under the receiver operating characteristic curve between the multivariable prediction models (1) without oliguria or mixed venous oxygen saturation ($SvO_2$) reduction, (2) with oliguria, and (3) with oliguria coupled with $SvO_2$ reduction. AUC of model with oliguria coupled with $SvO_2$ reduction was significantly greater than AUCs of model without $SvO_2$ reduction (AUC with oliguria coupled with $SvO_2$ reduction: 0.87, 95% CI 0.84–0.90 vs. AUC without oliguria or $SvO_2$ reduction: 0.68, 95% CI 0.64–0.72, $p < 0.0001$; vs. AUC with oliguria: 0.73, 95% CI 0.69–0.77, $p < 0.0001$).

## 4. Discussion

To our knowledge, the present study was the first to evaluate the association between intraoperative mean urine output, hemodynamic variables, and AKI after LDLT. Although there was a significant association between oliguria <1.0, <0.5 and <0.3 mL/kg/h and risk of AKI, the predictive ability of oliguria alone was relatively poor and did not add substantial additional discriminative power in multivariable prediction. However, when oliguria developed in association with decreased $SvO_2$, the AUC of a single predictor significantly increased, while oliguria coupled with mean arterial blood pressure or cardiac index failed to increase the AUC. These results suggested that oliguria accompanied by a reduction in $SvO_2$ during LDLT may be more strongly associated with the development of AKI than oliguria or reduction in $SvO_2$ alone. The AUC of multivariable prediction showed similar results and the model including oliguria coupled with decreased $SvO_2$ showed significantly higher performance in terms of AUC and Nagelkerke's $R^2$. Although oliguria alone is not specific and has little value in predicting AKI after LDLT, oliguria coupled with a decrease in cardiac output or $SvO_2$ could significantly increase the sensitivity and predictive ability for AKI after LDLT. However, our results should not be applied to the patients with poor baseline renal function including hepatorenal syndrome and the patients who received hydroxyethyl starch during surgery. Also, our results should be interpreted cautiously, because our oliguria was determined by the intraoperative mean value and the duration of oliguria was not considered.

The urine output criteria of the RIFLE criteria (Risk, Injury, Failure, Loss of function, and End-stage renal disease) and the AKIN (AKI network) criteria are widely used to diagnose AKI [7]. The clinical implications of the oliguria criteria have been validated in a critical care setting [27,28]. However, intraoperative oliguria is regarded as less predictive of postoperative AKI compared to non-surgical settings [29]. AKI determined by serum creatinine may develop without oliguria, and AKI may not develop despite the intraoperative oliguria. Furthermore, recent studies have suggested that the urine output criteria for AKI in surgical patients may be different from the previous commonly used value of 0.5 mL/kg/h [30,31].

Several studies have attempted to derive urine output thresholds that identify AKI in surgical patients [30–32]. Using a methodology that was similar to ours, one retrospective study in cardiac surgical patients undergoing cardiopulmonary bypass identified a urine flow rate of <1.5 mL/kg/h as a cutoff that was associated with AKI risk [30]. Another retrospective study involving major abdominal surgery reported that <0.3 mL/kg/h was the threshold of the risk of AKI [31]. As such, the threshold urine output to diagnose AKI may vary depending on the surgical setting. Therefore, we first identified the optimal cutoff of oliguria that is significantly associated with AKI after LDLT in our study sample. However, in these studies, the predictive ability of intraoperative oliguria has not been evaluated fully.

Along with the usual <0.5 or <0.3 mL/kg/h cutoff of oliguria, our analysis suggested significant associations between low urine flow rate of <1.0 mL/kg/h and risk of AKI after LDLT. We evaluated the cutoff of oliguria up to 3.0 mL/kg/h because previous studies reported different cutoffs of oliguria during surgery [30–32] (Supplemental Table S2). The significant threshold of <1.0 mL/kg/h may be influenced by the intraoperative diuretics use. More than 20% of our patients received diuretics before or intraoperatively. Our subgroup analysis after excluding all patients who administered diuretics pre- or intraoperatively ($n$ = 435) showed that <1.0 mL/kg/h was not significantly associated with postoperative AKI (Supplemental Table S3).

The performance of oliguria in predicting AKI defined by creatinine criteria was poor at any cutoff (Table 2). AUC was only between 0.55 to 0.60, with low sensitivity and specificity. Addition of oliguria <1.5 mL/kg/h did not significantly improve the predictive ability of multivariable prediction model for AKI. It seems that oliguria during LDLT is neither a sensitive nor specific marker of AKI—i.e., the patients with the same mean urine flow rate may or may not develop AKI. Although hemodynamic variables of $SvO_2$ showed a slightly better performance as a single predictor, the other hemodynamic variables did not. However, oliguria coupled with a decrease in $SvO_2$ showed a significantly better performance as a single predictor and enhanced the predictive ability of multivariable prediction when included in the multivariable logistic model.

A low $SvO_2$ may suggest poor oxygen delivery to the kidney [33]. During LDLT, decreased preload by intraoperative bleeding may decrease cardiac output and thereby impair renal perfusion. An ischemia/reperfusion injury of the kidney may develop especially during liver graft reperfusion [34]. A low $SvO_2$ during LDLT reflects decreased oxygen delivery by low cardiac output to the major organs including kidney. When oliguria developed in a patient who experienced a decrease in $SvO_2$, the oliguria of the patient is more likely to be caused by poor renal perfusion and oxygen delivery to the kidney. Meanwhile, the oliguria alone may not be associated with poor oxygen delivery to the kidney but associated with an extrarenal cause such as a transient decrease in preload or urinary tract obstruction.

However, decrease in cardiac index or mean arterial pressure combined with oliguria did not increase AUC to predict AKI after LDLT. Mean arterial pressure is not a sensitive marker to measure the cardiac output and oxygen delivery to the major organ especially in patients with significant cirrhosis or during and after reperfusion with unequal vasodilation [35]. Cardiac index could be more important than mean arterial pressure. However, in patients with liver cirrhosis, 20% decrease in cardiac index may not be meaningful in patients with cirrhosis and hyperdynamic hemodynamics with already elevated baseline cardiac output. Also, a previous study reported that there was a poor correlation between cardiac index and $SvO_2$ during liver transplantation [36].

Several urinary or serum biomarkers were reported to be sensitive to predict AKI after surgery [37–39]. The performance of neutrophil gelatinase-associated lipocalin (NGAL) to predict AKI after surgery in terms of AUC was reported to be 0.82 to 0.83 after cardiac surgery [40]. The AUC of urinary NGAL on postoperative day one to predict AKI after liver transplantation was 0.79 [41]. Considering these AUC, the performance of our multivariable prediction could be regarded as similar to that of NGAL. In addition to NGAL, many other promising biomarkers have been reported including kidney injury molecule-1 (KIM-1), interleukin-18, liver-type fatty-acid binding protein (L-FABP), angiotensinogen [42], tissue inhibitor of metalloproteinase-2 (TIMP-2), and insulin-like growth factor-binding protein-3 (IGFBP-3) [38,43]. Two recent studies reported that biomarker-guided implementation of KDIGO interventions could decrease the incidence of AKI after cardiac and major abdominal surgery [44,45]. However, the performance of these biomarkers are still controversial [46] and there seems to be a long way to go before incorporating the biomarkers into our routine perioperative practice.

Hemodynamic optimization may protect renal function in surgical patient [47]. Our results may suggest that hemodynamic goals should not be managed step-by-step—i.e., firstly, optimize preload; secondly, optimize contractility; thirdly, optimize afterload, and so on—and should be interpreted comprehensively. Goal-directed therapy algorithm usually establishes several hemodynamic goals first and do not pay attention to the remaining goals until the first goal, usually preload index, is achieved. However, hemodynamic goals including preload, afterload, and oxygenation index, as well as urine output, are associated with each other. Therefore, we suggest that intraoperative urine flow rate should be interpreted in conjunction with other hemodynamic parameters such as cardiac index or $SvO_2$. However, routine use of pulmonary artery catheter has been a subject of debate. A previous multicenter trial reported no difference in mortality in high-risk surgical patients with and without hemodynamic management guided by pulmonary artery catheter [48]. Pulmonary artery catheter was associated with higher risk of pulmonary embolism. The use of less invasive monitoring with central venous oxygen saturation may substitute the $SvO_2$ monitoring with pulmonary artery catheter [49].

There was a significant difference in gender distribution between the patients with and without AKI (Table 1). The incidence of female was significantly higher in the AKI group compared to the no-AKI group, which was consistent with a previous study [50], albeit not in other studies [1,20]. However, female was not an independent predictor in our multivariable analysis, suggesting that female gender is associated with other significant covariates. We compared the independent predictors identified in our multivariable analysis between male and female groups (Supplemental Table S3) and found that female was associated with significantly lower preoperative hemoglobin, and larger intraoperative crystalloid administration compared to male group in our study population.

The present study had several limitations. Firstly, it was a single-center retrospective analysis, and urine flow rate data collected from the medical records may have been inaccurate. Furthermore, our cutoff for urine output may not be extrapolated to other institutions with different fluid management strategy and different baseline medical conditions, although multivariable adjustment was performed in this study. The intraoperative urine output may differ markedly depending on the intraoperative goal of fluid management, transfusion amount and intraoperative diuretics or hydroxyethyl starch use. Secondly, in our analysis, we used a mean urine flow rate during surgery rather than hourly urine output. However, oliguria lasting for longer than 6 h is required for the KDIGO criteria. Furthermore, there may be critical periods during LDLT, such as the anhepatic or reperfusion period, which involve unstable hemodynamics and severe metabolic acidosis [34]. In future studies, duration of oliguria as well as phases of LDLT when oliguria developed should be considered when investigating the association of oliguria with AKI. Different oliguria cutoffs should be considered including 1.0 mL/kg/h. Thirdly, we did not consider the duration of a decrease in hemodynamic variables. We evaluated the association between the decrease in hemodynamic variables for at least one measurement and AKI. Our electronic record has data of most hemodynamic variables in 5-min intervals. Further studies may investigate the possible dose-response relationship between the duration of hemodynamic deterioration and the risk of AKI. Fourthly, since our study was a retrospective analysis and intraoperative mean urine output was used for analysis, the temporal relationship between oliguria and decrease in hemodynamic variables could not be identified. The risk of AKI may be different between oliguria following deterioration in hemodynamic variables and oliguria with no temporal relationship hemodynamic derangement.

## 5. Conclusions

Intraoperative oliguria alone could not accurately predict AKI after LDLT determined by creatinine criteria, although there were significant associations using a cutoff of oliguria <1.0, <0.5 and <0.3 mL/kg/h. However, when oliguria with these cutoffs was found with decreased intraoperative $SvO_2$, the performance to predict AKI improved significantly and the predictive ability of multivariable prediction model was significantly enhanced. Decrease in cardiac index or mean arterial blood pressure combined with oliguria did not significantly increase the AUC to predict AKI after LDLT. Intraoperative oliguria interpreted in conjunction with a decrease in $SvO_2$ may suggest the risk of AKI after LDLT more reliably in patients with normal baseline renal function and who did not receive hydroxyethyl starch during transplantation surgery.

**Supplementary Materials:**
Supplemental Table S1. Multivariable logistic regression analysis to predict acute kidney injury after liver transplantation without stepwise variable selection. Supplemental Table S2. Odds ratios (95% confidence intervals) and their P-values according to the categorized intraoperative urine flow rate with different cutoffs determined by both the univariable and multivariable logistic regression analysis for acute kidney injury. Supplemental Table S3. Subgroup analysis for the patients who had not received diuretics either before or during surgery ($n$ = 435). Odds ratios (95% confidence intervals) and their p-values according to the categorized intraoperative urine flow rate with different cutoffs determined by both the univariable and multivariable logistic regression analysis for acute kidney injury were shown. Supplemental Table S4. Comparisons of independent predictors of the multivariable logistic regression analysis of our study between male and female. Supplemental Figure S1. Distribution of mean urine flow rate during liver transplantation surgery in all patients (upper), and box and whisker plots of urine flow rate during liver transplantation surgery with and without postoperative acute kidney injury (lower).

**Author Contributions:** W.H.K.: conceptualization, data curation, formal analysis, investigation, methodology, visualization, writing—original draft; H.C.L.: data curation, formal analysis, writing—review and editing; C-W.J.: supervision, writing—review and editing; L.L., H.-G.R.: writing—review and editing.

## References

1. Utsumi, M.; Umeda, Y.; Sadamori, H.; Nagasaka, T.; Takaki, A.; Matsuda, H.; Shinoura, S.; Yoshida, R.; Nobuoka, D.; Satoh, D.; et al. Risk factors for acute renal injury in living donor liver transplantation: Evaluation of the RIFLE criteria. *Transpl. Int.* **2013**, *26*, 842–852. [CrossRef] [PubMed]
2. Zhu, M.; Li, Y.; Xia, Q.; Wang, S.; Qiu, Y.; Che, M.; Dai, H.; Qian, J.; Ni, Z.; Axelsson, J.; et al. Strong impact of acute kidney injury on survival after liver transplantation. *Transplant. Proc.* **2010**, *42*, 3634–3638. [CrossRef] [PubMed]
3. Ferreira, A.C.; Nolasco, F.; Carvalho, D.; Sampaio, S.; Baptista, A.; Pessegueiro, P.; Monteiro, E.; Mourão, L.; Barroso, E. Impact of RIFLE classification in liver transplantation. *Clin. Transplant.* **2010**, *24*, 394–400. [CrossRef] [PubMed]
4. Chen, J.; Singhapricha, T.; Hu, K.Q.; Hong, J.C.; Steadman, R.H.; Busuttil, R.W.; Xia, V.W. Postliver transplant acute renal injury and failure by the RIFLE criteria in patients with normal pretransplant serum creatinine concentrations: A matched study. *Transplantation* **2011**, *91*, 348–353. [CrossRef] [PubMed]
5. Lebron Gallardo, M.; Herrera Gutierrez, M.E.; Seller Perez, G.; Curiel Balsera, E.; Fernandez Ortega, J.F.; Quesada Garcia, G. Risk factors for renal dysfunction in the postoperative course of liver transplant. *Liver Transpl.* **2004**, *10*, 1379–1385. [CrossRef] [PubMed]
6. Barri, Y.M.; Sanchez, E.Q.; Jennings, L.W.; Melton, L.B.; Hays, S.; Levy, M.F.; Klintmalm, G.B. Acute kidney injury following liver transplantation: Definition and outcome. *Liver Transpl.* **2009**, *15*, 475–483. [CrossRef] [PubMed]
7. Thomas, M.E.; Blaine, C.; Dawnay, A.; Devonald, M.A.; Ftouh, S.; Laing, C.; Latchem, S.; Lewington, A.; Milford, D.V.; Ostermann, M. The definition of acute kidney injury and its use in practice. *Kidney Int.* **2015**, *87*, 62–73. [CrossRef]
8. Gameiro, J.; Agapito Fonseca, J.; Jorge, S.; Lopes, J.A. Acute Kidney Injury Definition and Diagnosis: A Narrative Review. *J. Clin. Med.* **2018**, *7*, 307. [CrossRef]

9. Paramesh, A.S.; Roayaie, S.; Doan, Y.; Schwartz, M.E.; Emre, S.; Fishbein, T.; Florman, S.; Gondolesi, G.E.; Krieger, N.; Ames, S.; et al. Post-liver transplant acute renal failure: Factors predicting development of end-stage renal disease. *Clin. Transplant.* **2004**, *18*, 94–99. [CrossRef]
10. Trinh, E.; Alam, A.; Tchervenkov, J.; Cantarovich, M. Impact of acute kidney injury following liver transplantation on long-term outcomes. *Clin. Transplant.* **2017**, *31*, e12863. [CrossRef]
11. Shin, S.R.; Kim, W.H.; Kim, D.J.; Shin, I.W.; Sohn, J.T. Prediction and Prevention of Acute Kidney Injury after Cardiac Surgery. *Biomed. Res. Int.* **2016**, *2016*, 2985148. [CrossRef] [PubMed]
12. Bellomo, R.; Kellum, J.A.; Ronco, C. Defining acute renal failure: Physiological principles. *Intensive Care Med.* **2004**, *30*, 33–37. [CrossRef] [PubMed]
13. Murray, P.T.; Le Gall, J.R.; Dos Reis Miranda, D.; Pinsky, M.R.; Tetta, C. Physiologic endpoints (efficacy) for acute renal failure studies. *Curr. Opin. Crit. Care* **2002**, *8*, 519–525. [CrossRef] [PubMed]
14. Alge, J.L.; Arthur, J.M. Biomarkers of AKI: A review of mechanistic relevance and potential therapeutic implications. *Clin. J. Am. Soc. Nephrol.* **2015**, *10*, 147–155. [CrossRef] [PubMed]
15. Chenitz, K.B.; Lane-Fall, M.B. Decreased urine output and acute kidney injury in the postanesthesia care unit. *Anesthesiol. Clin.* **2012**, *30*, 513–526. [CrossRef] [PubMed]
16. Katayama, S.; Koyama, K.; Goto, Y.; Koinuma, T.; Tonai, K.; Shima, J.; Wada, M.; Nunomiya, S. Body weight definitions for evaluating a urinary diagnosis of acute kidney injury in patients with sepsis. *BMC Nephrol.* **2018**, *19*, 101. [CrossRef] [PubMed]
17. Gaffney, A.M.; Sladen, R.N. Acute kidney injury in cardiac surgery. *Curr. Opin. Anaesthesiol.* **2015**, *28*, 50–59. [CrossRef] [PubMed]
18. Anderson, R.J.; Linas, S.L.; Berns, A.S.; Henrich, W.L.; Miller, T.R.; Gabow, P.A.; Schrier, R.W. Nonoliguric acute renal failure. *N. Engl. J. Med.* **1977**, *296*, 1134–1138. [CrossRef] [PubMed]
19. Klahr, S. Pathophysiology of obstructive nephropathy. *Kidney Int.* **1983**, *23*, 414–426. [CrossRef] [PubMed]
20. Park, M.H.; Shim, H.S.; Kim, W.H.; Kim, H.J.; Kim, D.J.; Lee, S.H.; Kim, C.S.; Gwak, M.S.; Kim, G.S. Clinical Risk Scoring Models for Prediction of Acute Kidney Injury after Living Donor Liver Transplantation: A Retrospective Observational Study. *PLoS ONE* **2015**, *10*, e0136230. [CrossRef] [PubMed]
21. Lee, H.C.; Yoon, S.; Yang, S.M.; Kim, W.; Ryu, H.G.; Jung, C.W.; Suh, K.S.; Lee, K. Prediction of Acute Kidney Injury after Liver Transplantation: Machine Learning Approaches vs. Logistic Regression Model. *J. Clin. Med.* **2018**, *7*, 428. [CrossRef] [PubMed]
22. Chen, Y.Y.; Wu, V.C.; Huang, W.C.; Yeh, Y.C.; Wu, M.S.; Huang, C.C.; Wu, K.D.; Fang, J.T.; Wu, C.J.; CAKS Group. Norepinephrine Administration Is Associated with Higher Mortality in Dialysis Requiring Acute Kidney Injury Patients with Septic Shock. *J. Clin. Med.* **2018**, *7*, 274. [CrossRef] [PubMed]
23. Selzner, M.; Kashfi, A.; Cattral, M.S.; Selzner, N.; McGilvray, I.D.; Greig, P.D.; Levy, G.A.; Renner, E.L.; Grant, D.R. Live donor liver transplantation in high MELD score recipients. *Ann. Surg.* **2010**, *251*, 153–157. [CrossRef] [PubMed]
24. Goren, O.; Matot, I. Perioperative acute kidney injury. *Br. J. Anaesth.* **2015**, *115* (Suppl. S2), ii3–ii14. [CrossRef] [PubMed]
25. Cockcroft, D.W.; Gault, M.H. Prediction of creatinine clearance from serum creatinine. *Nephron* **1976**, *16*, 31–41. [CrossRef] [PubMed]
26. DeLong, E.R.; DeLong, D.M.; Clarke-Pearson, D.L. Comparing the areas under two or more correlated receiver operating characteristic curves: A nonparametric approach. *Biometrics* **1988**, *44*, 837–845. [CrossRef] [PubMed]
27. Guerin, C.; Girard, R.; Selli, J.M.; Perdrix, J.P.; Ayzac, L. Initial versus delayed acute renal failure in the intensive care unit. A multicenter prospective epidemiological study. Rhone-Alpes Area Study Group on Acute Renal Failure. *Am. J. Respir. Crit. Care Med.* **2000**, *161*, 872–879. [CrossRef]
28. Teixeira, C.; Garzotto, F.; Piccinni, P.; Brienza, N.; Iannuzzi, M.; Gramaticopolo, S.; Forfori, F.; Pelaia, P.; Rocco, M.; Ronco, C.; et al. Fluid balance and urine volume are independent predictors of mortality in acute kidney injury. *Crit. Care* **2013**, *17*, R14. [CrossRef]
29. Alpert, R.A.; Roizen, M.F.; Hamilton, W.K.; Stoney, R.J.; Ehrenfeld, W.K.; Poler, S.M.; Wylie, E.J. Intraoperative urinary output does not predict postoperative renal function in patients undergoing abdominal aortic revascularization. *Surgery* **1984**, *95*, 707–711. [CrossRef]
30. Hori, D.; Katz, N.M.; Fine, D.M.; Ono, M.; Barodka, V.M.; Lester, L.C.; Yenokyan, G.; Hogue, C.W. Defining oliguria during cardiopulmonary bypass and its relationship with cardiac surgery-associated acute kidney injury. *Br. J. Anaesth.* **2016**, *117*, 733–740. [CrossRef]

31. Mizota, T.; Yamamoto, Y.; Hamada, M.; Matsukawa, S.; Shimizu, S.; Kai, S. Intraoperative oliguria predicts acute kidney injury after major abdominal surgery. *Br. J. Anaesth.* **2017**, *119*, 1127–1134. [CrossRef] [PubMed]
32. Kunst, G.; Ostermann, M. Intraoperative permissive oliguria - how much is too much? *Br. J. Anaesth.* **2017**, *119*, 1075–1077. [CrossRef] [PubMed]
33. Mayer, K.; Trzeciak, S.; Puri, N.K. Assessment of the adequacy of oxygen delivery. *Curr. Opin. Crit. Care* **2016**, *22*, 437–443. [CrossRef] [PubMed]
34. Adelmann, D.; Kronish, K.; Ramsay, M.A. Anesthesia for Liver Transplantation. *Anesthesiol. Clin.* **2017**, *35*, 491–508. [CrossRef] [PubMed]
35. Rudnick, M.R.; Marchi, L.D.; Plotkin, J.S. Hemodynamic monitoring during liver transplantation: A state of the art review. *World, J. Hepatol.* **2015**, *7*, 1302–1311. [CrossRef] [PubMed]
36. Acosta, F.; Sansano, T.; Palenciano, C.G.; Roqués, V.; Clavel, N.; González, P.; Robles, R.; Bueno, F.S.; Ramírez, P.; Parrilla, P. Does mixed venous oxygen saturation reflect the changes in cardiac output during liver transplantation? *Transplant. Proc.* **2002**, *34*, 277. [CrossRef]
37. De Geus, H.R.; Betjes, M.G.; Bakker, J. Biomarkers for the prediction of acute kidney injury: A narrative review on current status and future challenges. *Clin. Kidney, J.* **2012**, *5*, 102–108. [CrossRef] [PubMed]
38. Parikh, C.R.; Moledina, D.G.; Coca, S.G.; Thiessen-Philbrook, H.R.; Garg, A.X. Application of new acute kidney injury biomarkers in human randomized controlled trials. *Kidney Int.* **2016**, *89*, 1372–1379. [CrossRef] [PubMed]
39. Merchant, M.L.; Brier, M.E.; Slaughter, M.S.; Klein, J.B.; McLeish, K.R. Biomarker enhanced risk prediction for development of AKI after cardiac surgery. *BMC Nephrol.* **2018**, *19*, 102. [CrossRef] [PubMed]
40. Haase-Fielitz, A.; Haase, M.; Devarajan, P. Neutrophil gelatinase-associated lipocalin as a biomarker of acute kidney injury: A critical evaluation of current status. *Ann. Clin. Biochem.* **2014**, *51*, 335–351. [CrossRef] [PubMed]
41. Baron-Stefaniak, J.; Schiefer, J.; Miller, E.J.; Berlakovich, G.A.; Baron, D.M.; Faybik, P. Comparison of macrophage migration inhibitory factor and neutrophil gelatinase-associated lipocalin-2 to predict acute kidney injury after liver transplantation: An observational pilot study. *PLoS ONE* **2017**, *12*, e0183162. [CrossRef] [PubMed]
42. Yang, X.; Chen, C.; Tian, J.; Zha, Y.; Xiong, Y.; Sun, Z.; Chen, P.; Li, J.; Yang, T.; Ma, C.; et al. Urinary Angiotensinogen Level Predicts AKI in Acute Decompensated Heart Failure: A Prospective, Two-Stage Study. *J. Am. Soc. Nephrol.* **2015**, *26*, 2032–2041. [CrossRef] [PubMed]
43. Meersch, M.; Schmidt, C.; Van Aken, H.; Martens, S.; Rossaint, J.; Singbartl, K.; Görlich, D.; Kellum, J.A.; Zarbock, A. Urinary TIMP-2 and IGFBP7 as early biomarkers of acute kidney injury and renal recovery following cardiac surgery. *PLoS ONE* **2014**, *9*, e93460. [CrossRef] [PubMed]
44. Göcze, I.; Jauch, D.; Götz, M.; Kennedy, P.; Jung, B.; Zeman, F.; Gnewuch, C.; Graf, B.M.; Gnann, W.; Banas, B.; et al. Biomarker-guided Intervention to Prevent Acute Kidney Injury After Major Surgery: The Prospective Randomized BigpAK Study. *Ann. Surg.* **2018**, *267*, 1013–1020. [CrossRef] [PubMed]
45. Meersch, M.; Schmidt, C.; Hoffmeier, A.; Van Aken, H.; Wempe, C.; Gerss, J.; Zarbock, A. Prevention of cardiac surgery-associated AKI by implementing the KDIGO guidelines in high risk patients identified by biomarkers: The PrevAKI randomized controlled trial. *Intensive Care Med.* **2017**, *43*, 1551–1561. [CrossRef] [PubMed]
46. Meersch, M.; Schmidt, C.; Zarbock, A. Perioperative Acute Kidney Injury: An Under-Recognized Problem. *Anesth Analg.* **2017**, *125*, 1223–1232. [CrossRef] [PubMed]
47. Brienza, N.; Giglio, M.T.; Marucci, M.; Fiore, T. Does perioperative hemodynamic optimization protect renal function in surgical patients? A meta-analytic study. *Crit. Care Med.* **2009**, *37*, 2079–2090. [CrossRef]
48. Sandham, J.D.; Hull, R.D.; Brant, R.F.; Knox, L.; Pineo, G.F.; Doig, C.J.; Laporta, D.P.; Viner, S.; Passerini, L.; Devitt, H.; et al. A randomized, controlled trial of the use of pulmonary-artery catheters in high-risk surgical patients. *N. Engl. J. Med.* **2003**, *348*, 5–14. [CrossRef]
49. El-Masry, A.; Mukhtar, A.M.; el-Sherbeny, A.M.; Fathy, M.; el-Meteini, M. Comparison of central venous oxygen saturation and mixed venous oxygen saturation during liver transplantation. *Anaesthesia* **2009**, *64*, 378–382. [CrossRef]
50. Hilmi, I.A.; Damian, D.; Al-Khafaji, A.; Planinsic, R.; Boucek, C.; Sakai, T.; Chang, C.C.; Kellum, J.A. Acute kidney injury following orthotopic liver transplantation: Incidence, risk factors, and effects on patient and graft outcomes. *Br. J. Anaesth.* **2015**, *114*, 919–926. [CrossRef]

# 10

# General Anesthetic Agents and Renal Function after Nephrectomy

**Ho-Jin Lee [1], Jinyoung Bae [1], Yongsuk Kwon [1], Hwan Suk Jang [1], Seokha Yoo [1], Chang Wook Jeong [2], Jin-Tae Kim [1] and Won Ho Kim [1,*]**

1 Department of Anesthesiology and Pain Medicine, Seoul National University Hospital, Seoul National University College of Medicine, Seoul 03080, Korea; zenerdiode03@gmail.com (H-J.L.); baejy88@gmail.com (J.B.); ulsan-no8@hanmail.net (Y.K.); luminsishs@snu.ac.kr (H.S.J.); muroki22@gmail.com (S.Y.); jintae73@gmail.com (J-T.K.)

2 Department of Urology, Seoul National University Hospital, Seoul National University College of Medicine, Seoul 03080, Korea; drboss@korea.com

* Correspondence: wonhokim@snu.ac.kr

**Abstract:** The association between the choice of general anesthetic agents and the risk of acute kidney injury (AKI) and long-term renal dysfunction after nephrectomy has not yet been evaluated. We reviewed 1087 cases of partial or radical nephrectomy. The incidence of postoperative AKI, new-onset chronic kidney disease (CKD) and CKD upstaging were compared between general anesthetic agent groups (propofol, sevoflurane, and desflurane). Four different propensity score analyses were performed to minimize confounding for each pair of comparison (propofol vs. sevoflurane; propofol vs. desflurane; sevoflurane vs. desflurane; propofol vs. volatile agents). Study outcomes were compared before and after matching. Kaplan-Meier survival curve analysis was performed to compare renal survival determined by the development of new-onset CKD between groups up to 36 months after nephrectomy. Propofol was associated with a lower incidence of AKI (propofol 23.2% vs. sevoflurane 39.5%, $p = 0.004$; vs. propofol 21.0% vs. desflurane 34.3%, $p = 0.031$), a lower incidence of CKD upstaging (propofol 27.2% vs. sevoflurane 58.4%, $p < 0.001$; propofol 32.4% vs. desflurane 48.6%, $p = 0.017$) and better three-year renal survival after nephrectomy compared to sevoflurane or desflurane group (Log-rank test propofol vs. sevoflurane $p < 0.001$; vs. desflurane $p = 0.015$) after matching. Propofol was also associated with a lower incidence of new-onset CKD after nephrectomy compared to sevoflurane after matching ($p < 0.001$). There were no significant differences between sevoflurane and desflurane. However, subgroup analysis of partial nephrectomy showed a significant difference only in CKD upstaging. In conclusion, propofol, compared to volatile agents, could be a better general anesthetic agent for nephrectomy to attenuate postoperative renal dysfunction. However, limitations of the retrospective study design and inconsistent results of the subgroup analysis preclude firm conclusions.

**Keywords:** nephrectomy; acute kidney injury; chronic kidney disease; sevoflurane; desflurane; propofol

---

## 1. Introduction

Kidney cancer, more than 90% of which is renal cell carcinoma (RCC), is common in both men and women [1]. Although partial or radical nephrectomy is the standard treatment for localized RCC [2], postoperative acute kidney injury (AKI) remains a common complication with a risk of evolving chronic kidney disease (CKD) [3,4] and the distant organ dysfunction [5]. Postoperative AKI and CKD after nephrectomy result in the prolonged length of hospital stay, increased medical cost and mortality [4,6,7]. Since acute postoperative renal dysfunction is associated with other delayed morbidities, it would be important to identify and correct potentially reversible risk factors of AKI [8].

Previous studies investigated perioperative predictors for AKI and CKD after nephrectomy [9–12]. However, to our knowledge, previously reported risk factors were generally not modifiable except ischemic time during renal arterial clamping, cold ischemia during partial nephrectomy, and intraoperative hypotension [9,13–15]. Effective interventions to decrease the risk of renal functional decline after nephrectomy are still required [16]. As another modifiable risk factor, the choice of general anesthetic agents would be important. General anesthetic agents may affect the postoperative renal function by the following mechanisms. Propofol, a widely used intravenous anesthetic agent, could prevent renal ischemia/reperfusion injury by anti-oxidative effect and progression of renal fibrosis by downregulating inducible nitric oxide synthase expression [17,18]. Although there were concerns regarding compound A-associated nephrotoxicity, many previous studies demonstrated the safety of sevoflurane. [19]. Conversely, sevoflurane had a protective effect on acute renal injury due to its anti-inflammatory effect in a previous animal study [20]. Therefore, propofol or sevoflurane may be associated with better postoperative renal function compared to other general anesthetics after nephrectomy. However, there have been no previous reports regarding the effect of general anesthetic agents on the postoperative renal function and it is unknown whether the choice of general anesthetic agents influences the risk of AKI or long-term renal function after partial or radical nephrectomy.

Therefore, we attempted to investigate the association between the choice of general anesthetic agents and the risk of AKI and long-term renal function after nephrectomy [21]. We hypothesized that the incidences of AKI and new-onset CKD after general anesthesia with propofol may be lower than the incidences with sevoflurane or desflurane. To this aim, we conducted a retrospective cohort study to investigate the potential association between different anesthetic agents and the incidences of AKI and new-onset CKD after partial or radical nephrectomy.

## 2. Materials and Methods

### 2.1. Study Design

This retrospective observational study was approved by the institutional review board (IRB) of Seoul National University Hospital (1905-089-1034). The requirement for written informed consent was waived by the IRB due to the retrospective design of this study. Studies were conducted in accordance with the approved guidelines and regulations.

### 2.2. Data Collection

After approval from the IRB, we reviewed the electronic medical records of 1087 adult patients underwent radical or partial nephrectomy due to a renal mass at our hospital between 2010 and 2014. Demographic or perioperative variables known to be associated with AKI or CKD after nephrectomy were collected (Table 1) [9,10,12]. The cohort was divided into three groups according to the anesthetic agents commonly used for maintenance of general anesthesia; propofol, sevoflurane, and desflurane. The patients who received agents other than these ($n = 0$) or whose main agent was changed during surgery ($n = 0$) or whose renal function after surgery was not followed up at least two times after surgery three months apart were excluded from our analysis ($n = 0$).

**Table 1.** Patient characteristics and perioperative parameters.

| Characteristics | Propofol ($n$ = 130) | Sevoflurane ($n$ = 644) | Desflurane ($n$ = 313) | $p$-Value |
|---|---|---|---|---|
| **Demographic data** | | | | |
| Age, years | 55 (47–62) | 57 (48–67) | 58 (49–66) | 0.12 |
| Female, $n$ | 34 (26.2) | 199 (30.9) | 87 (27.8) | 0.42 |
| Body-mass index, kg/m$^2$ | 24.5 (22.4–26.6) | 24.5 (22.6–26.6) | 24.5 (22.5–26.6) | 0.98 |
| Current smoker, $n$ | 22 (16.9) | 85 (13.2) | 59 (18.8) | 0.06 |
| **Background medical status** | | | | |
| ASA 1/2/3/4 | 69 (53.1)/55 (42.3)/6 (4.6)/0 | 317 (49.2)/280 (43.5)/47 (7.3)/0 | 119 (38.0)/181 (57.8)/12 (3.8)/1 (0.3) | <0.001 |
| Hypertension, $n$ | 46 (35.4) | 292 (45.3) | 131 (41.9) | 0.10 |
| Diabetes mellitus, $n$ | 16 (12.3) | 99 (15.4) | 53 (16.9) | 0.47 |
| Cerebrovascular accident, $n$ | 4 (3.1) | 17 (2.6) | 4 (1.3) | 0.34 |
| Liver disease, $n$ | 11 (8.5) | 22 (3.4) | 13 (4.2) | 0.03 |
| Ischemic heart disease, $n$ | 2 (1.5) | 11 (1.7) | 2 (0.6) | 0.41 |
| Hyperlipidemia, $n$ | 8 (6.2) | 59 (9.2) | 34 (10.9) | 0.29 |
| Preoperative eGFR (mL/min/1.73 m$^2$) | 82 (73–89) | 81 (69–92) | 77 (68–90) | 0.068 |
| Preoperative stage of CKD | | | | 0.09 |
| 1 (eGFR ≥ 90 mL/min/1.73 m$^2$) | 29 (22.3) | 193 (30.0) | 79 (25.2) | 0.179 |
| 2 (60–89 mL/min/1.73 m$^2$) | 91 (71.0) | 365 (56.7) | 185 (59.1) | |
| 3a (45–59 mL/min/1.73 m$^2$) | 4 (3.1) | 47 (7.3) | 29 (9.3) | |
| 3b (30–44 mL/min/1.73 m$^2$) | 4 (3.1) | 13 (2.0) | 7 (2.2) | |
| 4 (15–30 mL/min/1.73 m$^2$) | 1 (0.8) | 3 (0.5) | 2 (0.6) | |
| 5 (< 15 mL/min/1.73 m$^2$) | 1 (0.8) | 23 (3.6) | 11 (3.5) | |
| Preoperative proteinuria, $n$ | 9 (6.9) | 43 (6.7) | 31 (9.9) | 0.20 |
| Preoperative hemoglobin, g/dL | 14.3 (12.8–15.1) | 13.7 (12.5–14.8) | 13.8 (12.5–14.9) | 0.04 |
| Preoperative albumin, g/dL | 4.4 (4.2–4.7) | 4.4 (4.1–4.6) | 4.4 (4.2–4.6) | 0.20 |
| ECOG performance status | | | | 0.001 |
| 0/1/2/3 | 121/6/3/0 | 536/82/23/2 | 285/25/1/2 | |
| Clinical stage | | | | |
| T 1a/1b | 103 (79.2)/ 14 (10.8) | 416 (64.6)/ 126 (19.6) | 231 (73.8)/ 25 (8.0) | 0.23 |
| T 2a/2b | 7 (5.4)/- | 65 (10.1)/ 15 (2.3) | 35 (11.2)/ 6 (1.9) | |
| T 3a/3b/3c | 3 (2.3)/2 (1.5)/1 (0.8) | 12 (1.9)/4 (0.6)/6 (0.9) | 4 (1.3)/6 (1.9)/6 (1.9) | |
| N 0/1 | 129 (99.2)/ 1 (0.8) | 616 (95.7)/ 28 (4.3) | 298 (95.2)/ 15 (4.8) | 0.10 |
| M 0/1 | 123 (94.6)/ 7 (5.4) | 619 (96.1)/ 25 (3.9) | 303 (96.8)/ 10 (3.2) | 0.30 |
| **Operation and anesthesia related** | | | | |
| Surgery type | | | | 0.07 |
| Radical nephrectomy, $n$ | 44 (33.8) | 286 (44.4) | 139 (44.4) | |
| Partial nephrectomy, $n$ | 86 (66.2) | 358 (55.6) | 174 (55.6) | |
| Surgical approach | | | | <0.001 |
| Laparoscopic, $n$ | 10 (7.7) | 130 (20.2) | 51 (16.3) | |
| Hand-assisted laparoscopic, $n$ | 2 (1.5) | 22 (3.4) | 11 (3.5) | |
| Robot-assisted, $n$ | 62 (47.7) | 40 (6.2) | 32 (10.2) | |
| Open, $n$ | 56 (43.1) | 452 (70.2) | 219 (70.0) | |
| Operation time, hour | 2.8 (2.3–3.3) | 2.2 (1.7–2.8) | 2.2 (1.7–2.9) | <0.001 |
| Renal ischemic time, min * | 27 (21.5–35.5) | 24.6 (20.0–31.0) | 22.4 (17.4–27.5) | <0.001 |
| Ischemia type * | | | | 0.13 |
| Cold ischemia | 1 (1.2) | 22 (6.1) | 7 (4.0) | |
| Warm ischemia | 85 (98.8) | 336 (93.9) | 167 (96.0) | |
| Intraoperative vasopressor use, $n$ | 5 (3.8) | 10 (1.6) | 7 (2.2) | 0.55 |
| pRBC transfusion, $n$ | 15 (11.5) | 68 (10.6) | 40 (12.8) | 0.59 |
| Crystalloid administration, mL/kg | 18.8 (12.3–24.9) | 18.7 (14.2–25.0) | 18.1 (12.5–25.2) | 0.17 |
| Colloid administration, mL/kg | 0 (0–5.8) | 0 (0–5.0) | 0 (0–5.5) | 0.78 |

The values are presented as the median (interquartile range) or number (%). * These values are for only partial nephrectomy. Liver disease includes hepatitis or liver cirrhosis. ASA = American society of Anesthesiologist physical classification, CKD = chronic kidney disease, ECOG performance status = Eastern Cooperative Oncology Group performance status, eGFR = estimated glomerular filtration rate, pRBC = packed red blood cell.

### 2.3. Anesthesia and Surgical Techniques

The anesthetic protocols of our hospital during the study period were as follows. In the propofol group, general anesthesia was induced and maintained with a target-controlled infusion of propofol using infusion pump (Orchestra®; Fresenius Vial, Brezins, France). In the volatile agent groups, anesthesia was induced with propofol 1–2 mg/kg and maintained with either sevoflurane (2–4 vol %) or desflurane (5–7 vol %). In all groups, remifentanil was continuously infused throughout the surgery for balanced anesthesia, adjusted to maintain arterial pressure within 20% of baseline ward pressure. If arterial pressure was less than 20% of baseline despite adequate fluid administration and urine output, vasopressor including phenylephrine or norepinephrine was infused. The choice of anesthetic agents for anesthetic maintenance was made according to the anesthesiologists' discretion. The decision was made according to the attending anesthesiologist's preference regardless of patients' comorbidity or baseline medical status. Patients were mechanically ventilated with a volume-controlled mode with a tidal volume of 6–8 mL/kg and a $FiO_2$ of 0.4 to 0.5. Nephrectomies were conducted by open, laparoscopic, or robot-assisted techniques. Decisions regarding the type of surgical approach were made based on tumor characteristics. For partial nephrectomy, surgical resection was performed after clamping the main renal artery or arteries. The renal vein was clamped selectively. Saline ice slush was used for cold ischemia. Mannitol was administered intraoperatively within 30 min prior to renal vascular clamping.

### 2.4. Outcome Variables

The primary outcome of our study was the incidence of AKI after nephrectomy. Postoperative AKI was diagnosed by the Kidney Disease: Improving Global Outcomes (KDIGO) criteria, which was determined by the maximal change of the serum creatinine level during the first seven postoperative days (Stage 1: 1.5–1.9; stage 2: 2–2.9; stage 3: More than 3-fold increase from baseline) [22,23]. The most recent preoperative serum creatinine level was defined as the baseline value.

The secondary outcomes included the incidence of new-onset CKD stage 3a or high (eGFR $< 60$ mL/min/1.73 $m^2$), CKD upstaging after nephrectomy, the incidence of postoperative complications, and length of hospital stay. Postoperative new-onset CKD was diagnosed by the creatinine criteria of KDIGO criteria, which was determined when the estimated glomerular filtration rate (eGFR) decreased below 60 mL/min/1.73 $m^2$ for three months or more [24]. We calculated eGFR from serum creatinine level using the Modification of Diet in Renal Disease (MDRD) study equation [25]. The most recent preoperative eGFR was defined as the baseline value. CKD upstaging was determined when the CKD stage follow-up was higher than the baseline until 3 years after nephrectomy.

### 2.5. Statistical Analysis

Statistical analyses were performed using SPSS software version 25.0 (IBM Corp., Armonk, NY, USA) and MedCalc Statistical Software version 18.6 (MedCalc Software bvba, Ostend, Belgium). A $p$-value of less than 0.05 was considered statistically significant. The Kolmogorov-Smirnov test was performed to determine the normality of the continuous variables. Continuous data are described as the mean (SD) or median (25 and 75 percentiles) and were compared by the independent $t$-test or the Mann-Whitney $U$ test or one-way analysis of variance (ANOVA). In the pairwise comparisons between two anesthetic groups, Bonferroni correction was used by dividing the critical $p$-value by the number of comparisons to minimize the chance of a type 1 error. $p$-value $< 0.017$ was considered statistically significant. Categorical data are described as number (%) and were compared by the chi-square test or Fisher's exact test. Missing data were less than 5% of the total records. We used simple imputation with median and mode. Missing values of continuous variables were replaced by the age-and sex-specific median values, and incidence data were assigned the most frequent age and sex-specific modes. The followings are main analyses of our study to evaluate the association between the general anesthetic agents and clinical outcomes.

Firstly, to reduce the influence of confounding variables, four different propensity score matching analyses were performed to adjust for intergroup differences; Propofol vs. Sevoflurane, Propofol vs. Desflurane, Sevoflurane vs. Desflurane, and Propofol vs. volatile agents. The following variables were used as contributors to the propensity score: Sex, age, body-mass index, current smoking, history of hypertension, diabetes mellitus, cerebrovascular disease, chronic hepatitis or cirrhosis, ischemic heart disease, dyslipidemia, preoperative hemoglobin, serum albumin, eGFR, TNM stage of renal cell carcinoma, year of surgery, open surgery (vs. laparoscopic surgery), radical nephrectomy (vs. partial nephrectomy), operation time, unit number of packed red cell transfusion, crystalloid and colloid administration and need for vasopressor infusion. All patients were matched at a 1:1 ratio using the nearest neighbor method with a caliper width of 0.2 of the pooled standard deviation of the logit of the propensity score. To evaluate the balance of the matched patients, the standardized mean difference for each contributor was compared before and after matching. In each propensity-matched cohort, we directly compared the incidences of postoperative AKI and other secondary outcomes.

Secondly, to evaluate the effect of general anesthetic agents on long-term renal function, Kaplan-Meier survival curve analyses were performed. Renal survival was determined by the development of new-onset CKD stage 3a or higher and the survival was compared between different anesthetic agent groups before and after matching. Patients were followed for up to 36 months and the log-rank test was used for inter-group comparison.

Thirdly, we performed a subgroup analysis for the patients who underwent partial nephrectomy. We compared our primary and secondary outcomes between the propofol and volatile agent groups.

Although power calculation was not conducted prior to analysis, available power was calculated with the number of patients used in our analysis. With 130 and 644 patients used to compare the incidence of AKI between propofol and sevoflurane group and incidences of AKI of the two groups observed in our study, there was about 84.7% power to detect the observed difference in AKI. However, power decreased to 76.0% in the matched cohort between propofol and sevoflurane.

## 3. Results

Among 1087 patients included in our analysis, 130 patients (12.0%) received propofol and 957 patients (88.0%: Sevoflurane 59.2%, Desflurane 28.8%) received volatile agent to maintain general anesthesia. After propensity score matching, 125 pairs of patients were matched between the propofol and sevoflurane group, 105 pairs between the propofol and desflurane group, and 307 pairs between the sevoflurane and desflurane group (Figure 1). Patient characteristics and perioperative parameters are summarized in Table 1. Histograms and covariate balance plots of the distribution of standardized differences of covariates between groups before and after matching are shown in Supplemental Figures S1–S4 according to the different pairs of matching.

There were significant differences in the incidences of postoperative AKI, new-onset CKD stage 3a or high and CKD upstaging between the propofol and volatile groups. (Tables 2 and 3) However, there was no significant difference between the sevoflurane and desflurane groups (Table 4). After propensity score matching, the propofol group still showed significantly less frequent postoperative AKI, new-onset CKD stage 3a or high, and CKD upstaging than the sevoflurane group (Table 2). The propofol group also showed significantly less frequent postoperative AKI and CKD upstaging than the desflurane group (Table 3). Between sevoflurane and desflurane groups, there was no significant difference (Table 4). When the sevoflurane and desflurane groups were combined into the volatile group, the propofol group showed significantly less frequent postoperative AKI and CKD upstaging than the volatile group before and after matching (Supplemental Table S1).

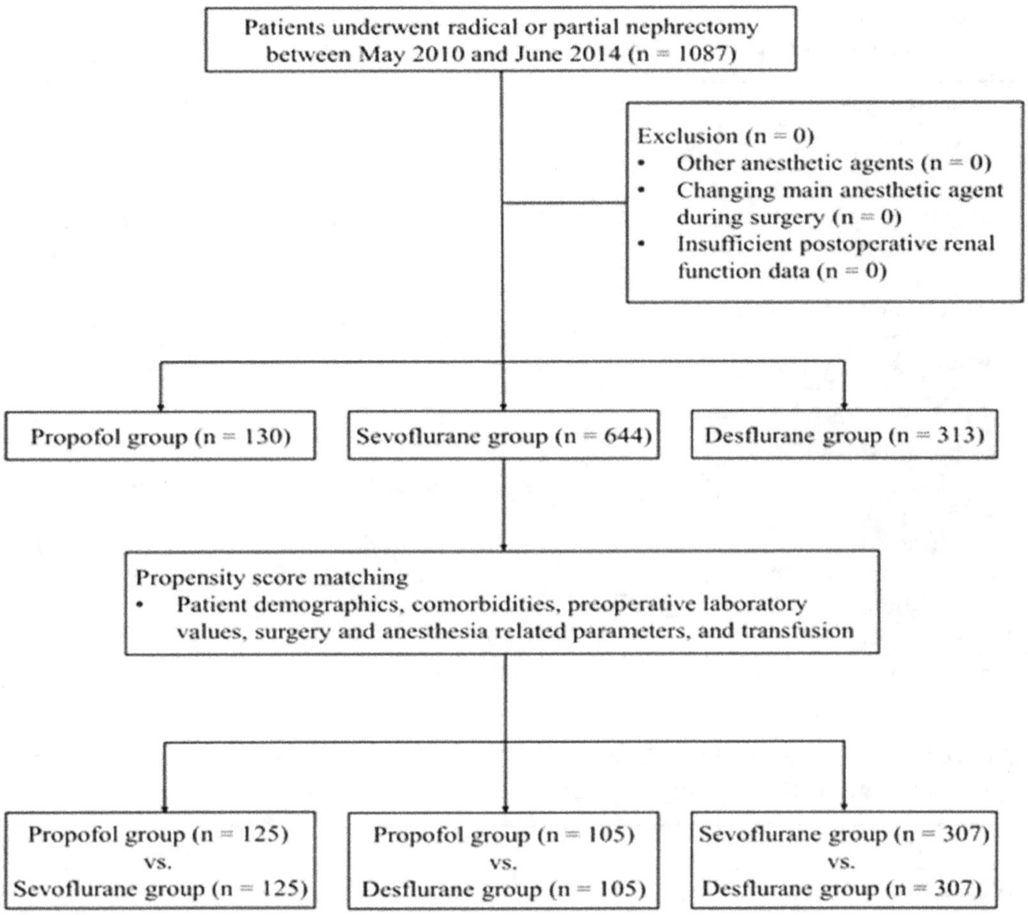


**Figure 1.** Flow diagram of the present study.

**Table 2.** Comparison of incidence of primary and secondary outcomes between patients according to the main anesthetic agents during surgery before and after propensity score matching.

| Outcomes | Propofol | Sevoflurane | Risk Difference, % | *p*-Value |
|---|---|---|---|---|
| Number of patients before matching | 130 | 644 | | |
| Postoperative AKI, *n* | 29 (22.3) | 229 (35.6) | −13 (−5 to −21) | 0.032 |
| Stage 1 | 24 (18.5) | 203 (31.5) | −13 (−5 to −21) | |
| Stage 2 | 1 (0.8) | 2 (0.3) | 0.5 (−1.1 to 2.0) | |
| Stage 3 | 4 (3.1) | 24 (3.7) | −0.6 (−3.9 to 2.7) | |
| Postoperative new-onset CKD stage 3a or high, *n* | 33 (25.4) | 296 (46.0) | −21 (−12 to −29) | <0.001 |
| CKD upstaging, *n* | 38 (29.2) | 307 (47.7) | −18 (−10 to −27) | <0.001 |
| Number of patients after matching | 125 | 125 | | |
| Postoperative AKI, *n* | 29 (23.2) | 50 (39.5) | −17 (−5 to −28) | 0.004 |
| Stage 1 | 24 (19.2) | 45 (36.0) | −17 (−6 to −28) | |
| Stage 2 | 1 (0.8) | - | - | |
| Stage 3 | 4 (3.2) | 5 (4.0) | −0.8 (−5.4 to 3.8) | |
| Postoperative new-onset CKD stage 3a or high, *n* | 33 (26.4) | 61 (48.8) | −22 (−11 to −34) | <0.001 |
| CKD upstaging, *n* | 34 (27.2) | 73 (58.4) | −31 (−20 to −43) | <0.001 |

The values are presented as the median (interquartile range) or number (%). AKI = acute kidney injury determined by KDIGO creatinine criteria, CKD = chronic kidney disease.

**Table 3.** Comparison of incidence of primary and secondary outcomes between patients according to the main anesthetic agents during surgery before and after propensity score matching.

| Outcomes | Propofol | Desflurane | Risk Difference, % | *p*-Value |
|---|---|---|---|---|
| Number of patients before matching | 130 | 313 | | |
| Postoperative AKI, *n* | 29 (22.3) | 113 (36.1) | −14 (−5 to −22) | 0.042 |
| Stage 1 | 24 (18.5) | 100 (31.9) | −13 (−5 to −22) | |
| Stage 2 | 1 (0.8) | 3 (1.0) | −0.2 (−2.0 to 1.7) | |
| Stage 3 | 4 (3.1) | 10 (3.2) | −0.1 (−3.7 to 3.4) | |
| Postoperative new-onset CKD stage 3a or high, *n* | 33 (25.4) | 131 (41.9) | −16 (−7 to −26) | 0.001 |
| CKD upstaging, *n* | 38 (29.2) | 141 (45.0) | −16 (−6 to −25) | 0.002 |
| Number of patients after matching | 105 | 105 | | |
| Postoperative AKI, *n* | 22 (21.0) | 36 (34.3) | −13 (−1 to −25) | 0.031 |
| Stage 1 | 19 (18.1) | 31 (29.5) | −11 (−0.1 to −23) | |
| Stage 2 | 1 (1.0) | - | - | |
| Stage 3 | 2 (1.9) | 5 (4.8) | −2.9 (−7.7 to 2.0) | |
| Postoperative new-onset CKD stage 3a or high, *n* | 24 (22.9) | 35 (33.3) | −10 (−23 to 2) | 0.09 |
| CKD upstaging, *n* | 34 (32.4) | 51 (48.6) | −16 (−29 to −3) | 0.017 |

The values are presented as the median (interquartile range) or number (%). AKI = acute kidney injury determined by KDIGO creatinine criteria, CKD = chronic kidney disease.

**Table 4.** Comparison of incidence of primary and secondary outcomes between patients according to the main anesthetic agents during surgery before and after propensity score matching.

| Outcomes | Sevoflurane | Desflurane | Risk Difference, % | *p*-Value |
|---|---|---|---|---|
| Number of patients before matching | 644 | 313 | | |
| Postoperative AKI, *n* | 229 (35.6) | 113 (36.1) | −0.5 (−7.0 to 5.9) | 0.98 |
| Stage 1 | 203 (31.5) | 100 (31.9) | −0.4 (−6.7 to 5.9) | |
| Stage 2 | 2 (0.3) | 3 (1.0) | −0.6 (−1.8 to 0.5) | |
| Stage 3 | 24 (3.7) | 10 (3.2) | 0.5 (−1.9 to 3.0) | |
| Postoperative new-onset CKD stage 3a or high, *n* | 296 (46.0) | 131 (41.9) | 4.1 (−2.6 to 10.8) | 0.23 |
| CKD upstaging, *n* | 307 (47.7) | 141 (45.0) | 2.7 (−4.1 to 9.4) | 0.45 |
| Number of patients after matching | 307 | 307 | | |
| Postoperative AKI, *n* | 103 (33.6) | 110 (35.8) | −2.3 (−9.8 to 5.2) | 0.55 |
| Stage 1 | 93 (30.3) | 99 (32.2) | −2.0 (−9.3 to 5.4) | |
| Stage 2 | - | 3 (1.0) | - | |
| Stage 3 | 10 (3.3) | 8 (2.6) | 0.7 (−2.0 to 3.3) | |
| Postoperative new-onset CKD stage 3a or high, *n* | 136 (44.3) | 127 (41.4) | 2.9 (−4.9 to 10.8) | 0.46 |
| CKD upstaging, *n* | 147 (47.9) | 139 (45.3) | 2.6 (−5.3 to 10.5) | 0.52 |

The values are presented as the median (interquartile range) or number (%). AKI = acute kidney injury determined by KDIGO creatinine criteria, CKD = chronic kidney disease.

Kaplan-Meier survival analyses of the entire cohort showed significant differences in renal survival between the propofol and other volatile groups (Log-rank test: vs. sevoflurane, $p < 0.001$; vs. desflurane, $p < 0.001$) (Figure 2). After matching, there were significant differences in survival between the propofol and volatile agent groups (vs. sevoflurane, $p < 0.001$; vs. desflurane, $p = 0.015$) (Figure 2). However, no significant difference was observed between the sevoflurane and desflurane groups before and after matching (Figure 2). Regarding combined volatile group, there was a significant difference in renal survival between the propofol and volatile group ($p < 0.001$) (Supplementary Figure S5). The significant difference was also observed after matching ($p = 0.032$).

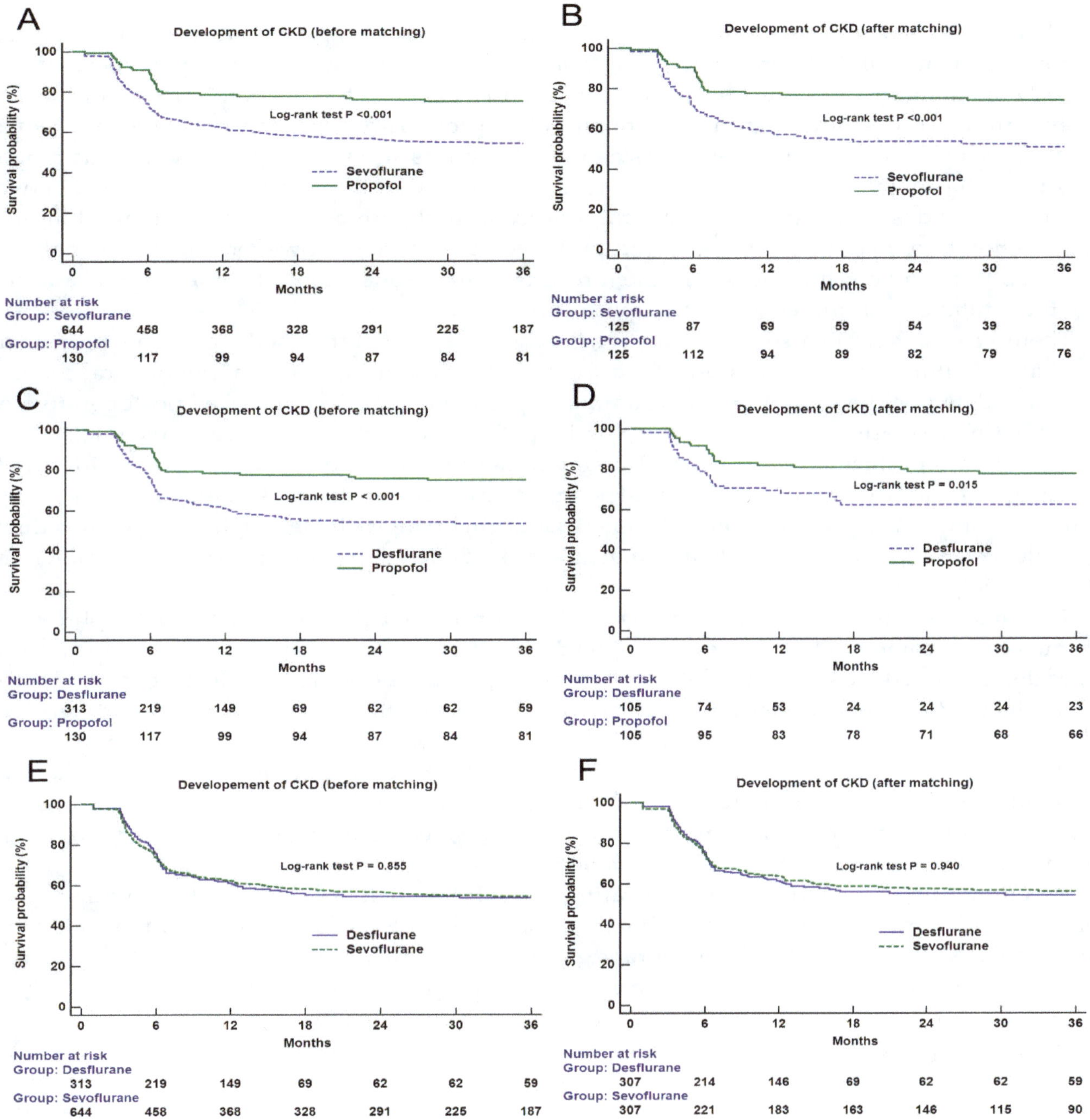


**Figure 2.** Kaplan-Meier survival curve analyses of new-onset chronic kidney disease stage 3a or high according to the main anesthetic agent groups (propofol vs. sevoflurane, upper, before (**A**) and after (**B**) matching; propofol vs. desflurane, middle, before (**C**) and after (**D**) matching; sevoflurane vs. desflurane, lower, before (**E**) and after (**F**) matching). The results of the log-rank test between groups are shown on the figure.

The results of the subgroup analysis of partial nephrectomy were shown in Supplemental Table S2 and Supplemental Figures S6 and S7. We also performed propensity score matching in the subgroup and obtained 67 pairs of matched cases. No significant difference in the incidence of postoperative AKI or new-onset CKD was found between the propofol and volatile groups. However, the propofol group showed significantly less frequent postoperative CKD upstaging than the volatile group.

## 4. Discussion

We investigated the association between general anesthetic agents and postoperative renal functional outcomes in patients undergoing nephrectomy. The incidences of postoperative AKI and CKD upstaging were significantly and consistently lower in the propofol group compared to the sevoflurane or desflurane group before and after propensity score matching. The three-year postoperative incidence of new-onset CKD stage 3a or high was also significantly lower in the propofol group than the sevoflurane group after matching. There was no significant difference between sevoflurane and desflurane groups. Propofol was associated with better both short- and long-term renal function after nephrectomy compared to the volatile agents. However, subgroup analysis of partial nephrectomy did not show consistent results. Our results should be interpreted cautiously given the limitations of single-center retrospective design.

There was a significant association between the choice of general anesthetic agent and the incidence of AKI after nephrectomy in our study, favoring the propofol group. Several possible mechanisms can be elucidated on the basis of previous animal experiments. Propofol reduced postoperative AKI by attenuating oxidative stress in a rat model [26]. Propofol conferred a protective effect against renal ischemia-reperfusion injury by modulating inflammatory cytokines [27,28]. Considering the mechanisms of renal dysfunction after partial nephrectomy involves the ischemia-reperfusion injury by vascular clamping [29], propofol could be beneficial to attenuate AKI after nephrectomy. By reducing the incidence of AKI, propofol could attenuate the risk of CKD subsequently, as AKI is a potent risk factor of postoperative CKD [3,30].

The safety issue of sevoflurane has been raised since its introduction due to potential nephrotoxicity of its metabolite, compound A. However, despite the nephrotoxicity proven in an animal study, clinical studies demonstrated the safety of sevoflurane regarding renal function [19,31]. In a recent randomized trial conducted in patients undergoing kidney transplantation, there was no significant difference in graft outcome between the sevoflurane and propofol groups [32]. Conversely, previous animal studies reported the renal protective effect of sevoflurane [33,34]. However, to our knowledge, there was no previous animal or clinical study comparing propofol and sevoflurane during nephrectomy. The influence of anesthetic agent on renal function may be greater during nephrectomy with frequent and significant postoperative renal functional decline [13,35].

Recent studies reported results advocating propofol, which are consistent with our findings. A previous randomized study reported that the propofol-based anesthesia reduced the incidence of postoperative AKI compared to the sevoflurane group after valvular heart surgery [36]. They measured plasma inflammatory markers and suggested the reno-protective effect was mediated by the anti-inflammatory action of propofol. Propofol-based anesthesia reduced postoperative urinary kidney-specific proteins and serum pro-inflammatory cytokines compared to sevoflurane-based anesthesia in patients undergoing open abdominal aortic aneurysm repair [37]. In addition, in a retrospective study conducted on 4320 patients undergoing colorectal surgery, propofol decreased the incidence of postoperative AKI when compared to sevoflurane [38].

There were also studies reporting no effect of general anesthetic agents on postoperative renal function in other surgical populations. However, the number of studies which reported neutral effect was small. Although study design was different, a previous randomized trial showed no significant differences in renal function between sevoflurane, desflurane, and propofol after elective surgery [39]. However, this study involved only a small number of patients and did not limit the type of surgery. There was also no significant difference in the incidence of postoperative AKI after lung surgery between the propofol and sevoflurane in a recent retrospective study [40]. However, the incidence of AKI after lung surgery was as low as 3.5% and larger number of patients are required for sufficient study power.

We performed propensity score analysis and used intraoperative vasopressor infusion as the contributor to the propensity score because vasopressor use could reflect intraoperative hypotension and was reported as an independent risk factor of postoperative AKI [41]. However, a recent retrospective study reported that intraoperative vasopressor infusion was not associated with AKI [42]. Vasopressor infusion during surgery could be a mediator to the development of AKI rather than a confounder because we infuse vasopressor to treat hypotension but vasopressor could also cause AKI [43].

The strength of our study is that we investigated the incidence of new-onset CKD after nephrectomy for 36 months after nephrectomy. Demographic and genetic factors, comorbidity, pre-existing renal disease, and surgical technique are associated with the development of CKD after nephrectomy [14]. However, there have been no reports of the association of anesthetic agents in the surgical population with long-term renal function. Although this was a single-center retrospective study, we demonstrated the possible benefit of propofol to mitigate the risk of CKD as well as AKI compared to volatile agents through rigorous adjustment of possible confounding factors. Matching was performed pairwise like a network analysis including matching for three different pairs of general anesthetics. The consistent results between different pair of network comparison supported our conclusion. However, we did not obtain significant difference in the incidence of AKI and new-onset CKD in the subgroup of partial nephrectomy. The incidence of AKI after partial nephrectomy is lower than the incidence after radical nephrectomy [11]. The incidences of AKI after partial and radical nephrectomy in our study were 16.0% and 58.0%, respectively. The incidences of new-onset CKD after partial and radical nephrectomy were 22.0% and 69.1%, respectively. As the incidences of AKI and CKD after partial nephrectomy are much lower than radical nephrectomy, a larger number of patients than our study would be required to detect any difference in the incidence of AKI or CKD after partial nephrectomy. Therefore, our subgroup analysis of partial nephrectomy may lack sufficient power.

The results of our study should be interpreted cautiously under several limitations. First, it was a single-center retrospective analysis. Unmeasured or unknown confounders may have affected our study results. However, the pair-wise propensity score matching was used to minimize confounding. Sensitivity analyses of secondary outcomes yielded consistent results. Secondly, we did not exclude the patients with pre-existing CKD stage 3a or high not to decrease the study power. This might affect the incidence of AKI because preoperative CKD is known to be an important risk factor of postoperative AKI [44]. Furthermore, acute-on-chronic kidney injury is a different disease entity from AKI [45]. However, to minimize confounding by the baseline renal function, we used preoperative eGFR and serum albumin as contributors to the propensity score analysis. Furthermore, our secondary outcome of CKD upstaging could detect the renal functional decline even in the patients with baseline CKD. Thirdly, we used only serum creatinine concentration except urine output to diagnose the AKI. However, urine output criteria may be inaccurate due to mannitol infusion during partial nephrectomy [11]. Fourthly, we included all types of surgical approach, which was reported to be associated with postoperative AKI [10]. However, we could not perform the subgroup analysis according to the type of surgical approach due to the small number of patients in each surgical category. We only performed a propensity score analysis using the type of surgical approach and operation time as contributors. Fifthly, mannitol was routinely administered in our patients undergoing partial nephrectomy, but a recent randomized trial showed no effect of mannitol infusion on postoperative renal function [46]. However, since mannitol infusion did not affect postoperative eGFR [46] and we did not use the urine output criteria of AKI, the effect of mannitol on our study results would be insignificant. Sixthly, in the volatile groups, propofol bolus dose was used to induce anesthesia and this might have some residual effect in the volatile groups. However, propofol is distributed and eliminated rapidly after single bolus injection [47]. Therefore, the dose of propofol (1–2 mg/kg) used during anesthesia induction would not be a significant confounder for our analysis. Lastly, we performed post hoc power analysis instead of prior power analysis due to the limited number of patients. A sufficient number of patients were not included for the primary outcome according to our post hoc power calculation.

## 5. Conclusions

In our propensity score-matched comparison of the general anesthetic agents in patients undergoing radical and partial nephrectomy, propofol was associated with a lower incidence of postoperative AKI and CKD upstaging compared to sevoflurane or desflurane. The three-year renal survival after nephrectomy was also significantly better for propofol compared to volatile agents. Therefore, in patients receiving nephrectomy, propofol may be the reasonable general anesthetic agent to mitigate postoperative renal functional deterioration compared to volatile agents. However, inconsistent subgroup analysis of partial nephrectomy and significant limitations of our study design preclude a firm conclusion.

**Supplementary Materials:**
Table S1: Comparison of incidence of primary and secondary outcomes between patients according to the main anesthetic agents (propofol vs. volatile agents) during surgery before and after propensity score matching, Table S2: Comparison of incidence of primary and secondary outcomes between patients according to the main anesthetic agents (propofol vs. volatile agents) before and after propensity score matching in the subgroup of partial nephrectomy, Figure S1: Histograms (left) and covariate balance plot (right) of distribution of standardized differences of covariates between the patients who received propofol and sevoflurane during surgery in all cohort, Figure S2: Histograms (left) and covariate balance plot (right) of distribution of standardized differences of covariates between the patients who received propofol and desflurane during surgery in all cohort, Figure S3: Histograms (left) and covariate balance plot (right) of distribution of standardized differences of covariates between the patients who received sevoflurane and desflurane during surgery in all cohort, Figure S4: Histograms (left) and covariate balance plot (right) of distribution of standardized differences of covariates between the patients who received propofol and volatile agents during surgery in all cohort, Figure S5: Kaplan-Meier survival curve analysis of new-onset chronic kidney disease according to the main anesthetic agents (TIVA vs. volatile agents) before (A) and after (B) propensity score matching in all cohort, Figure S6: Histograms (left) and covariate balance plot (right) of distribution of standardized differences of covariates between the patients who received propofol and volatile agents during surgery in the subgroup of partial nephrectomy, Figure S7: Kaplan-Meier survival curve analysis of new-onset chronic kidney disease according to the main anesthetic agents (TIVA vs. volatile agents) before (A) and after (B) propensity score matching in the subgroup of partial nephrectomy.

**Author Contributions:** Data curation, formal analysis, investigation, visualization, writing-original draft, H-J.L.; writing review and editing, J.B., Y.K., H.S.J., S.Y.; supervision, writing review and editing, J-T.K.; data curation, writing—review and editing, C.W.J.; conceptualization, data curation, formal analysis, investigation, methodology, visualization, writing-original draft, W.H.K.

## References


1. Znaor, A.; Lortet-Tieulent, J.; Laversanne, M.; Jemal, A.; Bray, F. International variations and trends in renal cell carcinoma incidence and mortality. *Eur. Urol.* **2015**, *67*, 519–530. [CrossRef] [PubMed]
2. Ljungberg, B.; Albiges, L.; Abu-Ghanem, Y.; Bensalah, K.; Dabestani, S.; Fernández-Pello, S.; Giles, R.H.; Hofmann, F.; Hora, M.; Kuczyk, M.A.; et al. European Association of Urology Guidelines on Renal Cell Carcinoma, the 2019 Update. *Eur. Urol.* **2019**, *75*, 799–810. [CrossRef] [PubMed]
3. Garofalo, C.; Liberti, M.E.; Russo, D.; Russo, L.; Fuiano, G.; Cianfrone, P.; Conte, G.; De Nicola, L.; Minutolo, R.; Borrelli, S. Effect of post-nephrectomy acute kidney injury on renal outcome, a retrospective long-term study. *World J. Urol.* **2018**, *36*, 59–63. [CrossRef] [PubMed]
4. Schmid, M.; Krishna, N.; Ravi, P.; Meyer, C.P.; Becker, A.; Dalela, D.; Sood, A.; Chun, F.K.H.; Kibel, A.S.; Menon, M.; et al. Trends of acute kidney injury after radical or partial nephrectomy for renal cell carcinoma. *Urol. Oncol.* **2016**, *34*, 293-e1–293-e10. [CrossRef] [PubMed]
5. Grams, M.E.; Rabb, H. The distant organ effects of acute kidney injury. *Kidney Int.* **2012**, *81*, 942–948. [CrossRef] [PubMed]
6. Weight, C.J.; Larson, B.T.; Fergany, A.F.; Gao, T.; Lane, B.R.; Campbell, S.C.; Kaouk, J.H.; Klein, E.A.; Novick, A.C. Nephrectomy induced chronic renal insufficiency is associated with increased risk of cardiovascular death and death from any cause in patients with localized cT1b renal masses. *J. Urol.* **2010**, *183*, 1317–1323. [CrossRef] [PubMed]
7. Hobson, C.; Ozrazgat-Baslanti, T.; Kuxhausen, A.; Thottakkara, P.; Efron, P.A.; Moore, F.A.; Moldawer, L.L.; Segal, M.S.; Bihorac, A. Cost and Mortality Associated with Postoperative Acute Kidney Injury. *Ann. Surg.* **2015**, *261*, 1207–1214. [CrossRef]
8. Bellomo, R.; Kellum, J.A.; Ronco, C. Acute kidney injury. *Lancet* **2012**, *380*, 756–766. [CrossRef]

9. Rajan, S.; Babazade, R.; Govindarajan, S.R.; Pal, R.; You, J.; Mascha, E.J.; Khanna, A.; Yang, M.; Marcano, F.D.; Singh, A.K.; et al. Perioperative factors associated with acute kidney injury after partial nephrectomy. *Br. J. Anaesth.* **2016**, *116*, 70–76. [CrossRef]
10. Schmid, M.; Gandaglia, G.; Sood, A.; Olugbade, K., Jr.; Ruhotina, N.; Sammon, J.D.; Varda, B.; Chang, S.L.; Kibel, A.S.; Chun, F.K.; et al. Predictors of 30-day acute kidney injury following radical and partial nephrectomy for renal cell carcinoma. *Urol. Oncol.* **2014**, *32*, 1259–1266. [CrossRef]
11. Hur, M.; Park, S.K.; Yoo, S.; Choi, S.N.; Jeong, C.W.; Kim, W.H.; Kim, J.T.; Kwak, C.; Bahk, J.H. The association between intraoperative urine output and postoperative acute kidney injury differs between partial and radical nephrectomy. *Sci. Rep.* **2019**, *9*, 760. [CrossRef] [PubMed]
12. Kim, N.Y.; Hong, J.H.; Koh, D.H.; Lee, J.; Nam, H.J.; Kim, S.Y. Effect of Diabetes Mellitus on Acute Kidney Injury after Minimally Invasive Partial Nephrectomy, A Case-Matched Retrospective Analysis. *J. Clin. Med.* **2019**, *8*, 468. [CrossRef] [PubMed]
13. Mir, M.C.; Ercole, C.; Takagi, T.; Zhang, Z.; Velet, L.; Remer, E.M.; Demirjian, S.; Campbell, S.C. Decline in renal function after partial nephrectomy, etiology and prevention. *J. Urol.* **2015**, *193*, 1889–1898. [CrossRef] [PubMed]
14. Li, L.; Lau, W.L.; Rhee, C.M.; Harley, K.; Kovesdy, C.P.; Sim, J.J.; Jacobsen, S.; Chang, A.; Landman, J.; Kalantar-Zadeh, K. Risk of chronic kidney disease after cancer nephrectomy. *Nat. Rev. Nephrol.* **2014**, *10*, 135–145. [CrossRef] [PubMed]
15. Salmasi, V.; Maheshwari, K.; Yang, D.; Mascha, E.J.; Singh, A.; Sessler, D.I.; Kurz, A. Relationship between intraoperative hypotension, defined by either reduction from baseline or absolute thresholds, and acute kidney and myocardial injury after noncardiac SurgeryA retrospective cohort analysis. *Anesthesiology* **2017**, *126*, 47–65. [CrossRef] [PubMed]
16. Kil, H.; Kim, J.; Choi, Y.; Lee, H.; Kim, T. Effect of Combined Treatment of Ketorolac and Remote Ischemic Preconditioning on Renal Ischemia-Reperfusion Injury in Patients Undergoing Partial Nephrectomy, Pilot Study. *J. Clin. Med.* **2018**, *7*, E470. [CrossRef] [PubMed]
17. Song, L.; Shi, S.; Jiang, W.; Liu, X.; He, Y. Protective role of propofol on the kidney during early unilateral ureteral obstruction through inhibition of epithelial-mesenchymal transition. *Am. J. Transl. Res.* **2016**, *8*, 460. [PubMed]
18. Li, Y.; Zhong, D.; Lei, L.; Jia, Y.; Zhou, H.; Yang, B. Propofol prevents renal ischemia-reperfusion injury via inhibiting the oxidative stress pathways. *Cell. Physiol. Biochem.* **2015**, *37*, 14–26. [CrossRef] [PubMed]
19. Gentz, B.A.; Malan, T.P. Renal toxicity with sevoflurane. *Drugs* **2001**, *61*, 2155–2162. [CrossRef]
20. Kong, H.Y.; Zhu, S.M.; Wang, L.Q.; He, Y.; Xie, H.Y.; Zheng, S.S. Sevoflurane protects against acute kidney injury in a small-size liver transplantation model. *Am. J. Nephrol.* **2010**, *32*, 347–355. [CrossRef]
21. Chawla, L.S.; Eggers, P.W.; Star, R.A.; Kimmel, P.L. Acute kidney injury and chronic kidney disease as interconnected syndromes. *N. Engl. J. Med.* **2014**, *371*, 58–66. [CrossRef] [PubMed]
22. Thomas, M.E.; Blaine, C.; Dawnay, A.; Devonald, M.A.; Ftouh, S.; Laing, C.; Latchem, S.; Lewington, A.; Milford, D.V.; Ostermann, M. The definition of acute kidney injury and its use in practice. *Kidney Int.* **2015**, *87*, 62–73. [CrossRef] [PubMed]
23. Shin, S.R.; Kim, W.H.; Kim, D.J.; Shin, I.W.; Sohn, J.T. Prediction and Prevention of Acute Kidney Injury after Cardiac Surgery. *BioMed Res. Int.* **2016**, *2016*, 2985148. [CrossRef] [PubMed]
24. Eknoyan, G.; Lameire, N.; Eckardt, K.; Kasiske, B.; Wheeler, D.; Levin, A.; Stevens, P.E.; Bilous, R.W.; Lamb, E.J.; Coresh, J.; et al. Kidney Disease, Improving Global Outcomes (KDIGO) CKD Work Group. KDIGO 2012 clinical practice guideline for the evaluation and management of chronic kidney disease. *Kidney Int. Suppl.* **2013**, *3*, 1–150.
25. Levey, A.S.; Coresh, J.; Greene, T.; Stevens, L.A.; Zhang, Y.L.; Hendriksen, S.; Kusek, J.W.; Van Lente, F. Using standardized serum creatinine values in the modification of diet in renal disease study equation for estimating glomerular filtration rate. *Ann. Intern. Med.* **2006**, *145*, 247–254. [CrossRef] [PubMed]
26. Luo, C.; Yuan, D.; Li, X.; Yao, W.; Luo, G.; Chi, X.; Li, H.; Irwin, M.G.; Xia, Z.; Hei, Z. Propofol attenuated acute kidney injury after orthotopic liver transplantation via inhibiting gap junction composed of connexin 32. *Anesthesiology* **2015**, *122*, 72–86. [CrossRef] [PubMed]
27. Hsing, C.-H.; Chou, W.; Wang, J.-J.; Chen, H.-W.; Yeh, C.-H. Propofol increases bone morphogenetic protein-7 and decreases oxidative stress in sepsis-induced acute kidney injury. *Nephrol. Dial. Transplant.* **2010**, *26*, 1162–1172. [CrossRef] [PubMed]

28. Sánchez-Conde, P.; Rodriguez-Lopez, J.M.; Nicolás, J.L.; Lozano, F.S.; García-Criado, F.J.; Cascajo, C.; González-Sarmiento, R.; Muriel, C. The comparative abilities of propofol and sevoflurane to modulate inflammation and oxidative stress in the kidney after aortic cross-clamping. *Anesth. Analg.* **2008**, *106*, 371–378. [CrossRef] [PubMed]
29. Zabell, J.R.; Wu, J.; Suk-Ouichai, C.; Campbell, S.C. Renal ischemia and functional outcomes following partial nephrectomy. *Urol. Clin.* **2017**, *44*, 243–255. [CrossRef]
30. Cho, A.; Lee, J.E.; Kwon, G.Y.; Huh, W.; Lee, H.M.; Kim, Y.G.; Kim, D.J.; Oh, H.Y.; Choi, H.Y. Post-operative acute kidney injury in patients with renal cell carcinoma is a potent risk factor for new-onset chronic kidney disease after radical nephrectomy. *Nephrol. Dial. Transplant.* **2011**, *26*, 3496–3501. [CrossRef]
31. Kharasch, E.D.; Frink, E.J.; Artru, A., Jr.; Michalowski, P.; Rooke, G.A.; Nogami, W. Long-duration low-flow sevoflurane and isoflurane effects on postoperative renal and hepatic function. *Anesth. Analg.* **2001**, *93*, 1511–1520. [CrossRef] [PubMed]
32. Nieuwenhuijs-Moeke, G.J.; Nieuwenhuijs, V.B.; Seelen, M.A.J.; Berger, S.P.; Van Den Heuvel, M.C.; Burgerhof, J.G.M.; Ottens, P.J.; Ploeg, R.J.; Leuvenink, H.G.D.; Struys, M.M.R.F. Propofol-based anaesthesia versus sevoflurane-based anaesthesia for living donor kidney transplantation, results of the VAPOR-1 randomized controlled trial. *Br. J. Anaesth.* **2017**, *118*, 720–732. [CrossRef] [PubMed]
33. Lee, H.T.; Chen, S.W.; Doetschman, T.C.; Deng, C.; D'Agati, V.D.; Kim, M. Sevoflurane protects against renal ischemia and reperfusion injury in mice via the transforming growth factor-β1 pathway. *Am. J. Physiol. Renal Physiol.* **2008**, *295*, F128–F136. [CrossRef] [PubMed]
34. Lee, H.T.; Kim, M.; Song, J.H.; Chen, S.W.; Gubitosa, G.; Emala, C.W. Sevoflurane-mediated TGF-β1 signaling in renal proximal tubule cells. *Am. J. Physiol. Renal Physiol.* **2008**, *294*, F371–F378. [CrossRef] [PubMed]
35. Scosyrev, E.; Messing, E.M.; Sylvester, R.; Campbell, S.; Van Poppel, H. Renal function after nephron-sparing surgery versus radical nephrectomy, results from EORTC randomized trial 30904. *Eur. Urol.* **2014**, *65*, 372–377. [CrossRef]
36. Yoo, Y.C.; Shim, J.K.; Song, Y.; Yang, S.Y.; Kwak, Y.L. Anesthetics influence the incidence of acute kidney injury following valvular heart surgery. *Kidney Int.* **2014**, *86*, 414–422. [CrossRef]
37. Ammar, A.; Mahmoud, K. Comparative effect of propofol versus sevoflurane on renal ischemia/reperfusion injury after elective open abdominal aortic aneurysm repair. *Saudi J. Anaesth.* **2016**, *10*, 301.
38. Bang, J.Y.; Lee, J.; Oh, J.; Song, J.G.; Hwang, G.S. The Influence of Propofol and Sevoflurane on Acute Kidney Injury after Colorectal Surgery, A Retrospective Cohort Study. *Anesth. Analg.* **2016**, *123*, 363–370. [CrossRef]
39. Ebert, T.J.; Arain, S.R. Renal responses to low-flow desflurane, sevoflurane, and propofol in patients. *Anesthesiology* **2000**, *93*, 1401–1406. [CrossRef]
40. Oh, T.K.; Kim, J.; Han, S.; Kim, K.; Jheon, S.; Ji, E. Effect of sevoflurane-based or propofol-based anaesthesia on the incidence of postoperative acute kidney injury, A retrospective propensity score-matched analysis. *Eur. J. Anaesthesiol.* **2019**, *36*, 649–655.
41. Kheterpal, S.; Tremper, K.K.; Englesbe, M.J.; O'Reilly, M.; Shanks, A.M.; Fetterman, D.M.; Rosenberg, A.L.; Swartz, R.D. Predictors of postoperative acute renal failure after noncardiac surgery in patients with previously normal renal function. *Anesthesiology* **2007**, *107*, 892–902. [CrossRef] [PubMed]
42. Farag, E.; Makarova, N.; Argalious, M.; Cywinski, J.B.; Benzel, E.; Kalfas, I.; Sessler, D.I. Vasopressor infusion during prone spine surgery and acute renal injury, A retrospective cohort analysis. *Anesth. Analg.* **2019**, *219*, 896–904. [CrossRef] [PubMed]
43. Mascha, E.J.; Dalton, J.E.; Kurz, A.; Saager, L. Statistical grand rounds, understanding the mechanism, mediation analysis in randomized and nonrandomized studies. *Anesth. Analg.* **2013**, *117*, 980–994. [CrossRef]
44. Kheterpal, S.; Tremper, K.K.; Heung, M.; Rosenberg, A.L.; Englesbe, M.; Shanks, A.M.; Campbell, D.A. Development and validation of an acute kidney injury risk index for patients undergoing general surgery, results from a national data set. *Anesthesiology* **2009**, *110*, 505–515. [CrossRef]
45. Stucker, F.; Ponte, B.; De la Fuente, V.; Alves, C.; Rutschmann, O.; Carballo, S.; Vuilleumier, N.; Martin, P.Y.; Perneger, T.; Saudan, P. Risk factors for community-acquired acute kidney injury in patients with and without chronic kidney injury and impact of its initial management on prognosis, a prospective observational study. *BMC Nephrol.* **2017**, *18*, 380. [CrossRef] [PubMed]
46. Spaliviero, M.; Power, N.E.; Murray, K.S.; Sjoberg, D.D.; Benfante, N.E.; Bernstein, M.L.; Wren, J.; Russo, P.; Coleman, J.A. Intravenous mannitol versus placebo during partial nephrectomy in patients with normal

kidney function, a double-blind, clinically-integrated, randomized trial. *Eur. Urol.* **2018**, *73*, 53–59. [CrossRef] [PubMed]

47. Cockshott, I.D.; Briggs, L.P.; Douglas, E.J.; White, M. Pharmacokinetics of propofol in female patients, studies using single bolus injections. *Br. J. Anaesth.* **1987**, *59*, 1103–1110. [CrossRef] [PubMed]

# 11

# Preoperative Albuminuria and Intraoperative Chloride Load: Predictors of Acute Kidney Injury Following Major Abdominal Surgery

**Diamantina Marouli [1,2], Kostas Stylianou [3,*], Eleftherios Papadakis [1], Nikolaos Kroustalakis [3], Stavroula Kolyvaki [4], Georgios Papadopoulos [5], Christos Ioannou [5], Alexandra Papaioannou [1], Eugene Daphnis [3], Dimitris Georgopoulos [2] and Helen Askitopoulou [1]**

1 Departments of Anaesthesiology, University Hospital of Heraklion, 71110 Crete, Greece; marouli_matina@yahoo.gr (D.M.); elepapadakis@gmail.com (E.P.); alpapa@med.uoc.gr (A.P.); askitop@gmail.com (H.A.)
2 Intensive Care, University Hospital of Heraklion, 71110 Crete, Greece; georgop@med.uoc.gr
3 Nephrology, University Hospital of Heraklion, 71110 Crete, Greece; nkroustalakis@yahoo.gr (N.K.); eugenedaphnis@yahoo.gr (E.D.)
4 Clinical Biochemistry, University Hospital of Heraklion, 71110 Crete, Greece; s.kolyvaki@gmail.com
5 Vascular Surgery, University Hospital of Heraklion, 71110 Crete, Greece; gpamd2003@yahoo.gr (G.P.); ioannou@med.uoc.gr (C.I.)
* Correspondence: kstylianu@gmail.com

**Abstract:** Background: Postoperative Acute Kidney Injury (AKI) is a common and serious complication associated with significant morbidity and mortality. While several pre- and intra-operative risk factors for AKI have been recognized in cardiac surgery patients, relatively few data are available regarding the incidence and risk factors for perioperative AKI in other surgical operations. The aim of the present study was to determine the risk factors for perioperative AKI in patients undergoing major abdominal surgery. Methods: This was a prospective, observational study of patients undergoing major abdominal surgery in a tertiary care center. Postoperative AKI was diagnosed according to the Acute Kidney Injury Network criteria within 48 h after surgery. Patients with chronic kidney disease stage IV or V were excluded. Logistic regression analysis was used to evaluate the association between perioperative factors and the risk of developing postoperative AKI. Results: Eleven out of 61 patients developed postoperative AKI. Four intra-operative variables were identified as predictors of AKI: intra-operative blood loss ($p = 0.002$), transfusion of fresh frozen plasma ($p = 0.004$) and red blood cells ($p = 0.038$), as well as high chloride load ($p = 0.033$, cut-off value > 500 mEq). Multivariate analysis demonstrated an independent association between AKI development and preoperative albuminuria, defined as a urinary Albumin to Creatinine ratio $\geq$ 30 mg·g$^{-1}$ (OR = 6.88, 95% CI: 1.43–33.04, $p = 0.016$) as well as perioperative chloride load > 500 mEq (OR = 6.87, 95% CI: 1.46–32.4, $p = 0.015$). Conclusion: Preoperative albuminuria, as well as a high intraoperative chloride load, were identified as predictors of postoperative AKI in patients undergoing major abdominal surgery.

**Keywords:** albuminuria; chloride; postoperative acute kidney injury

---

## 1. Introduction

Postoperative acute kidney injury (AKI) represents a common, yet under-recognized, perioperative complication, with a reported incidence varying between 1% and 36%, depending on the type of surgery and the definition of kidney failure [1–4]. AKI represents a leading cause of morbidity and mortality in surgical patients [5–7], and an increased risk for chronic kidney disease (CKD) and hemodialysis after discharge, factors associated with increased cost and resource utilization [8]. Even minor postoperative creatinine increases not fulfilling AKI criteria are independently associated with a two-fold risk of in-hospital death and a three-day longer hospital stay [9]. Although risk factors for postoperative AKI in patients undergoing cardiac surgery have been extensively studied [10,11], there is a relative paucity of available data regarding perioperative risk factors associated with major non-cardiac surgery.

The aim of this prospective observational study was to determine the incidence and to identify the pre- and intra-operative risk factors associated with the development of postoperative AKI, using the Acute Kidney Injury Network (AKIN) criteria [12], in patients undergoing elective major abdominal surgery.

## 2. Methods

### 2.1. Study Population

This was a single-center, prospective cohort study conducted at a tertiary academic hospital. Between February 2012 and December 2016 all adult patients undergoing elective major abdominal (including vascular) surgery were enrolled. All subjects gave their informed consent for inclusion before they participated in the study. The study was conducted in accordance with the Declaration of Helsinki, and the protocol was approved by the local institutional Ethics Committee (Approval-Nr. 5985, 14.07.2011)

On admission to hospital, the following patient variables were recorded: Age, sex, body mass index, preoperative medications, American Society of Anesthesiologists (ASA) physical status [13], and co-morbidities (arterial hypertension, coronary artery disease, congestive heart failure, chronic obstructive pulmonary disease, and diabetes mellitus). Perioperative evaluation of renal function included measurements of the following laboratory parameters: Serum creatinine and cystatin C, as well as urine albumin and creatinine at predefined time points. The times of measurements were: Preoperatively (Pre-op), in the recovery room (RR), and on postoperative days (POD) 1, 3, 5 and 7 (POD1, POD3, POD5, POD7). The calculated parameters were: Estimated glomerular filtration rate (eGFR), urine albumin to creatinine ratio (UACR), fractional excretion of sodium (FeNa), and fractional excretion of urea (FeUr). An eGFR $< 90$ mL·min·m$^{-2}$ and a UACR value $\geq 30$ mg·g$^{-1}$ were considered abnormal. Serum and urine samples were centrifuged at 3000 rpm for 10 min and at 1500 rpm for 5 min, respectively, and stored at $-80$ °C until analysis. Exclusion criteria included: ASA 5 (moribund, not expected to live 24 h irrespective of procedure), chronic kidney disease (CKD) stage IV or V [14], preoperative (within the prior month) use of drugs with known nephrotoxic activity, and emergency surgery.

The recorded intra-operative surgical and anesthetic parameters were: Type of surgery, volume and type of intravenous fluids, transfusions of red blood cells, fresh frozen plasma or platelets, vasopressor administration, mean arterial blood pressure, urine output, and blood loss. The total chloride ion content of intra-operatively administered crystalloids and colloids was estimated. Patients were followed until the 7th postoperative day or hospital discharge, whatever occurred first. Preoperative patient demographics, laboratory values and intra-operative variables were evaluated for their association with perioperative AKI development.

### 2.2. Outcomes

The primary outcome of the study was the development of perioperative AKI, defined by the AKIN criteria using the maximal change in serum creatinine and eGFR within 48 h after surgery (Table 1). The eGFR was estimated by using the Chronic Kidney Disease Epidemiology (CKD-EPI) Creatinine Equation [15].

**Table 1.** AKI * diagnosis based on AKIN ** creatinine criteria. (Patients receiving RRT *** are considered to have met criteria for Stage 3, irrespective of the stage they were at the commencement of RRT).

| AKI Staging | Definition |
|---|---|
| Stage 1 | 1.5-fold increase in sCr or increase of $\geq$0.3 mg·dL$^{-1}$ |
| Stage 2 | 2-fold increase in sCr |
| Stage 3 | 3-fold increase in sCr or sCr $\geq$ 4 mg·dL$^{-1}$, with acute rise of $\geq$0.5 mg·dL$^{-1}$ |

* AKI = acute kidney injury; ** AKIN = Acute Kidney Injury Network; sCr = serum creatinine; *** RRT = renal replacement therapy.

### 2.3. Statistical Analysis

Data were analyzed using SPSS for Windows (version 22.0; SPSS Inc., Chicago, IL, USA). Continuous variables were expressed as medians with range or means ± SD and were analyzed using an independent *t*-test or the Mann-Whitney test. Numerical data, expressed as counts and % proportions, were analyzed using the Pearson's chi-square or the Fisher's exact test. Simple logistic regression models were applied to determine odds ratios (ORs) and 95% confidence intervals (CIs), for the perioperative risk factors associated with postoperative AKI development. Multiple logistic regression was applied to establish a model for AKI prediction with prediction variables UACR > 30 mg·g$^{-1}$ and intraoperative chloride load > 500 mEq.

For graphical representation, data box and whisker plots were used. For all analyses, a $p$ value < 0.05 was considered statistically significant.

## 3. Results

Between February 2012 and December 2016, 61 patients (47 males and 14 females) with a mean age of 67.1 ± 10.2 years underwent major elective abdominal surgery. Eleven patients (18%) developed postoperative AKI (AKI group), while 50 did not (Non-AKI group). The baseline clinical and demographic characteristics of both groups are presented in Table 2, while preoperative laboratory values and intraoperative variables are presented in Tables 3 and 4, respectively. The two groups were comparable in terms of sex, age, body mass index, co-morbidities, major drug categories prescription, pre-operative CKD stage, and ASA score. However, a significant association between type of surgery and development of perioperative AKI was detected, with vascular surgery patients experiencing a significantly higher AKI incidence (31.8% vs. 10.3% in non-vascular surgery patients).

**Table 2.** Baseline clinical and demographic characteristics according to AKI status.

| | Non-AKI Group ($n$ = 50) | AKI Group ($n$ = 11) | $p$ Value | Odd's Ratio (95% CI) |
|---|---|---|---|---|
| | **Demographics** | | | |
| Mean age, (years ± SD) | 66.9 ± 10 | 68.2 ± 10.4 | 0.699 | 1.01 (0.95–1.08) |
| Male gender, ($n$) | 33 | 8 | 0.67 | 1.02 (0.92–1.13) |
| Mean BMI, kg·m$^{-2}$ | 27.2 ± 4.2 | 27.7 ± 5.6 | 0.721 | 1.03 (0.89–1.19) |
| | **ASA Classification, ($n$)** | | | |
| ASA II | 27 | 4 | 0.087 | 1.0 |
| ASA III | 20 | 6 | 0.076 | 3.9 (0.73–33.80) |
| ASA IV | 3 | 1 | 0.249 | 4.8 (0.33–70.40) |
| | **Comorbidities, ($n$)** | | | |
| Hypertension | 31 | 6 | 0.738 | 1.4 (0.20–2.75) |
| CKD | 34 | 9 | 0.481 | 2.1 (0.41–10.95) |
| Stage I | 4 | 2 | 0.226 | 4 (0.42–37.78) |
| Stage II | 25 | 5 | 0.600 | 1.6 (0.28–9.26) |
| Stage III | 5 | 2 | 0.301 | 3.2 (0.35–28.94) |
| CAD | 14 | 4 | 0.717 | 1.5 (0.37–5.81) |
| CHF | 11 | 5 | 0.067 | 3.8 (0.98–14.70) |

**Table 2.** *Cont.*

| | Non-AKI Group ($n$ = 50) | AKI Group ($n$ = 11) | $p$ Value | Odd's Ratio (95% CI) |
|---|---|---|---|---|
| DM | 14 | 5 | 0.137 | 3 (0.76–11.54) |
| COPD | 19 | 6 | 0.174 | 3.1 (0.80–12.09) |
| **Surgical Procedures, ($n$)** | | | | |
| Other abdominal Surgery | 35 (89.7%) | 4 (10.3%) | 0.079 | |
| Vascular surgery | 15 (68.2%) | 7 (31.8%) | 0.035 | 4.1 (1.04–16.06) |

Mean (SD): mean and standard deviation (in brackets), $n$: number of patients OR (95% CI): Odd's ratio with 95% confidence intervals (in brackets), $p$-values from Pearson's chi-square or Fisher's exact test. Abbreviations: AKI: Acute Kidney Injury; BMI: Body Mass Index; CKD: Chronic Kidney Disease; CAD: Coronary Artery Disease; CHF: Congestive Heart Failure; DM: Diabetes Mellitus; COPD: Chronic Obstructive Pulmonary Disease.

**Table 3.** Baseline laboratory values according to AKI status (expressed as mean ± SD, except UACR which is expressed in numbers of patients).

| | Non-AKI Group ($n$ = 50) | AKI Group ($n$ = 11) | $p$ Value | Odd's Ratio (95% CI) |
|---|---|---|---|---|
| Serum Creatinine, mg·dL$^{-1}$ | 0.87 (±0.23) | 1.02 (±0.21) | 0.063 | 12.6 (0.80–198.7) |
| Serum Cystatin C, mg·L$^{-1}$ | 0.76 (±0.19) | 0.82 (±0.28) | 0.319 | 5.20 (0.21–126.7) |
| eGFR, mL·min$^{-1}$ 1.73 m$^{-2}$ | 83.92 (±15.15) | 75.27 (±15.97) | 0.095 | 0.97 (0.93–1.01) |
| Urine Albumin, mg·L$^{-1}$ | 24.1 (±50.7) | 325 (±729.9) | 0.042 | 1.01 (1.00–1.01) |
| Urine Creatinine, g·L$^{-1}$ | 1.1 (±0.6) | 1.2 (±0.7) | 0.344 | 1.66 (0.58–4.66) |
| UACR > 30 mg·gr$^{-1}$, ($n$) | 9 (18.0) | 6 (54.5) | 0.011 | 5.47 (1.36–21.92) |
| FeNa, % | 0.8 (±0.7) | 0.8 (±0.8) | 0.919 | 1.05 (0.40–2.75) |
| FeUrea, % | 41.4 (±12.7) | 37.2 (±10.5) | 0.303 | 0.97 (0.92–1.03) |

Mean (SD): mean and standard deviation (in brackets), $n$: number of patients. OR (95% CI): Odd's ratio with 95% confidence intervals (in brackets), $p$-values from Pearson's chi-square or Fisher's exact test. Abbreviations: AKI: Acute Kidney Injury; eGFR: estimated Glomerular Filtration Rate; UACR: Urine Albumin to Creatinine Ratio; FeNa: Fractional Excretion of Sodium; FeUrea: Fractional Excretion of Urea.

**Table 4.** Intraoperative variables according to AKI status (expressed as mean ± SD, except Vasopressors which are expressed in numbers of patients).

| | Non-AKI Group ($n$ = 50) | AKI Group ($n$ = 11) | $p$ Value | Odd's Ratio (95% CI) |
|---|---|---|---|---|
| **Intraoperative Variables(mean±SD)** | | | | |
| Urine output (mL·kg$^{-1}$·hr$^{-1}$) | 2.1 (±2.0) | 1.1 (±0.8) | 0.151 | 0.37 (0.13–1.1) |
| Mean Arterial Pressure (mmHg) | 78.7 (±6.9) | 79.6 (±10.5) | 0.734 | 1.01 (0.93–1.10) |
| Vasopressor administration, ($n$) | 32 (64.0) | 8 (72.7) | 0.581 | 1.67 (0.86–2.65) |
| Blood loss (mL) | 479 (±508.5) | 1345.5 (±1336.7) | 0.002 | 1.06 (1.02–1.1) |
| **Intraoperative Fluids(mean ± SD)** | | | | |
| Total crystalloids (mL) | 2441 (±1195) | 3018 (±1497) | 0.171 | 1.00 (1.00–1.00) |
| Total colloids (mL) | 865 (±354) | 1046 (±611) | 0.191 | 1.00 (1.00–1.00) |
| RBC transfusion (units) | 1.1 (±1.4) | 2.3 (±2.4) | 0.042 | 1.49 (1.03–2.01) |
| FFP transfusion (units) | 1.2 (±1.4) | 2.6 (±2.1) | 0.006 | 1.69 (1.11–2.56) |
| PLT transfusion (units) | 0.04 (±0.28) | 0.4 (±1.2) | 0.088 | 2.04 (0.73–5.71) |
| Chloride load (mEq) | 458.6 (±179.8) | 583.9 (±191.5) | 0.043 | 1.03 (1.01–1.05) |

Mean (SD): mean and standard deviation (in brackets), $n$: number of patients; OR (95%CI): Odd's ratio with 95% confidence intervals (in brackets); $p$-values from Pearson's chi-square or Fisher's exact test. AKI: Acute Kidney Injury; RBC: Red Blood Cells; FFP: Fresh Frozen Plasma; PLT: Platelets.

There was no statistically significant difference in the preoperative eGFR between AKI and non-AKI patients (75.3 ± 16 vs. 83.9 ± 15.2 mL·min$^{-1}$·m$^{-2}$). However, in the AKI group, the eGFR was significantly lower in the recovery room (69.5 ± 18.7 vs. 85.7 ± 15.6 mL·min$^{-1}$·m$^{-2}$, $p$ = 0.001) and remained so throughout the entire follow-up period (Figure 1).

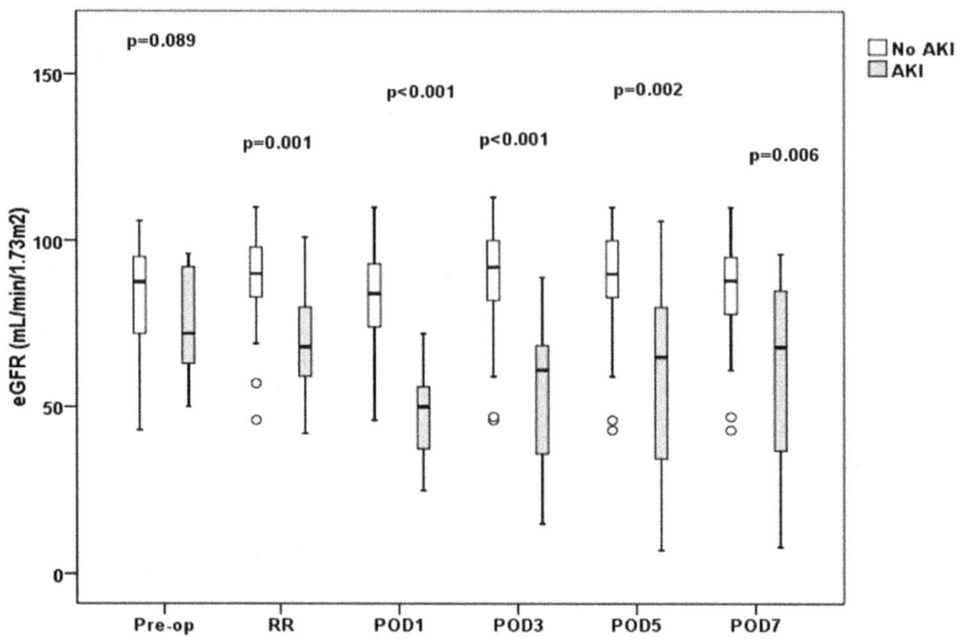


**Figure 1.** Estimated glomerular filtration rate (eGFR) at predefined time-points. Open boxes represent non-AKI patients, shaded boxes AKI patients. Boxes and whiskers show interquartile ranges and total observed ranges, respectively. eGFR: estimated Glomerular Filtration Rate; Pre-op: preoperatively; RR: recovery room; POD1: postoperative day 1; POD3: postoperative day 3; POD5: postoperative day 5; POD7: postoperative day 7.

Differences between AKI and non-AKI patients regarding serum creatinine and cystatin C concentrations are shown in Figures 2 and 3, respectively.

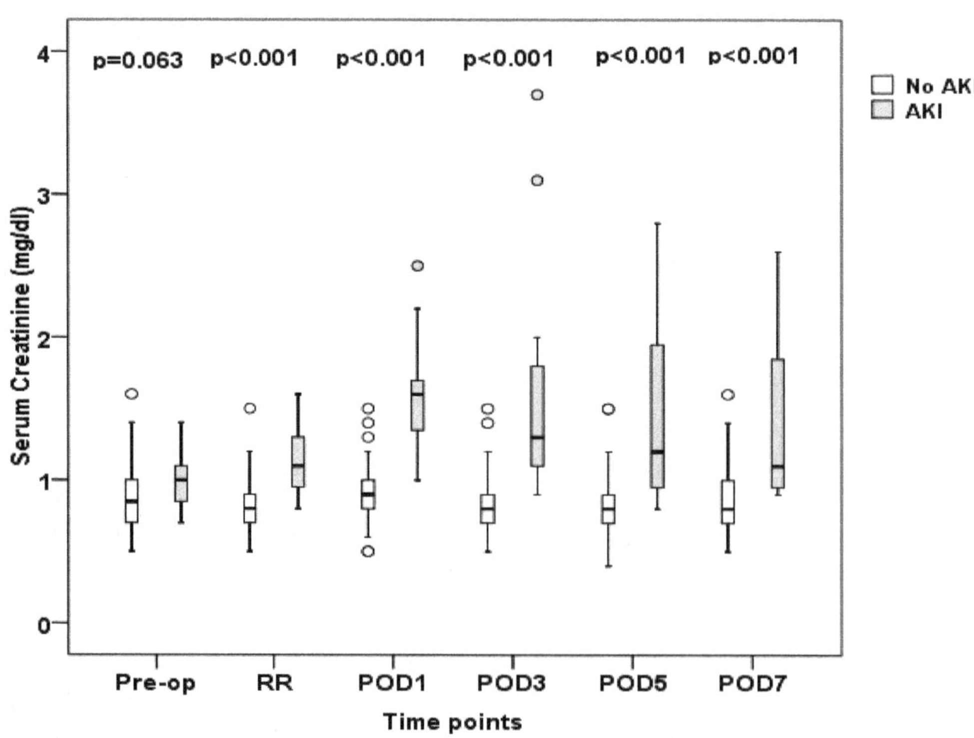


**Figure 2.** Serum creatinine measurements at predefined time-points. Open boxes represent non-AKI patients, shaded boxes AKI patients. Boxes and whiskers show interquartile ranges and total observed ranges, respectively. Pre-op: preoperatively; RR: recovery room; POD1: postoperative day 1; POD3: postoperative day 3; POD5: postoperative day 5; POD7: postoperative day 7.

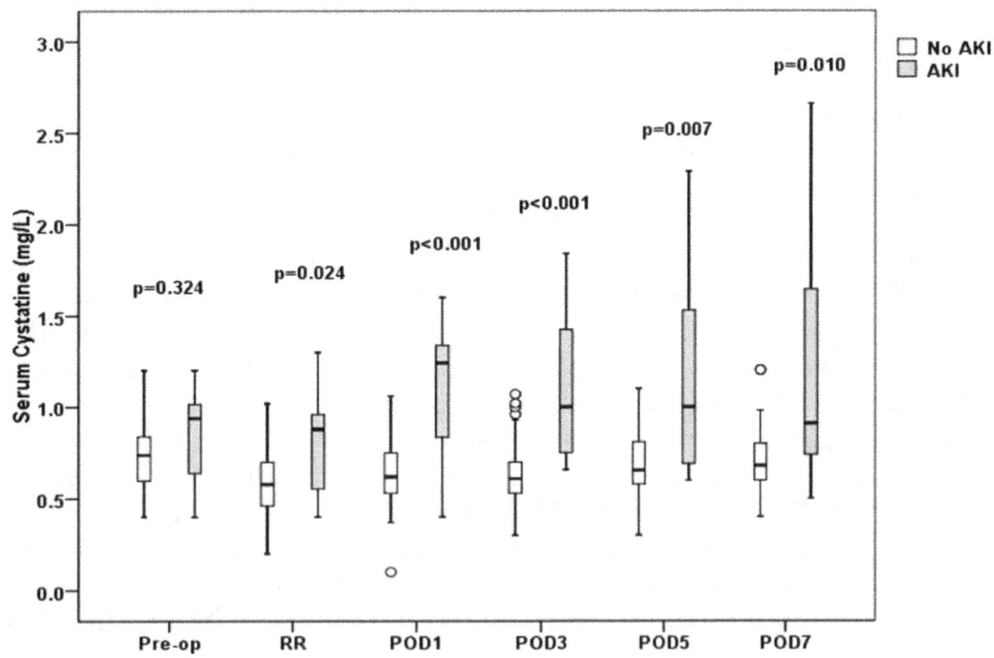


**Figure 3.** Serum cystatin C measurements at predefined time-points. Open boxes represent non-AKI patients, shaded boxes AKI patients. Boxes and whiskers show interquartile ranges and total observed ranges, respectively. Pre-op: preoperatively; RR: recovery room; POD1: postoperative day 1; POD3: postoperative day 3; POD5: postoperative day 5; POD7: postoperative day 7.

Univariate analysis showed that an abnormal *preoperative* UACR was strongly associated with postoperative AKI development (OR = 5.47, 95% CI: 1.36–21.92, $p = 0.019$). Four *intra-operative* variables were also identified as significant predictors of postoperative AKI (Table 4): intra-operative blood loss, transfusion of RBCs and FFP, and intraoperative chloride load. Receiver operating curve analysis showed that an intraoperative chloride load > 500 mEq (AUC 0.715 $\pm$ 0.095, $p = 0.033$) had a sensitivity of 70% and a specificity of 77% in predicting the development of AKI. There was a strong correlation between blood losses and transfusion of RBCs and FFP. Thus, due to co-linearity, only the total amount of intraoperative fluids, along with chloride load and UACR were introduced in the multivariate model. Multivariate regression analysis confirmed that a UACR $\geq$ 30 mg·g$^{-1}$ (OR = 6.88, 95% CI: 1.43–33.04, $p = 0.016$) and chloride load > 500 mEq (OR = 6.87, 95% CI: 1.46–32.4, $p = 0.015$) were independent predictors of postoperative AKI. The remaining intra-operative variables did not differ significantly between the two groups.

## 4. Discussion

The present prospective study of postoperative acute kidney injury following elective major abdominal surgery showed an incidence of 18%. The development of AKI, defined by the AKIN creatinine criteria, was strongly associated with an abnormal (i.e., $\geq$30 mg·g$^{-1}$) preoperative urine albumin to creatinine ratio. Furthermore, four intra-operative variables were identified as independent AKI predictors: Intra-operative blood loss, transfusion of red blood cells and fresh frozen plasma, and intraoperative chloride load >500 mEq.

The incidence of postoperative AKI and its association with perioperative risk factors has been extensively studied in the cardiac surgery population [16]. In the majority of these studies, postoperative AKI was defined as deterioration in renal function requiring renal replacement therapy in patients without pre-existing kidney dysfunction. However, risk factors for AKI following major abdominal surgery have received less attention. According to a recent systematic review of risk prediction models for AKI following non-cardiac surgery, seven models were identified from six studies [17], with only two studies focusing on general surgery patients. Kheterpal et al. [18] studied the incidence and risk factors for postoperative AKI in a general population of non-cardiac (mainly thoracic, intraperitoneal, and suprainguinal vascular) surgery patients with normal renal function (defined as a calculated preoperative creatinine clearance of $\geq$80 mL·min$^{-1}$). They found an AKI incidence of 0.8% and identified seven independent preoperative AKI risk factors: Age, body mass index, liver disease, peripheral vascular disease, chronic obstructive pulmonary disease, high-risk surgery, and emergent surgery. The low incidence of postoperative AKI in that study was probably related to the definition of AKI as a drop in estimated creatinine clearance below 50 mL·min$^{-1}$, within the first 7 postoperative days. Biteker et al. [19] studied postoperative AKI, as defined by the RIFLE [20] AKI staging criteria in elective non-cardiac major surgery patients without preoperative renal dysfunction (serum creatinine <1.6 mg·dL$^{-1}$ for men and <1.4 mg·dL$^{-1}$ for women, respectively). They found a postoperative AKI incidence of 6.7% and identified four independent AKI predictors (age, diabetes, Revised Cardiac Risk Index [21], and ASA physical status).

In the present study, the incidence of AKI was 18%, significantly higher compared to the aforementioned studies. This could be partly explained by the different definitions used for the diagnosis of AKI. It is well known that the AKIN classification (by "broadening" the stage I AKI criteria) increases the sensitivity of AKI diagnosis. In fact, Joannidis et al. [22] showed that by using the AKIN classification, an additional 9% of cases not fulfilling RIFLE criteria could be identified. Furthermore, the present study excluded only patients with stage IV and V chronic kidney disease and patients receiving drugs with established nephrotoxic effects [23]. In fact, 49.2% and 11.5% of the studied population had CKD stage II and III, respectively. This factor should be considered when interpreting our results, since a well-defined graded association exists between severity of reduction in baseline eGFR and progressively higher risk of AKI [24]. Furthermore, it should be noted that 22 of the total 61 patients underwent vascular surgery, mainly open abdominal aneurysm repair, a procedure known to be associated with a postoperative AKI incidence of up to 26% depending on the AKI definition [25].

It is noteworthy that in the AKI group, a significant decline in eGFR with a concomitant rise in serum creatinine and cystatin C was already evident at the recovery room, immediately following surgery. This finding is in line with previous observations in cardiac surgery patients [26], as well as surgical ICU patients [27], where an immediate postoperative elevation in serum creatinine and cystatin C has also been described. However, one should keep in mind that in the early stages of AKI, the diagnostic value of serum creatinine is limited for several well-known reasons [28]. More importantly, the various eGFR equations that have been developed are intended for diagnosing and staging CKD patients in steady-state conditions rather than estimating creatinine clearance during an AKI episode [29].

The most interesting finding of the present study was the significant association between an abnormal preoperative UACR and the development of postoperative AKI, regardless of preoperative renal function or other comorbidities. In fact, the presence of a UACR >30 mg·gr$^{-1}$ resulted in a five-fold higher risk of AKI development. In recent years, albuminuria has been identified as a significant risk factor for AKI and adverse long-term outcomes, both in the general population [30,31] and in cardiac surgery patients [32,33]. Our findings are in line with the results of a large prospective study in the general population (the Atherosclerosis Risk in Communities (ARIC) study) [24], showing a significant risk of hospitalizations and/or death from AKI in people with increased baseline UACR. Preoperative proteinuria, independent of preoperative eGFR, was not only associated with the risk of AKI, but was also a powerful independent risk factor for long-term all-cause mortality and end stage renal disease (ESRD) after cardiac surgery [32,33]. However, to the best of our knowledge, this is the first study reporting a strong relationship between pre-operative albuminuria and postoperative AKI after non-cardiac surgery, a factor that has been overlooked in existing predictive models.

CKD is the most consistent pre-existing condition associated with a high risk of AKI in almost every relevant study. While the definition of CKD includes many parameters, with the most prevalent being albuminuria, this parameter has been largely neglected in most studies where data on urine albumin were generally lacking [12]. Albuminuria represents a state of generalized endothelial dysfunction and is recognized as one of the most important risk factors for cardiovascular and renal events [34,35]. It is not surprising that baseline UACR was identified as an independent prognostic factor for postoperative AKI for two reasons: First, the recognition of increased UACR reclassifies patients with normal eGFR to stage I CKD, which increases the risk for AKI; and second, it unmasks an already existing renal pathology that is not detected by serum creatinine alone. In this context, angiotensin converting enzyme inhibitors (ACEi(s)), an established anti-proteinuric therapy, have been shown to reduce the incidence of postoperative AKI and all-cause mortality by 17% and 9%, respectively [36]. Thus, we can hypothesize that the protective effect of ACEi(s) may be mediated not only via the intra-renal hemodynamic effects, but also due to their anti-proteinuric properties. Nevertheless, since this is an observational study, we can only report associations and cannot claim causality.

Blood loss and the need for intraoperative transfusion of red blood cells and fresh frozen plasma were found to be associated with the development of postoperative AKI. These factors represent well-known risks for AKI [37]. A meta-analysis of 20 randomized controlled trials on perioperative hemodynamic optimization identified several interventions associated with significant reduction in the incidence of postoperative AKI [38], including optimization of intravascular volume, cardiac output, and oxygen delivery, emphasizing the importance of intraoperative preservation of renal perfusion. Furthermore, multiple studies have found an association between RBC transfusion and renal dysfunction in patients undergoing cardiac and vascular surgery. It is known that stored RBCs undergo changes known as "storage lesion", i.e., irreversible changes in RBC deformity causing stronger adherence to vascular endothelium with a resulting decreased microvascular flow [38,39].

Regarding preservation of renal perfusion, intraoperative blood pressure management is regarded as a key element. Recent observational studies identified episodes of intraoperative hypotension as an independent risk factor for AKI development [40,41]. This observation has been further strengthened by a multi-center randomized controlled trial [42], where an intraoperative strategy targeting an individualized systolic blood pressure (within 10% of patient baseline values) achieved an absolute AKI risk reduction of 16% compared to standard management, emphasizing the importance of individualized patient care. We were not able to reproduce these findings in our study population, where according to anesthetic charts, time-averaged mean arterial pressure was higher than 65 mmHg and did not differ between the two groups. However, a larger proportion of patients in the AKI group required intraoperative vasopressor support, which might be regarded as an indirect indicator of severe intraoperative hypotensive episodes.

Another intraoperative factor significantly and independently associated with development of postoperative AKI was the intraoperative infusion of a high chloride load. This finding is in line with experimental, as well as clinical data, showing that chloride infusion-induced hyperchloremia causes renal vasoconstriction resulting in cortical hypoperfusion [43,44]. A growing body of evidence from observational studies suggests that volume loading with chloride-rich solutions is associated with kidney dysfunction, as compared with the use of balanced solutions [45–47]. A recent meta-analysis including more than 6000 patients concluded that the perioperative use of chloride-rich crystalloids, as compared to the use of balanced solutions, increased the risk of AKI [48].

## 5. Conclusions

In conclusion, the present study showed that in patients developing postoperative AKI, a reduction of the eGFR can be detected very early in the postoperative period. An intraoperative chloride load higher than 500 mEq, as well as a pre-operative urine albumin to creatinine ratio >30 $mg{\cdot}g^{-1}$, were significantly and independently associated with postoperative AKI development. However, since the study patients had several comorbidities and some degree of pre-existing renal dysfunction rendering them more susceptible to future renal injury, the implications of these results might be limited to patients with similar comorbidities and not be applicable to otherwise healthy surgical patients. Nevertheless, the presence of preoperative albuminuria seems to be a significant, yet neglected, independent risk factor for postoperative AKI. Bearing in mind that the strength of association and degree of external validity of this risk association needs further evaluation. We suggest that albuminuria should be included in the routine preoperative patient evaluation for major abdominal surgery and considered as a possible prognostic factor in future AKI risk prediction models.

**Author Contributions:** Conceptualization, K.S., A.P., E.D., and D.G.; Data curation, D.M., N.K., S.K., and G.P.; Formal analysis, D.M., E.P., and N.K.; Investigation, D.M., E.P., N.K., S.K., and G.P.; Methodology, K.S.; Project administration, D.G. and H.A.; Resources, N.K., S.K., G.P., C.I., A.P., E.D., and D.G.; Supervision, A.P. and E.D.; Validation, G.P., C.I., E.D., and D.G.; Writing—original draft, D.M.; Writing—review & editing, K.S., C.I., A.P., D.G., and H.A.

## References

1. Ishani, A.; Nelson, D.; Clothier, B.; Schult, T.; Nugent, S.; Greer, N.; Slinin, Y.; Ensrud, K.E. The magnitude of acute serum creatinine increase after cardiac surgery and the risk of chronic kidney disease, progression of kidney disease, and death. *Arch. Intern. Med.* **2011**, *171*, 226–233. [CrossRef] [PubMed]
2. Bihorac, A.; Delano, M.J.; Schold, J.D.; Lopez, M.C.; Nathens, A.B.; Maier, R.V.; Layon, A.J.; Baker, H.V.; Moldawer, L.L. Incidence, clinical predictors, genomics, and outcome of acute kidney injury among trauma patients. *Ann. Surg.* **2010**, *252*, 158–165. [CrossRef] [PubMed]
3. Shaw, A. Update on acute kidney injury after cardiac surgery. *J. Thorac. Cardiovasc. Surg.* **2012**, *143*, 676–681. [CrossRef] [PubMed]
4. Grams, M.E.; Sang, Y.; Coresh, J.; Ballew, S.; Matsushita, K.; Zolnar, M.Z.; Szabo, Z.; Kalantar-Zadeh, K.; Covesdy, C.P. Acute kidney injury after major surgery: A retrospective analysis of Veterans Health Administration data. *Am. J. Kidney Dis.* **2016**, *67*, 872–880. [CrossRef] [PubMed]
5. Borthwick, E.; Ferguson, A. Perioperative acute kidney injury: Risk factors, recognition, management and outcomes. *BMJ* **2010**, *341*, c3365. [CrossRef] [PubMed]
6. Bihorac, A.; Yavas, S.; Subbiah, S.; Hobson, C.E.; Schold, J.D.; Gabrielli, A.; Layon, A.J.; Segal, M.S. Long-term risk of mortality and acute kidney injury during hospitalization after major surgery. *Ann. Surg.* **2009**, *249*, 851–858. [CrossRef] [PubMed]
7. Hobson, C.E.; Yavas, S.; Segal, M.S.; Schold, J.D.; Tribble, C.G.; Layon, A.J.; Bihorac, A. Acute kidney injury is associated with increased long-term mortality after cardiothoracic surgery. *Circulation* **2009**, *119*, 2444–2453. [CrossRef] [PubMed]
8. Hobson, C.E.; Ozrazgat-Baslanti, T.; Kuxhausen, A.; Thottakara, P.; Efron, P.A.; Moore, F.A.; Moldawer, L.L.; Segal, M.S.; Bihorac, A. Cost and mortality associated with postoperative acute kidney injury. *Ann. Surg.* **2015**, *261*, 1207–1214. [CrossRef] [PubMed]
9. Kork, F.; Balzer, F.; Spies, C.D.; Wernecke, K.D.; Ginde, A.A.; Jankowski, J.; Eltzschik, H.K. Minor postoperative increases of creatinine are associated with higher mortality and longer hospital length of stay in surgical patients. *Anesthesiology* **2015**, *123*, 1301–1311. [CrossRef] [PubMed]
10. Thakar, C.V.; Arrigain, S.; Worley, S.; Yared, J.P.; Paganini, E.P. A clinical score to predict acute renal failure after cardiac surgery. *J. Am. Soc. Nephrol.* **2005**, *16*, 162–168. [CrossRef] [PubMed]
11. Mehta, R.H.; Grab, J.D.; O'Brien, S.M.; Bridges, C.R.; Gammie, J.S.; Haan, C.K.; Ferguson, T.B.; Peterson, E.D. Society of thoracic surgeons national cardiac surgery database investigators. Bedside tool for predicting the risk of postoperative dialysis in patients undergoing cardiac surgery. *Circulation* **2006**, *114*, 2208–2216. [CrossRef] [PubMed]
12. Khwaja, A. KDIGO clinical practice guidelines for acute kidney injury. *Nephron Clin. Pract.* **2012**, *120*, 179–184. [CrossRef] [PubMed]
13. American Society of Anesthesiologists. New classification of physical status. *Anesthesiology* **1963**, *24*, 111.
14. National kidney Foundation. K/DOQI clinical practice guidelines for chronic kidney disease: Evaluation, classification, and stratification. *Am. J. Kidney Dis.* **2002**, *39*, S1–S266.
15. Inker, L.A.; Schmid, C.H.; Tighiouart, H.; Eckfeldt, J.H.; Feldman, H.I.; Greene, T.; Kusek, J.W.; Manzi, J.; Van Lente, F.; Zhang, Y.L.; et al. Estimating glomerular filtration rate from serum creatinine and cystatin C. *N. Engl. J. Med.* **2012**, *367*, 20–29. [CrossRef] [PubMed]
16. Huen, S.C.; Parikh, C.R. Predicting acute kidney injury after cardiac surgery: A systematic review. *Ann. Thorac. Surg.* **2012**, *93*, 337–347. [CrossRef] [PubMed]

17. Wilson, T.; Quan, S.; Cheema, K.; Zarnke, K.; Quinn, R.; de Koning, L.; Dixon, E.; Pannu, N.; James, M.T. Risk prediction models for acute kidney injury following major noncardiac surgery: Systematic review. *Nephrol. Dial. Transplant.* **2016**, *31*, 231–240. [CrossRef] [PubMed]
18. Kheterpal, S.; Tremper, K.K.; Englesbe, M.J.; O'Reilly, M.; Shanks, A.M.; Fetterman, D.M.; Rosenberg, A.L.; Swartz, R.D. Predictors of postoperative acute renal failure after noncardiac surgery in patients with previously normal renal function. *Anesthesiology* **2007**, *107*, 892–902. [CrossRef] [PubMed]
19. Biteker, M.; Dayan, A.; Tekkesin, A.I.; Can, M.M.; Tayci, I.; Ilhan, E.; Gülizar, S. Incidence, risk factors, and outcomes of perioperative acute kidney injury in noncardiac and nonvascular surgery. *Am. J. Surg.* **2014**, *207*, 53–59. [CrossRef] [PubMed]
20. Bellomo, R.; Ronco, C.; Kellum, J.A.; Mehta, R.L.; Palevsky, P. Acute renal Failure: Definition, outcome measures, animal models, fluid therapy and information technology needs. The second international consensus conference of the Acute Dialysis Quality Initiative (ADQI) Group. *Crit. Care* **2004**, *8*, R204–R212. [CrossRef] [PubMed]
21. Lee, T.H.; Marcantonio, E.R.; Mangione, C.M.; Thomas, E.J.; Polanczyk, C.A.; Cook, E.F.; Sugarbaker, D.J.; Donaldson, M.C.; Poss, R.; Ho, K.K.; et al. Derivation and prospective validation of a simple index for prediction of cardiac risk of major noncardiac surgery. *Circulation* **1999**, *100*, 1043–1049. [CrossRef] [PubMed]
22. Joannidis, M.; Metnitz, B.; Bauer, P.; Schusterschitz, N.; Moreno, R.; Druml, W.; Metnitz, P.G. Acute kidney injury in critically ill patients classified by AKIN versus RIFLE using the SAPS 3 database. *Intensive Care Med.* **2009**, *35*, 1692–1702. [CrossRef] [PubMed]
23. Hosohata, K.; Ando, H.; Fujimura, A. Early detection of drug-induced kidney injury by vanin-1. *J. Pharmacol. Exp. Ther.* **2012**, *341*, 656–662. [CrossRef] [PubMed]
24. Grams, M.E.; Astor, B.C.; Bash, L.D.; Matsushita, K.; Wang, Y.; Coresh, J. Albuminuria and estimated glomerular filtration rate independently associate with acute kidney injury. *J. Am. Soc. Nephrol.* **2010**, *21*, 1757–1764. [CrossRef] [PubMed]
25. Dariane, C.; Coscas, R.; Boulitrop, C.; Javerliat, I.; Vilaine, E.; Goeau-Brissonierre, O.; Coggia, M.; Massy, Z.A. Acute kidney injury after open repair of intact abdominal aortic aneurysms. *Ann. Vasc. Surg.* **2017**, *39*, 294–300. [CrossRef] [PubMed]
26. Haase-Fielitz, A.; Bellomo, R.; Devarajan, P.; Story, D.; Matalanis, G.; Dragun, D.; Haase, M. Novel and conventional serum biomarkers predicting acute kidney injury in adult cardiac surgery—A prospective cohort study. *Crit. Care Med.* **2009**, *37*, 553–560. [CrossRef] [PubMed]
27. Dewitte, A.; Joannes-Boyau, O.; Sidobre, C.; Fleureau, C.; Bats, M.L.; Derarche, P.; Leuillet, S.; Ripoche, J.; Combe, C.; Ouattara, A. Kinetic eGFR and novel AKI biomarkers to predict renal recovery. *Clin. J. Am. Soc. Nephrol.* **2015**, *10*, 1900–1910. [CrossRef] [PubMed]
28. Wasung, M.E.; Chawla, L.S.; Madero, M. Biomarkers of renal function, which and when? *Clin. Chim. Acta* **2015**, *438*, 350–357. [CrossRef] [PubMed]
29. Levey, A.S.; Inker, L.A.; Coresh, J. GFR estimation: From physiology to public health. *Am. J. Kidney Dis.* **2014**, *63*, 820–834. [CrossRef] [PubMed]
30. Levey, A.S.; de Jongh, P.E.; Coresh, J.; El Nahas, M.; Astor, B.C.; Matsushita, K.; Gansevoort, R.T.; Kasiske, B.L.; Eckardt, K.U. The definition, classification, and prognosis of chronic kidney disease: A KDIGO controversies conference report. *Kidney Int.* **2011**, *80*, 17–28. [CrossRef] [PubMed]
31. Mikkelsen, M.; Andersen, L.; Christensen, T.; Hansen, T.K.; Eiskjaer, H.; Gjedsted, J.; Johnsen, S.P.; Hjortdal, V.E. Microalbuminuria is associated with high adverse event rate following cardiac surgery. *Eur. J. Cardiothorac. Surg.* **2011**, *39*, 932–938. [CrossRef] [PubMed]
32. Huang, T.; Wu, V.; Young, G.; Lin, Y.F.; Shiao, C.C.; Wu, P.C.; Li, W.Y.; Yu, H.Y.; Hu, F.C.; Lin, J.W.; et al. Preoperative proteinuria predicts adverse renal outcomes after coronary artery bypass grafting. *J. Am. Soc. Nephrol.* **2010**, *22*, 156–163. [CrossRef] [PubMed]
33. Hobson, C.E.; Singhania, G.; Bihorac, A. Acute kidney injury in the surgical patient. *Crit. Care Clin.* **2015**, *31*, 705–723. [CrossRef] [PubMed]
34. Seliger, S.L.; Salimi, S.; Pierre, V.; Giffuni, G.; Katzel, L.; Parsa, A. Microvascular endothelial dysfunction is associated with albuminuria and CKD in older adults. *BMC Nephrol.* **2016**, *17*, 82. [CrossRef] [PubMed]
35. Brienza, N.; Giglio, M.T.; Marucci, M.; Fiore, T. Does perioperative hemodynamic optimization protect renal function in surgical patients? A meta-analytic study. *Crit. Care Med.* **2009**, *37*, 2079–2090. [CrossRef] [PubMed]

36. Shah, M.; Jain, A.K.; Brunelli, S.M.; Coca, S.G.; Devereaux, P.J.; James, M.T.; Luo, J.; Molnar, A.O.; Mrkobrada, M.; Pannu, N.; et al. Association between angiotensin converting enzyme inhibitor or angiotensin receptor blocker use prior to major elective surgery and the risk of acute dialysis. *BMC Nephrol.* **2014**, *15*, 53. [CrossRef] [PubMed]
37. Hobson, C.; Ruchi, R.; Bihorac, A. Perioperative acute kidney injury: Risk factors and predictive strategies. *Crit. Care Clin.* **2017**, *33*, 379–396. [CrossRef] [PubMed]
38. Habib, R.H.; Zacharias, A.; Schwann, T.A.; Riordan, C.J.; Engoren, M.; Durham, S.J.; Shah, A. Role of hemodilutional anemia and transfusion during cardiopulmonary bypass in renal injury after coronary revascularization: Implications on operative outcome. *Crit. Care Med.* **2005**, *33*, 1749–1756. [CrossRef] [PubMed]
39. O'Keefe, S.D.; Davenport, D.L.; Minion, D.J.; Sorial, E.E.; Endean, E.D.; Xenos, E.S. Blood transfusion is associated with increased morbidity and mortality after lower extremity revascularization. *J. Vasc. Surg.* **2010**, *51*, 616–621. [CrossRef] [PubMed]
40. Salmasi, V.; Maheshwari, K.; Yang, D.; Mascha, E.J.; Singh, A.; Sessler, D.I.; Kurz, A. Relationship between intraoperative hypotension, defined by either reduction from baseline or absolute thresholds, and acute kidney and myocardial injury after noncardiac surgery. A retrospective cohort analysis. *Anesthesiology* **2017**, *126*, 47–65. [CrossRef] [PubMed]
41. Hallqvist, L.; Granath, F.; Huldt, E.; Bell, M. Intraoperative hypotension is associated with acute kidney injury in noncardiac surgery. An observational study. *Eur. J. Anaesthesiol.* **2017**, *35*, 273–279.
42. Futier, E.; Lefrant, J.Y.; Guinot, P.G.; Godet, T.; Lorne, E.; Cuvillon, P.; Bertran, S.; Leone, M.; Pastene, B.; Piriou, V.; et al. Effect of individualized vs. standard blood pressure management strategies on postoperative organ dysfunction among high-risk patients undergoing major surgery. *JAMA* **2017**, *318*, 1346–1357. [CrossRef] [PubMed]
43. Hansen, P.B.; Jensen, B.L.; Skott, O. Chloride regulates afferent arteriolar contraction in response to depolarization. *Hypertension* **1998**, *32*, 1066–1070. [CrossRef] [PubMed]
44. Chowdhury, A.H.; Cox, E.F.; Francis, S.T.; Lobo, D.N. A randomized, controlled, double-blind crossover study on the effects of 2-L infusions of 0.9% saline and Plasmalyte (R) 148 on renal blood flow velocity and renal cortical tissue perfusion in healthy volunteers. *Ann. Surg.* **2012**, *256*, 18–24. [CrossRef] [PubMed]
45. Shaw, A.D.; Bagshaw, S.M.; Goldstein SL Scherer, L.A.; Duan, M.; Schermer, C.R.; Kellum, J.A. Major complications, mortality and resource utilization after open abdominal surgery: 0.9% Saline compared to plasma-lyte. *Ann. Surg.* **2012**, *255*, 821–829. [CrossRef] [PubMed]
46. Yunos, N.M.; Bellomo, R.; Hegarty, C.; Story, D.; Ho, L.; Bailey, M. Association between a chloride-liberal vs. chloride-restrictive intravenous fluid administration strategy and kidney injury in critically ill adults. *JAMA* **2012**, *308*, 1566–1572. [CrossRef] [PubMed]
47. McCluskey, S.A.; Karkouti, K.; Wijeysundera, D.; Minkovich, L.; Tait, G.; Beattie, W.S. Hyperchloremia after noncardiac surgery is independently associated with increased morbidity and mortality: A propensity-matched cohort study. *Anesth. Analg.* **2013**, *117*, 412–421. [CrossRef] [PubMed]
48. Krajewski, M.; Raghunathan, K.; Paluscкiewicz, S.M.; Schermer, C.R.; Shaw, A.D. Meta-analysis of high-versus low-chloride content in perioperative and critical care fluid resuscitation. *Br. J. Surg.* **2015**, *102*, 24–36. [CrossRef] [PubMed]

# 12

# A Narrative Review on C3 Glomerulopathy: A Rare Renal Disease

**Francesco Paolo Schena [1,2,*], Pasquale Esposito [3] and Michele Rossini [1]**

[1] Department of Emergency and Organ Transplantation, Renal Unit, University of Bari, 70124 Bari, Italy; michelerossini@libero.it
[2] Schena Foundation, European Center for the Study of Renal Diseases, 70010 Valenzano, Italy
[3] Department of Internal Medicine, Division of Nephrology, Dialysis and Transplantation, University of Genoa and IRCCS Ospedale Policlinico San Martino, 16132 Genova, Italy; p.esposito@smatteo.pv.it
* Correspondence: paolo.schena@uniba.it

**Abstract:** In April 2012, a group of nephrologists organized a consensus conference in Cambridge (UK) on type II membranoproliferative glomerulonephritis and decided to use a new terminology, "C3 glomerulopathy" (C3 GP). Further knowledge on the complement system and on kidney biopsy contributed toward distinguishing this disease into three subgroups: dense deposit disease (DDD), C3 glomerulonephritis (C3 GN), and the CFHR5 nephropathy. The persistent presence of microhematuria with or without light or heavy proteinuria after an infection episode suggests the potential onset of C3 GP. These nephritides are characterized by abnormal activation of the complement alternative pathway, abnormal deposition of C3 in the glomeruli, and progression of renal damage to end-stage kidney disease. The diagnosis is based on studying the complement system, relative genetics, and kidney biopsies. The treatment gap derives from the absence of a robust understanding of their natural outcome. Therefore, a specific treatment for the different types of C3 GP has not been established. Recommendations have been obtained from case series and observational studies because no randomized clinical trials have been conducted. Current treatment is based on corticosteroids and antiproliferative drugs (cyclophosphamide, mycophenolate mofetil), monoclonal antibodies (rituximab) or complement inhibitors (eculizumab). In some cases, it is suggested to include sessions of plasma exchange.

**Keywords:** C3 glomerulopathy; Dense deposits disease; C3 glomerulonephritis; CFHR5 nephropathy

---

## 1. Introduction

Membranoproliferative or mesangiocapillary glomerulonephritis (MPGN) has been traditionally classified based on the light and electron microscopy (EM) findings; here, there are three categories: type I, characterized by the presence of immune deposits in the subendothelial space and mesangium of glomeruli; type II, characterized by C3 deposits within the mesangium and in the basement membranes highly osmiophilic on electron microscopy (dense deposits disease; DDD); and type III, which is a variant of type I [1].

In August 2012, a group of experts in renal pathology, nephrology, complementology, and complement therapeutics organized a consensus conference on the C3 glomerulopathy (C3 GP), meeting in Cambridge, UK [2]. Subsequently, new information on the complement system has increased our understanding of the MPGN, which has been divided into two groups: (i) MPGN caused by immune complexes (IC-MPGN) that can be caused by polyclonal or monoclonal IgG and (ii) complement-mediated glomerulonephritis (Figure 1).

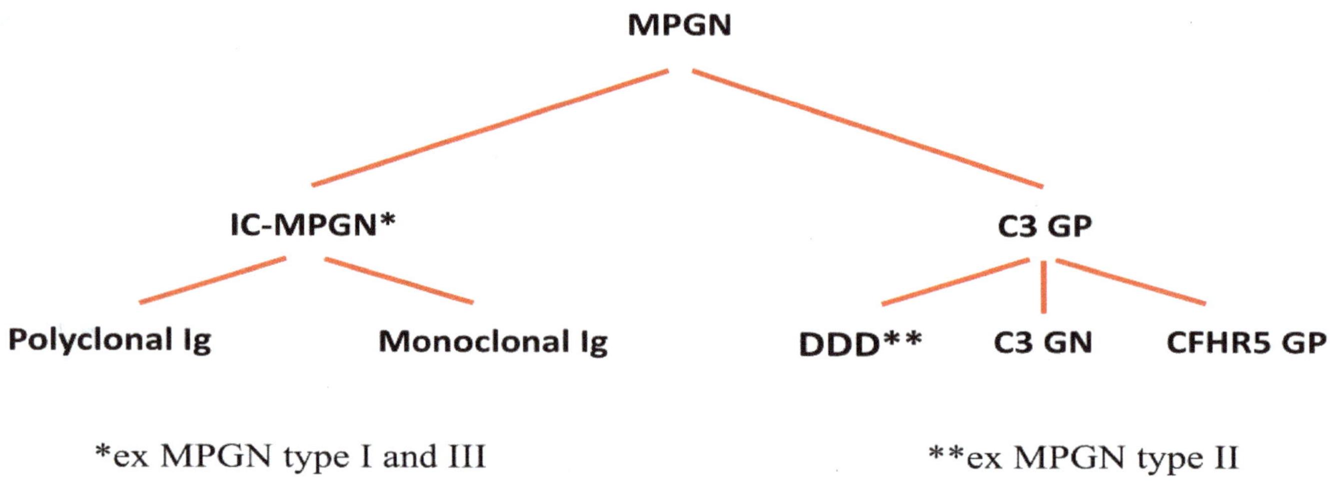


**Figure 1.** Classification of the membranoproliferative glomerulonephritis (MPGN). Abbreviations: IC-MPGN (immune complex MPGN); Ig (immunoglobulin); C3 GP (C3 glomerulopathy); DDD (dense deposits disease); C3 GN (C3 glomerulonephrits); CFHR5 GP (complement factor H-related protein 5 glomerulopathy).

The term C3 GP includes a group of nephritides based on the abnormal control of the alternative pathway of the complement system that causes a dominant accumulation of C3 fragments in glomeruli, as evidenced by an intense staining of C3 with absence or low presence of immunoglobulins and components of the classical complement pathway in the immunofluorescence pattern of a kidney biopsy [3]. This form of nephritis can be detected in individuals with defects in the complement activation that is induced by circulating factors or the presence of rare gene variants in complement components of the alternative pathway.

In a recent classification proposed by Cook and Pickering [4], C3 GP was shown to be principally composed of three major subgroups (Figure 1): (i) *DDD* is characterized by intramembranous glomerular deposits of dense osmophilic material; (ii) *C3 glomerulonephritis* (C3 GN) is based on the presence of less dense deposits of C3 in the mesangial, subendothelial, and subepithelial areas of glomeruli; it also appears with the presence of circulating auto-antibodies against C3bBb, factor B (FB), and factor H (FH); (iii) *complement factor H-related 5 glomerulopathy* (CFHR5 GP) is caused by genetic variants of CFHR5. Differences in these three nephritides are based on the interpretation of data obtained by light microscopy, immunofluorescence/immunohistochemistry and EM, laboratory complement findings, and clinical data. However, in some cases, there is an overlap of clinical data and laboratory findings, suggesting the possibility of a disease continuum based on the dysregulation of the complement alternative pathway; this would be caused by acquired factors (autoantibodies) or genetic variants of some complement components of the alternative pathway.

## 2. Pathogenesis

The complement system is the first cornerstone of innate immunity, and in the presence of various infections, it induces the lysis of agents through the generation of the membrane attack complex (MAC) [5]. Moreover, the system modulates adaptive immunity.

The complement system can be activated through three different pathways, as illustrated in Figure 2.

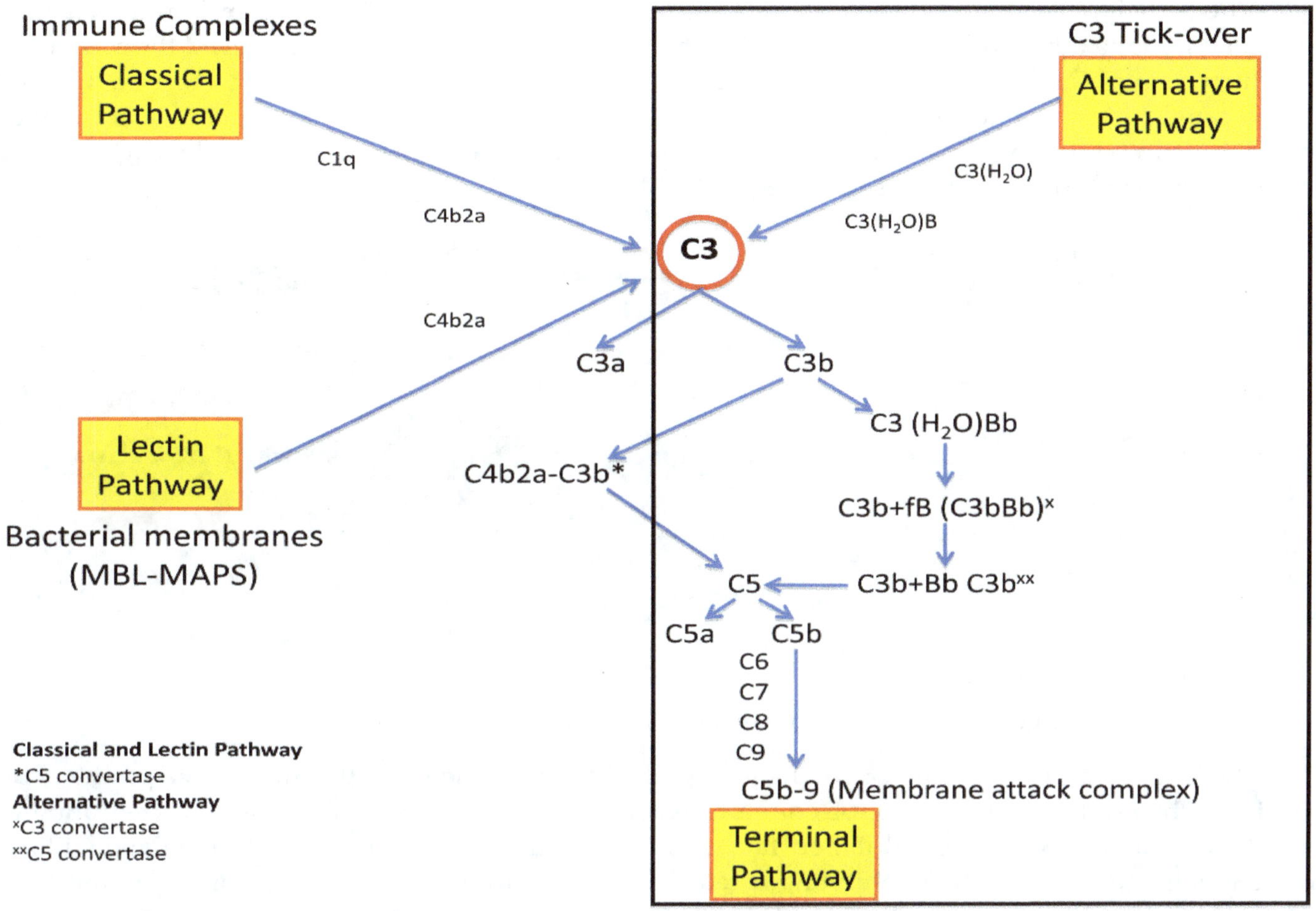


**Figure 2.** Complement system pathways.

The *classical pathway* is activated by circulating immune complexes, whereas the *lectin pathway* is activated by bacteria or their membrane fragments. Both pathways cleave C3 into C3a and C3b. C3a is an anaphylatoxin with a proinflammatory effect, whereas C3b binds a fragment of factor B (Bb), thus forming the C3 convertase (C3bBb). Additional production of C3b promotes the formation of the complex C3bBbC3b (C5 convertase), which cleaves C5 into C5a and C5b and combines with C6, C7, C8, and C9, thus forming the membrane attack complex (C5b-9) that induces the lysis of cellular membranes and the glomerular basement membrane (GBM).

The *alternative pathway* is continuously activated by the C3 tick-over at a low rate with the constant generation of C3b, which here is rapidly degraded. In this physiological process, C3 is hydrolyzed to C3($H_2O$) and combines with fB the complex C3($H_2O$)B. Then, this complex cleaves C3, generating C3b, which combines with Bb and forms the C3 convertase of the alternative pathway (C3bBb). In the presence of further C3b, the formed C5 convertase (C3bBbC3b) activates C5 with the sequential induction of the *terminal complement pathway* (C5b-9).

The three pathways of the complement system are modulated by proteins that regulate the system in the blood (fluid phase) and on the surface of cells (surface phase). In the fluid phase, the C1-inhibitor (C1-INH) downregulates the classical and lectin pathways; the C4 binding protein (C4bp) downregulates the classical pathway; clusterin and vimentin regulate C5b-9. The regulators of the complement in the surface phase system are the membrane cofactor protein (MCP, named CD46), CD59 that is a regulator of MAC formation, the decay accelerating factor (DAF, named CD55), and the complement receptor 1 (CR1).

The alternative pathway is regulated by properdin, FB, FI, FH, and FH-related proteins. Properdin enhances the formation of C3 convertase and stabilizes it; thus, properdin prevents the action of FH.

FH is the principal regulator of the alternative pathway both in the fluid phase and on the cellular surface; it inhibits the binding of C3b with FB, enhances C3 convertase dissociation, and the activity of FI, which cleaves C3b into inactivated C3b (iC3b). A dysregulated control of C3 convertase (C3bBb) can be caused by the abnormal activity of FH, as illustrated in Figure 3. The regulatory activity of this factor can be inhibited by the presence of genetic FH deficiency or autoantibodies against FH, which have been found in patients with C3 GP [6–9].

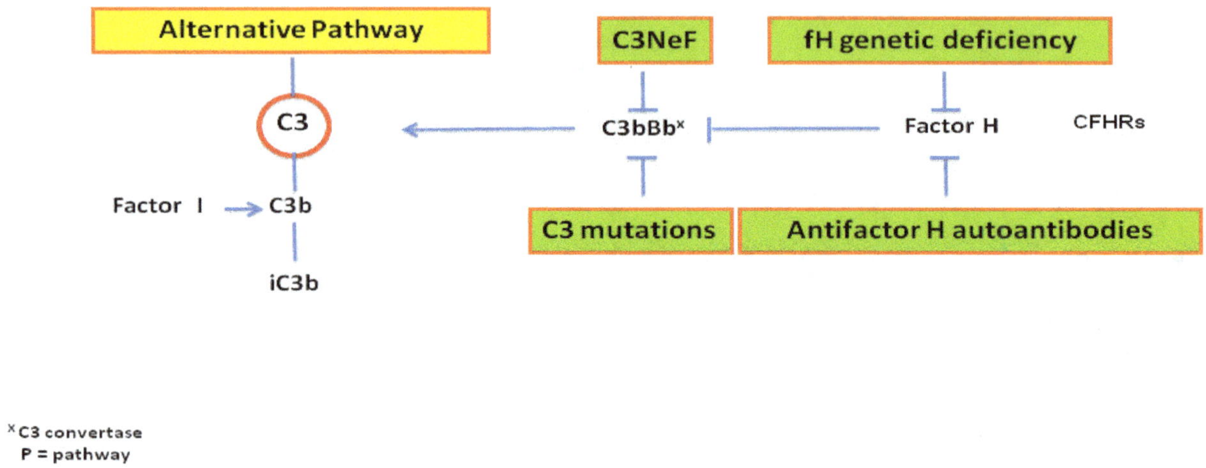


**Figure 3.** Schematic dysregulation of the C3 activation in C3 GP.

The activity of FH is regulated by the group of CFHRs that activate the alternative pathway by binding C3b and the activity of C3bBb convertase. CFHRs also compete with FH when attempting to bind to C3b deposited on the cellular surfaces. Therefore, the competition between FH and CFHRs influences the degree of C3b by inhibiting (predominant FH binding) or allowing (predominant FHR binding) to this process. The CFHR system is composed of five proteins that are coded by genes (CFHR1 to CFHR5) located near the CFH gene. CFHR genes may have rearrangements because the deletion or duplication of the first two consensus repeats with the presence of altered activity of CFHR proteins. Abnormal rearrangements include intragenic duplication in CFHR1 and CFHR5 and the presence of hybrid CFHR2-CFHR5 and CFHR3-CFHR1 genes. A deletion of the CFHR1 gene is associated with the abnormal activity of FH and reduced control of the activation of the alternative complement pathway in the circulation system.

CFHR5 interacting with CFHR1 and CFHR2 may generate abnormal CFHR proteins that impact the function of C3 and/or C5 convertases in the fluid phase or on the glomeruli, causing C3 GP. More than 20 different mutations have been identified in the CFH-CFHR gene family of patients affected by C3 GP, as reported by Xiao et al. [10] and Merinero et al. [11]. A recent review on the process of CFH deregulation that is responsible for the C3 activation has been published by Barbour et al. [12].

An excessive activation of the alternative pathway may be caused by the presence of autoantibodies against the C3 convertase of the alternative pathway (C3NeF) and C3 convertase of the classical pathway (C4NeF) (Figure 3). In 1969, NeF was detected for the first time in a case of MPGN with persistent hypocomplementemia [13]. The serum of this patient was able to break down into C3 when it was incubated with normal human serum. The activity of NeF was attributed to the stabilization of the alternative complement pathway convertase (C3bBb), and it was named C3NeF [13,14]. Then, further studies [15–18] described various types of NeF stabilizing different convertases, thus preventing their cleavage and causing continuous activation of the complement system. Marinozzi et al. [19] detected a C3NeF that stabilizes the C5 convertase of the alternative pathway (C5NeF). C4NeF was first detected in a case of patients with postinfection glomerulonephritis and who had persistent low levels of C3 and C5 [20], and it was also discovered in a case of MPGN. C3NeF and C4NeF may coexist in the same patient [21], but plasma C3, consumption, and disease severity do not always correlate with the presence and activity of C3NeF in individuals with MPGN [22]. Other autoantibodies related to complement components, such as FB, FH, and C3b have been detected in a smaller percentage of patients [23]. A recent review regarding the use of diagnostic tools to detect and characterize NeFs was published by Donadelli et al. [24].

In conclusion, various autoantibodies enhance the activity of the alternative pathway in different ways. C3NeF binds and stabilizes the C3 convertase in the presence of properdin. C4NeF binds and stabilizes C3 convertase (C4bC2a) of the classical pathway, thus causing more production of C3b and C3bBb. Autoantibodies against factor H eliminate the regulatory function of this factor [25], whereas autoantibodies against factor B stabilize the enhancing function of factor B [26,27]. The presence of one of these autoantibodies is responsible for the development of C3 GP caused by an abnormal control of alternative complement pathway activation with reduced C3 degradation and increased C3 fragment deposition in the GBM.

## 3. Epidemiology

C3 GP is a rare disease, so its frequency can only be approximately calculated. Cohort studies and an analysis of data from C3 GP registry have estimated an annual incidence of biopsy-proven DDD and C3 GN of one to two cases per million, with both sexes being affected equally [28]. The prevalence has been calculated as less than five cases per 1,000,000 in the United States and ~0.2–1.0 cases per 1,000,000 among the European population [25,29].

Instead, for CFHR5 GP, which was first observed in patients from Cyprus, data of incidences are lacking, while the prevalence value has been estimated at 140 cases per 1,000,000 Cypriot individuals [30].

## 4. Clinical Manifestations

Because of the low frequency of C3 GP, patient cohort studies are important and can provide valuable information regarding clinical presentation, pathological and laboratory features, and their correlation with disease outcomes.

Table 1 shows the clinical and laboratory data of patients affected by C3 GP in different cohorts, as described by many investigators [23,25,29,31–36]. C3 GP involves mainly children and young people and may develop after an infectious episode (i.e., streptococcal infection) of the upper respiratory tract. However, the presence of rare variants linked to C3 and other components of the alternative pathway predisposes an individual to C3 GP susceptibility.

The onset of the disease is characterized by micro- or macroscopic hematuria, light or heavy proteinuria, and a progressive reduction of renal function. Microhematuria is present in 90% of individuals, and episodes of gross hematuria may occur in 20% of patients in concomitance with upper respiratory tract infections. At the beginning of the disease and mainly in adults, light proteinuria may be present, which then becomes heavy over the course of the disease. The impairment of renal function is more frequent in adults and elderly subjects.

These clinical manifestations are common in all subtypes of C3 GP based on the aberrant control of the alternative complement pathway and sequential deposition of C3 in glomeruli. Therefore, renal biopsy remains the main approach for diagnosis.

In **DDD**, the onset is characterized by nephrotic syndrome in 50% of the patients and acute nephritic syndrome in the other 50%. Hypertension may be present at the onset of the disease or detected during the course of the disease. These clinical manifestations are preceded by an acute episode of upper respiratory tract infection.

In a few cases, DDD shows at the fundus oculi drusen bodies that are electron-dense deposits of complement factors between the Bruch's membrane and the retinal epithelium. This abnormality may be present at all ages and comes with a modest risk of progressive visual loss.

In some cases, patients with DDD may show acquired partial lipodistrophy that is characterized by the absence of subcutaneous fat in the face, but can also be present in the arms and upper portions of the trunk. However, partial lipodistrophy is more frequent in MPGN.

**Table 1.** Clinical and laboratory characteristics of patients affected by C3 GP enrolled in cohort studies.

| Study Population | | | | | | Clinical Findings | | | Histology | Complement Findings § | | | | |
|---|---|---|---|---|---|---|---|---|---|---|---|---|---|---|
| Author-Year (Ref. No.) | Country | C3 GP Class | N | Age at Diagnosis (Years) | Male Sex (%) | Median SCr at Diagnosis (mg/dL) | Median UP at Diagnosis (g/24 h) | Main Clinical Presentation (%) | Main Histological Patterns (%) | Low C3 (%) | Low C4 (%) | C3Nef No. (%) | Complement Gene Variant Identified No. (%) | Other Complement Antibodies No. (%) |
| Athanasiou, 2011 [31] | Cyprus | CFHR5 GP | 91 | Range 12–88 | 47 | N/A | N/A | H 90 Pu 38 | MES | 0 | 0 | N/A | 91/91 (100) | N/A |
| Servais, 2012 [32] | France | C3 GN | 56 | 30 | 58.6 | 1.3 | 3.6 | H 64 NS 27 | MPGN (71), MES (29) | 40 | 0 | 25 (45) | 10 (18) | N/A |
| | | DDD | 29 | 12 | 43 | 1.6 | 5.6 | H 76 NS 30 | | 59 | 4 | 25 (86) | 5 (17) | N/A |
| Mejeral-Thomas, 2014 [25] | UK/ Ireland | C3 GN | 59 | 26 | 54 | 1.4 | 3 | H 87 NS 44 | MPGN (52), MES (24), Crescentic (5) | 48 | 36 | N/A | N/A | N/A |
| | | DDD | 21 | 12 | 43 | 0.9 | 3 | H 86 NS 43 | MPGN (62), MES (14), Crescentic (19) | 79 | 15 | N/A | N/A | N/A |
| Rabasco, 2015 [33] | Spain | C3 GN | 60 | 27 | 57 | 1.4 | 3.8 | NS 52 H 49 | MPGN (75), MES (15) | 63 | N/A | 11/23 (48) | 3/23 (13) | 0 |
| Iatropoulos, 2016 [34] | Italy | C3 GN | 52 | 14.6 | 42 | N/A | N/A | H 86 NS 29 | N/A | 69 | N/A | 23/52 (44) | 10/52 (20) | N/A |
| | | DDD | 21 | 15.9 | 38 | N/A | N/A | H 90 NS29 | | 86 | N/A | 16/21 (78) | 3/21 (14) | N/A |
| Caliskan, 2017 [35] | Turkey | C3 GN (no subclass) | 66 | 36 | 54 | 1.6 | 3.8 | H 89 NS 48 | MPGN (75), MES (24) | 41 | 4 | N/A | N/A | N/A |
| Bomback, 2018 [29] | USA | C3 GN | 87 | 28.3 | 63.2 | 2 | 3.7 | H 59 NS 33 | MPGN (68.8), MES (17.5) | 65 | 14 | 13/42 (31) | 12/42 (28) | 3/42 (7) |
| | | DDD | 24 | 40 | 67 | 2.1 | 4.4 | H 82 NS 17 | MPGN (45.8), MES (29.3) | 64 | 14 | 1/9 (11) | 3/9 (33) | 1/9 (11) |
| Le Quintec, 2018 [36] | France | C3 GN (no subclass) | 26 | 17.5 | 48 | 1 | 4.1 | NS 73 | MPGN (62) | 88 | N/A | 16/24 (67) | 5/22 (23) | 2/22 (9) |
| Ravindran, 2018 [23] | USA * | C3 GN | 102 | 41.5 | 59 | 1.6 | 2.5 | H 87 Pu 38 | MPGN (52), MES (34), Crescentic (7) | 42 | 12 | 27/60 (46) | 21/61 (39) | 8/60 (13) |
| | | DDD | 12 | 31.5 | 25 | 1.4 | 6.5 | H 92 Pu 75 | MPGN (45), MES (27), Crescentic (16) | 58 | 8 | 3/10 (30) | 2/9 (22) | 1/8 (12) |

Abbreviations: C3G = C3 glomerulopathy; CeGN = C3 glomerulonephritis; DDD = dense deposition disease; CFHR5N = CFHR5 nephropathy; SCr = serum creatinine; UP = urinary protein; H = hematuria, Pu = proteinuria; NS = nephrotic syndrome; MPGN = Membrano-Proliferative Glomerulonephritis; MES = Mesangial expansion; C3Nef = C3 Nephritic factors; N/A = data not available from the study. Notes: * including 36 patients with Monoclonal immunoglobulin; § complement findings were often evaluated only in a part of the studied patients.

The outcome of DDD patients is poor, given that 50% of individuals progress to end-stage kidney disease (ESKD) within 10 years of diagnosis.

In **C3 GN**, the onset of the disease is characterized by microhematuria associated with hypertension in one-third of patients and nephritic syndrome in another third. The percentage of patients with ESKD is similar to that of patients with DDD. The disease involves mainly children and young adults. Microhematuria is present in 90% of individuals, and episodes of gross hematuria may occur in 20% of patients, along with upper respiratory tract infections. At the beginning of the disease light proteinuria that becomes heavy during the course of the disease is present but mainly in adults. The impairment of renal function is more frequent in adults.

**CFHR5 glomerulopathy** (CHFR5 GP) has been described in family studies; here, the abnormal activity of the complement factor H-related (CFHR) proteins or deregulation of CFH caused by CFH gene polymorphisms segregates in some members of the family [33,37,38]. Individuals with these genomic abnormalities show persistent microscopic hematuria that may be associated with proteinuria. The development of chronic renal failure progressing to ESKD is more frequent in men with proteinuria. In other patients, the usual presentation may be macroscopic hematuria in the concomitance of upper respiratory tract infection, as in IgA nephropathy, which mainly occurs in children.

However, familial cases of C3 GP have been observed in the presence of CFHR3-1 protein abnormalities [39] or the internal duplication of CFHR1 [40] or CFHR5, specifically in members of a Cypriot family [41].

## 5. Renal Biopsy

A renal biopsy is essential to identify C3 GP because it is the correct approach for distinguishing the different subtypes of MPGN.

### *5.1. Immunofluorescence Microscopy*

The diagnosis of C3 GP is based on an immunofluorescence (IF) technique, which reveals C3 dominant staining, with C3 being the only positive immunoreactant or with others (IgG, IgA, IgM, C1q) but C3 at least 2 + stronger [42].

In DDD, C3 deposits are arranged in a ribbon-like ("garland") pattern in the glomerular basement membranes with sometimes ring-shaped mesangial deposits (Figure 4a). Broad linear tubular basement membranes (~60%) (Figure 4b) and Bowman capsule deposits (~30%) can also be present in DDD.

In C3 GN, prominent granular C3 deposits are seen in the mesangium and/or glomerular basement membranes (Figure 4c,d).

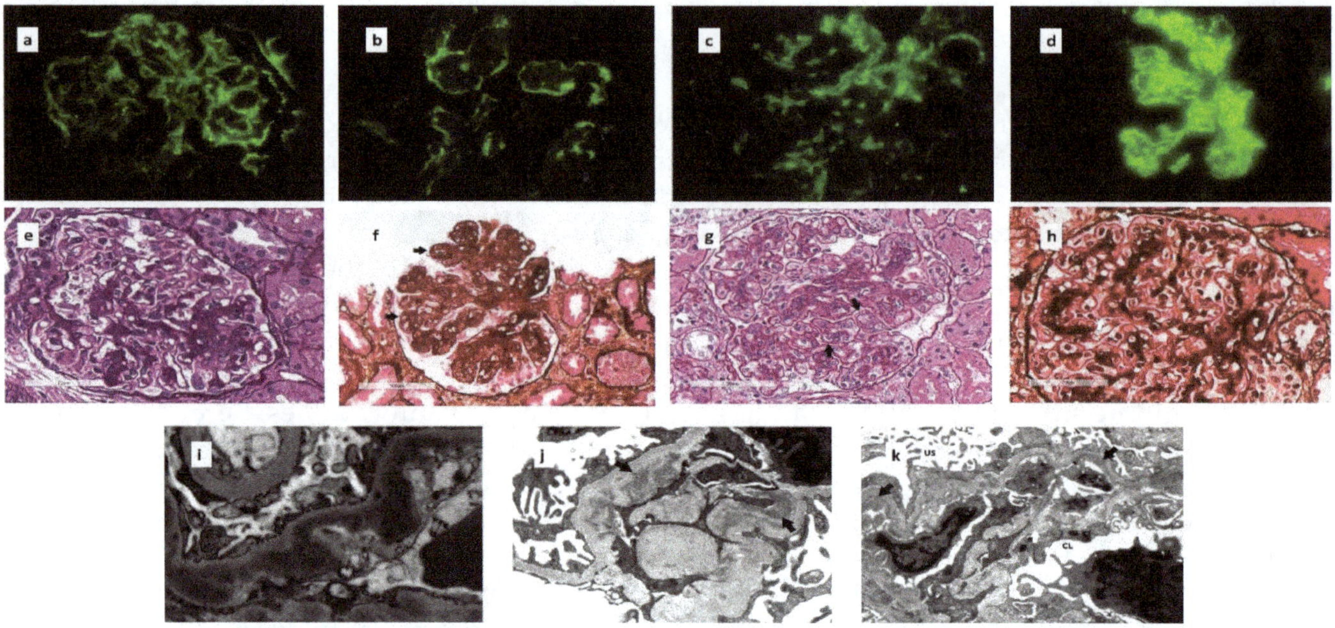

**Figure 4.** (**a**) Ribbon like pattern of C3 deposition along glomerular basement membrane in a patient with DDD (×400). (**b**) Linear C3 deposition along tubular basement membrane in DDD (×400). (**c**) Granular mesangial C3 deposits in a patient with a mesangial proliferative C3 GN (×400). (**d**) Coarsely granular mesangial and glomerular capillary wall C3 deposits in a patient with membranoproliferative pattern of C3 GN (×400). (**e**) Glomerulus with segmental mesangial proliferation in a patient with C3 GN (PAS). (**f**) Glomerulus with global membranoproliferative pattern of injury in a patient with C3 GN. Several aspects of glomerular basement membrane double contours (black arrows) are present (Jones silver stain). (**g**) Glomerulus with thickened strongly PAS positive glomerular basement membranes with several double contours (black arrows) (PAS) in a patient with DDD. (**h**) Silver negative glomerular basement membrane in a patient with DDD (white arrows). Glomerular basement membranes appear eosinophilic and refractile (Jones silver stain). (**i**) Highly osmiophilic electron dense deposits permeating lamina densa in a patient with DDD (TEM, ×8900). (**j**) Mesangial electron dense deposits (black arrows) in a patient with mesangial proliferative C3 GN (TEM, ×11000). (**k**) Subendothelial electron dense deposits (black arrows) with newly formed lamina densa (i.e., double contours) and cellular interposition (white arrow) in a patient with membranoproliferative patter of C3 GN (US: urinary space, CL: capillary lumen) (TEM, ×8900).

The absence of C4d in the kidney biopsy from proliferative GN has been found to be helpful, as noted by Sethi et al. [43], in distinguishing C3 GP from Ig complex-mediated and postinfection glomerulonephritis. Although helpful, this feature has been questioned by other studies [44].

C3 GP has now been included among the possible manifestations of monoclonal gammopathy of renal significance (MGRS) because 30–50% of patients >50 years of age with C3 GP have a detectable monoclonal Ig [45]. For this reason, careful examination of a renal biopsy and searching for a monoclonal Ig or light chain is mandatory. Failing to detect a monoclonal protein using an immunofluorescence technique from fresh frozen tissue should prompt reprocessing to formalin-fixed-paraffin-embedded tissue after pronase digestion. Actually, 10–20% of patients with a serum monoclonal component and finding of C3 GP on immunofluorescence have a proliferative GN with masked monoclonal deposits [45].

It is important to distinguish C3 deposition in C3 GN from other forms of glomerulonephritis, such as postinfection glomerulonephritis, in which immunoglobulin deposition occurs in the first phase of the disease and then disappears. In this case, persistence of heavy proteinuria and/or double contours on light microscopy (LM) may suggest the occurrence of C3 GP.

### 5.2. *Light Microscopy*

LM can vary greatly, presenting with different morphologic patterns. Mesangial proliferative glomerulonephritis (Figure 4e) and membranoproliferative glomerulonephritis (Figure 4f) are the most common patterns found, respectively, 33.3% and 50.8% of a cohort of 114 patients with C3 GP from the Mayo Clinic [23]. The membrane proliferative pattern in light microscopy is not different from that seen in idiopathic forms with Ig deposits. It is characterized by the thickening of glomerular basement membranes with double contours and cellular interposition. The features of exudative glomerulonephritis with endocapillary hypercellularity with or without polymorphonucleates are observed in 10–20% of cases. Extracellular proliferation with a crescent formation can also be present. In chronic phases of injury focal, segmental and/or global glomerulosclerosis and a fibrous crescent can be found. Fibrinoid necrosis is uncommon.

In DDD, glomerular basement membranes appear eosinophilic and refractile and stain brightly with periodic acid-Schiff (PAS) and poorly with a Jones silver stain (Figure 4g,h).

### 5.3. *Electron Microscopy*

EM studies have refined the G3 GP classification into further categories (DDD and C3 GN) based on the appearance of deposits.

In DDD (formerly MPGN type II), EM shows highly osmiophilic dense deposits in the lamina densa of the glomerular basement membranes, resulting in an electron-dense appearance (Figure 4i). These deposits can also be found in the mesangium, Bowman capsule, tubular basement membranes, and small vessel walls.

In C3 GN, the "usual" electron-dense deposits are found in various locations: the mesangial (Figure 4j), subendothelial (Figure 4k), and intramembranous areas. Subepithelial humps can be found both in DDD and C3 GN.

## 6. Diagnosis

A single algorithm cannot define the diagnostic approach to C3 GP, which is based on the interpretation of individual cases through the integration of the information provided by the renal biopsy together with clinical, serological, and genetic assessments.

Because the clinical presentation of C3 GP in its different forms may vary from asymptomatic hematuria to nephrotic syndrome and acute kidney injury, a diagnosis of C3 GP should be taken into consideration virtually in all patients presenting features of glomerulonephritis (proteinuria, hematuria, renal failure, or active urine sediment).

The clinical and laboratory work-up for the diagnosis of C3 GP is illustrated in Figure 5. After collecting the medical history and providing an accurate examination of the physical status, the patient usually undergoes general laboratory evaluation, looking at immunity (measurement of the serum levels of immunoglobulins and detection of serum cryoglobulins) and the complement system (hemolytic assay of the classical and alternative pathway). In the presence of the specific activation of the alternative complement pathway (i.e., reduced C3 and normal C4 serum levels) C3 GP is highly suspected although not yet determined. The diagnosis of C3 GP is exclusively made based on renal histological findings. In particular, as previously shown, LM is not specific enough for C3 GP, but IF and EM are necessary to make a diagnosis of C3 GP and to distinguish between C3 GN and DDD.

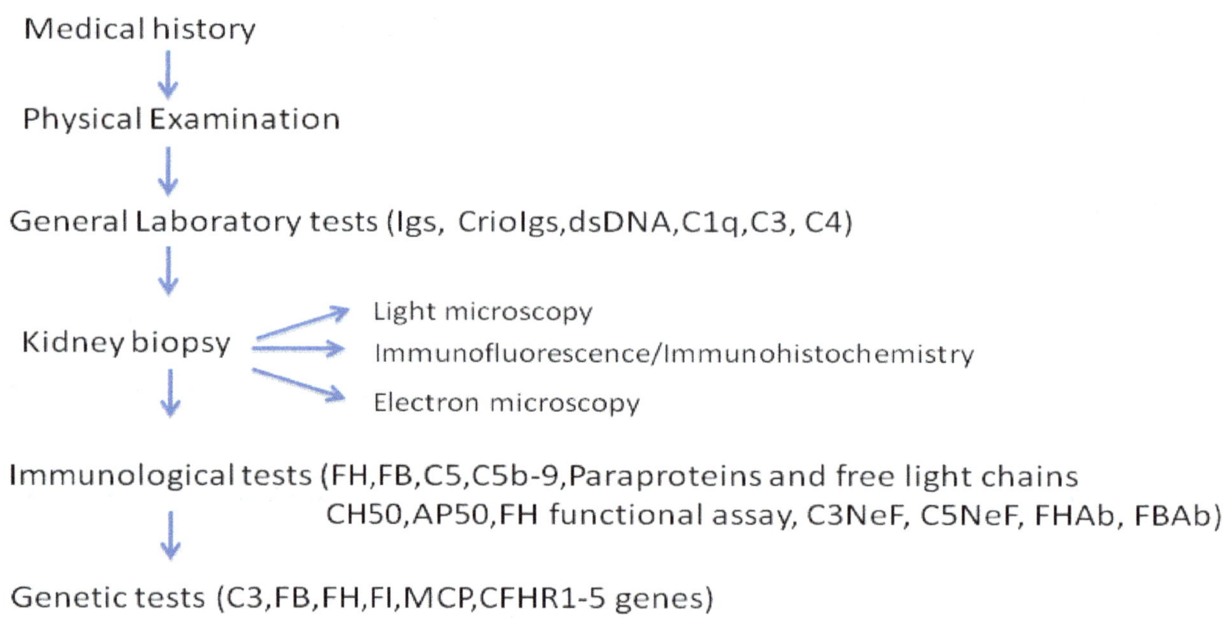


**Figure 5.** Clinical and Laboratory Work-up for diagnosis of C3 glomerulopathy.

C3-dominant glomerulonephritis is defined as C3 deposition in renal tissue of at least two orders of magnitude greater than that for any other immunoreactant (including Ig, C4, C1q, etc.). However, even when a C3 prevailing deposition is found, only a suspected diagnosis of C3 GP may be formulated, while the definitive diagnosis might require an ultra-structural analysis by EM.

Once the histological diagnosis of C3 GP has been realized, additional laboratory tests should be done to evaluate the serum levels of other components of the complement system, such as FH, FB, C5, and other complement regulatory proteins. Then, the work-up proceeds to a differential diagnosis and excludes secondary forms of glomerulonephritis. Investigations of the medical history should include a possible familial story of glomerulonephritis, unclear renal insufficiency, prior episodes of hematuria and/or proteinuria, and secondary causes, such as infections, autoimmune diseases, and paraproteinemia. Particular attention should be paid to recent infective episodes that may represent a trigger for complement activation. Moreover, all patients (especially if the age is more than 50 years) should be screened for the presence of paraproteins by serum electrophoresis-immunofixation and serum-free light chain measurement. Indeed, it has been shown that monoclonal gammopathy may be common in patients with a histological diagnosis of C3 GP [46]. If paraproteins are present, the patient should be referred to hematology consultation because in these cases, a clone-guided treatment might improve renal outcomes.

If secondary forms of complement activation are unlikely or excluded, all patients with C3 GP should undergo a comprehensive evaluation of the complement system, which includes measurements of the complement hemolytic activity, screening for circulating autoantibodies and genetic studies, which can help in defining the diagnosis and choosing the therapeutic approach [47].

The evaluation of the overall complement activity may be performed by evaluating the total complement hemolytic activity (CH50), the complement alternative pathway activity (AP50), or the complement FH functional activity [48]. Although functional tests may be considered the gold standard for studying the complement activity, they may actually have a significant rate of false-negative results, and their use still needs to be validated.

Moving to the specific details, serological studies of the complement AP should include the quantification of individual complement components, here bearing in mind that the results of these studies may change over the course of the disease. The most important complement components to evaluate are C3 and C4. Low C3 is found in a substantial number of patients with C3 GN (40–75%) and DDD (60%), while serum C4 levels are usually normal [23]. Moreover, serum FB, FH, FI, properdin, and membrane cofactor proteins (MCP or CD46) should also be tested, considering that a deficiency of these factors, often accompanied by low C3 levels, can be associated with altered AP activation [49]. However, complement activation may also be detected by measuring the decay products of complement activation; when elevated, they may reflect an increased turnover of C3 (C3a, C3d), C5 (C5a), and FB (Bb) [50]. Finally, considering that the activation of all complement pathways leads to the generation of the membrane attack complex (C5b-9), soluble levels of C5b-9 should be evaluated as an additional marker of complement activation [49]. Interestingly, it should be noted that small differences in complement biomarkers between C3 GN and DDD exist. For example, in C3 GN, the plasma properdin reduction and soluble C5b-9 elevation tend to be higher than in DDD. Thus, a complement component evaluation may also provide an indication of the disease in the differential diagnosis between C3GN and DDD.

Serological studies in patients with C3 GP should also include screening for autoantibodies, which may constitute the acquired causes of C3 GP. C3NeF and C5NeF are the most frequently identified autoantibodies (Figure 5). Various diagnostic tools can be used to detect NeFs [51]. Three of these tools are functional and hemolytic assays. The first method consists of the measurement of C3 fragments in the serum's patient by two-dimensional immunoelectrophoresis, immunofixation electrophoresis, or Western blotting. The second test is based on a hemolytic assay that measures the lysis of sheep or rabbits erythrocytes after incubation with the serum or plasma of the patient. Finally, the presence of NeFs can be detected through the quantification of C3a and C5a anaphylotoxins. NeFs can be measured by binding assays that detect C3NeF by various ELISA techniques. Actually, they encompass a heterogeneous group of IgG and IgM autoantibodies that stabilize the alternative pathway of C3 and C5 convertase (C3bBb and C3bBbC3b, respectively), prolonging their survival and promoting massive C3 or C5 consumption [51]. C3NeF is found in 80% of patients affected by DDD and in 50% of patients affected by C3 GN. Detecting C3NeF can be done in many different ways, including ELISA, C3 convertase surface assay, and electrophoresis [52]. In addition, C4 nephritic factor (C4NeF), which stabilizes the C3 convertase of the classical and lectin pathways, has been identified in a small subset of patients with C3 GP, even if its role remains unclear [53]. Antifactor H antibodies are another group of auto-antibodies described in patients affected by C3 GP; they may be detected using an enzyme-linked immunosorbent assay and have been related to the presence of monoclonal gammopathy [54]. Finally, anti-FB antibodies have rarely been described, but their detection remains confined to research laboratories [26].

Because genetic factors have been reported in cohorts of patients with C3 GP, genetic testing should be considered in these patients [32] (Figure 5). In particular, genetic screening should include the evaluation of the C3, FB, FH, MCP, CFHR1-5, and FI genes to detect single nucleotide changes, small insertions and deletions, or more complex rearrangements, such as copy number variations [34]. However, the interpretation of a genetic analysis in C3 GP is often difficult for several reasons. First, genetic defects have been identified only in a small number of patients with C3 GP. Second, the actual pathogenetic and functional meaning of many mutations is still not defined. Finally, most genetic variants have a low penetrance, and combined variants may coexist, which also involves other genes, such as thrombomodulin (THBD) and diacylglycerol kinase-epsilon (DGKE) [55]. Thus, it is necessary to cautiously analyze the detected gene alterations to determine if they are specifically disease associated.

A different situation is found in the familial forms of C3 GP, where disease-specific gene mutations have been characterized. This is the case of patients affected by CFHR5 GP and who are of Cypriot origin, in which an internal duplication in the CFHR5 gene has been described as causative [37]. Interestingly, other forms of familial C3 GP have been related to rearrangements of the CFHR2-CFHR5 hybrid gene and abnormalities in CFHR1 and CFHR5 [39,40], suggesting that the CFHR1-5 gene family should be carefully assessed in all C3 GP cases. A detailed description of the methods to quantify the CFHR proteins in the serum and detect circulating autoantibodies has recently been published by Sanchez-Corral et al. [56].

In any case, although the precise value of genetic testing remains to be defined in a general clinical setting for C3 GP, a genetic cause of the disease should be taken into consideration, and genetic screening should be offered to all the family members of affected patients who carry a potentially causative mutation.

## 7. Differential Diagnosis

A differential diagnosis should be done in the presence of diagnosed C3 GP on either a native or transplanted kidney. In this case, it is necessary to investigate the concomitant presence of low plasma levels of C4, occurrence of C4NeF (C4bC2a), and paraproteins (i.e., monocolonal gammopathy) because in this case, the patient is affected by MPGN type 1.

C3 GP must be differentiated from other types of glomerulonephritides that have excessive activation of the C system in the presence of circulating immune complexes, causing postinfection glomerulonephritis or secondary glomerulonephritides (lupus nephritis, essential cryoglobulinemia, and others) [1]. Because the clinical presentation in these cases is similar, it is suggested that an accurate study of the complement system and genetic tests in specialized laboratories be carried out. However, a kidney biopsy is diriment in these patients because it shows a prevalent deposition of immunoglobulins, which is the characteristic pattern of these nephritides. In addition, postinfection glomerulonephritis should be differentiated from C3 GP when there is no spontaneous resolution of the disease within one to two months.

G3 GP can be diagnosed in the presence of false-negative staining for immunoglobulins by immunofluorescence on the frozen renal tissue sections of patients with essential cryoglobulinemia. In these cases, it is suggested to investigate the presence of C4 in a kidney biopsy to discover the potential occurrence of the low serum levels of circulating immune complexes or cryoglobulins.

In many cases, the prognosis of C3 GP is severe when it comes to the progression of renal damage to ESKD [28,32]. It is less severe in CFHR5 GP.

## 8. Recurrence or De Novo C3 GP after Kidney Transplatation

Patients with C3 GP are at high risk to develop the disease after kidney transplantation. Therefore, post-transplant monitoring and available optional therapies are necessary for improving the outcome of the patients. The recurrence is at high rate for both DDD and C3 GN. The recurrence of CHFR5 GP has been observed in the kidney allograft of patients, allowing for a family with CFHR gene abnormalities [57]. C3 GP occurs in over 50% of patients with native C3 GP [58]. The timing and clinical presentation may be different with DDD recurrence in later post-transplant time. The appearance of hematuria, proteinuria and reduction of eGFR is a strong indicator of C3 GP recurrence. However, LM, IF, and EM studies are necessary for a correct diagnosis. A recent report [59] suggests that aggressive renal lesions in native kidney and hybrid CFHR3 1 gene-related C3 GN contribute to more recurrence of the disease in the post-transplant time.

The approach to therapy has not been established because different treatments have been used in these patients. Recent data from Bomback et al. [60] in a prospective open-label, uncontrolled trial and by other investigators [61–63] suggest the administration of eculizumab which induces reduction of proteinuria and stabilization of the renal function. However, the heterogeneous treatment response suggests the opportunity to design a larger multicenter study in C3 GP patients after kidney transplantation. For this reason in 2017, a group of researchers across Europe and North and South America initiated the post-TrANsplant GlOmerular (TANGO) disease study, an observational multicenter cohort study with the aim to enroll patients who arrived to ESKD for different forms of glomerulonephritis, mainly C3 GP [64].

If eculizumab represents a successful therapy in atypical hemolytic uremic syndrome (AHUS) [65], the response rate is heterogeneous in patients with C3 GP [66]. The different response is due to the correct blockage of the terminal complement pathway in AHUS, whereas this therapy is questionable in patients with C3 GP because the disease is characterized by abnormal activation of the alternative complement pathway, abnormal cleavage of C3 and continuous deposition of C3 split products in glomeruli. This provides different response rate between the two diseases.

Some considerations should be done on the use of anti-CD 20 (rituximab) that has been used in a small number of cases with different response to the treatment. This drug is correctly indicated in patients with kidney graft who develop MPGN with monoclonal IgG deposits caused by dysregulated B cells or plasma cells alone without hematologic malignancy [67]. However, sporadic use of rituximab in association with immunosuppressive drugs has shown failure in the treatment of many cases [62,68,69].

Recurrence or *de novo* C3 GP may receive other therapies that are under trough evaluation as (i) compostatin that is a C3 inhibitory peptide; (ii) CP40 is a compostatin analog [70]; (iii) monoclonal antibodies against C3b [71], FB [72] and properdin [73]. Moreover, soluble complement receptor 1(CR1)) may prevent the dysregulated alternative pathway caused by abnormal production of C3 convertase.

All these drugs can block the dysregulated alternative complement pathway induced by autoantibodies or genetic mutations.

## 9. Therapy

The current gap in the treatment of C3 GP derives from the absence of a robust understanding of its natural outcomes. Therefore, a specific treatment for different types of C3 GP has not been established. Recommendations have been obtained from case series and observational studies [12] because there are no randomized clinical trials for treatments. Current treatment is based on the inhibition of factors that activate the complement pathways, which is done by administering the available drugs as corticosteroids and antiproliferative drugs (cyclophoshamide, mycophenolate mofetil), monoclonal antibodies (rituximab), or complement inhibitors (eculizumab).

Children and adults with C3 GP in presence of mild or moderate proteinuria should receive supportive therapy with angiotensin-converting enzyme inhibitors or angiotensin receptor blockers. Patients with nephrotic syndrome and a decline in renal function should receive oral CYC or MMF plus a low dose of daily or alternate-day corticosteroids [33]. If despite this treatment nephrotic syndrome persists or the renal function impairs, tacrolimus or RTX can be considered although the percentage of its beneficial effect is very low [35,70].

Treatment with chemotherapeutic agents, immune-suppressive drugs, and complement inhibitors confer infection risks. Indeed, Koopman et al. [71] suggest vaccination prophylaxis against Streptococcus pneumonia, Neisseria meningitis, and Hemophilus influenzae.

In patients with C3 GN with abnormal deposition of C3 because of persistent activation of the alternative complement pathway, it is suggested that treatment with eculizumab (monoclonal anti-C5 antibody) may be administered. A prospective clinical trial in which six patients with native or post-transplant recurrent DDD or C3 GN received eculizumab therapy was the first clinical study to evaluate the benefit of this monoclonal antibody [60]. Other case reports described by Barbour et al. [12] have shown complete or partial remission of the clinical findings (significant reduction of serum creatinine and/or proteinuria). Recently, Le Quintrec et al. [36] evaluated a cohort of 26 patients (13 children/adolescents) with C3 GP who were treated with eculizumab. At the initiation of eculizumab, 40% of the patients had chronic kidney disease, while about 30% had a rapidly progressive disease. After eculizumab treatment, six (23%) patients achieved a complete clinical response, defined as a >50% decrease in serum creatinine and proteinuria, while six (23%) and 14 (54%) had partial or no response, respectively. Interestingly, at the time of diagnosis, patients who had a complete clinical response, when compared with others, presented a more severe disease associated with more extracapillary proliferation on kidney biopsy, suggesting that different response profiles to eculizumab treatment among C3 GP patients could be recognized.

In individuals with monoclonal gammopathy that causes C3 GP (proteinuria and decline of renal function), a retrospective study of 50 patients with various types of monoclonal gammopathy [72] demonstrated that chemotherapy reduced proteinuria and improved renal function in 74% of patients, mainly in patients who had a reduction of gammopathy. Moreover, the hazard of ESRD was 83% lower in patients with reduced gammopathy. The same improvement was observed in other patients who received chemotherapy [23] in the presence of gammopathy because of lymphoproliferative disorders [73,74]. Many patients have shown an improvement in the clinical course, which is characterized by a reduction of proteinuria and improvement of renal function. However, the role of eculizumab remains to be defined. C3 GP remains the ideal disease in which anticomplement drugs (compostatin, monoclonal antibodies against C3, FB, properdin) can be tested [75–78].

Plasma exchange removes autoantibodies such as NeFs and mutated proteins, but it must be associated with immunosuppressive therapy for blocking antibody production. This approach has been used successfully in patients with CFH mutations [79–81]. The Consensus Report on C3 GP [2] concluded that an international pathology registry is necessary to define the different spectra of this disease and to divide patients into appropriate subgroups. Thus, the combination of well-defined clinical studies associated with a robust complement study would be ideal before enrolling patients in clinical trials. The final aim will be to treat homogenous cohorts before enrolling patients in clinical trials.

## 10. Conclusions

C3 GPs are orphan diseases of which the understanding of the pathophysiology of the complement system has improved laboratory and clinical diagnosis. However, a multidisciplinary approach that involves nephrologists, renal pathologists, and geneticists is helpful for a correct diagnosis and for choosing optimum therapeutic plans. More comprehensive genetic and biomarker studies are needed to refine our diagnostic approach. We should continue to improve the clinicopathological phenotype for designing correct multicenter trials that will give more information on the clinical course of the disease and the effect of new drugs. Treatment with a combination of immune-suppressive drugs or anticomplement agents can induce complete or partial remission in 50% of patients. Remission is more frequent in C3 GN than in DDD, whereas spontaneous remission is very rare. These diseases lead to ESKD in 50% of patients; some of them have persistent heavy proteinuria that is nonresponsive to therapy, ranging from ACEi-ARB to immunosuppressive drugs. Older age reduced renal function, and nephrotic syndrome at presentation are unfavorable prognostic factors. The recurrence of these diseases in patients after kidney transplantation is very frequent; therefore, post-transplant monitoring and available treatment options should be taken into consideration. Newer therapies such as monoclonal antibodies and recombinant proteins may be promising strategies in the near future.

**Author Contributions:** The authors contributed equally to the conception of the work and to the acquisition, analysis and interpretation of data from the literature. All authors have read and agreed to the published version of the manuscript.

## References

1. Schena, F.P.; Alpers, G.E. Membranoproliferative glomerulonephritis and cryoglobulinemic glomerulonephritis. In *Comprehensive Clinical Nephrology*, 5th ed.; Elsevier: Sanders, PA, USA, 2015; pp. 253–260.
2. Pickering, M.C.; D'Agati, V.D.; Nester, C.M.; Smith, R.J.; Haas, M.; Appel, G.B.; Alpers, C.E.; Bajema, I.M.; Bedrosian, C.; Braun, M.; et al. C3 glomerulopathy: Consensus report. *Kidney Int.* **2013**, *84*, 1079–1089. [CrossRef]
3. Fakhouri, F.; Frémeaux-Bacc, V.; Noël, L.H.; Cook, H.T.; Pickering, M.C. C3 glomerulopathy: A new classification. *Nat. Rev. Nephrol.* **2010**, *6*, 494–499. [CrossRef]
4. Cook, H.T.; Pickering, M.C. Clusters Not Classifications: Making Sense of Complement-Mediated Kidney Injury. *J. Am. Soc. Nephrol.* **2019**, *29*, 9–12. [CrossRef]

5. Ricklin, D.; Mastellos, D.C.; Reis, E.S.; Lambris, J.D. The renaissance of complement therapeutics. *Nat. Rev. Nephrol.* **2018**, *14*, 26–47. [CrossRef]
6. Jokiranta, T.S.; Solomon, A.; Pangburn, M.K.; Zipfel, P.F.; Meri, S. Nephritogenic lambda light chain dimer: A unique human miniautoantibody against complement factor H. *J Immunol.* **1999**, *163*, 4590–4596.
7. Goodship, T.H.; Pappworth, I.Y.; Toth, T.; Denton, M.; Houlberg, K.; McCormick, F.; Warland, D.; Moore, I.; Hunze, E.M.; Staniforth, S.J.; et al. Factor H autoantibodies in membranoproliferative glomerulonephritis. *Mol. Immunol.* **2012**, *52*, 200–206. [CrossRef]
8. Nozal, P.; Strobel, S.; Ibernon, M.; López, D.; Sánchez-Corral, P.; Rodríguez de Córdoba, S.; Józsi, M.; López-Trascasa, M. Anti-factor H antibody affecting factor H cofactor activity in a patient with dense deposit disease. *Clin. Kidney J.* **2012**, *5*, 133–136. [CrossRef] [PubMed]
9. Blanc, C.; Togarsimalemath, S.K.; Chauvet, S.; Le Quintrec, M.; Moulin, B.; Buchler, M.; Jokiranta, T.S.; Roumenina, L.T.; Fremeaux-Bacchi, V.; Dragon-Durey, M.A. Anti-factor H autoantibodies in C3 glomerulopathies and in atypical hemolytic uremic syndrome: One target, two diseases. *J. Immunol.* **2015**, *194*, 5129–5138. [CrossRef] [PubMed]
10. Xiao, X.; Pickering, M.C.; Smith, R.J. C3 glomerulopathy: The genetic and clinical findings in dense deposit disease and C3 glomerulonephritis. *Semin. Thromb. Hemost.* **2014**, *40*, 465–471. [CrossRef] [PubMed]
11. Merinero, H.M.; García, S.P.; García-Fernández, J.; Arjona, E.; Tortajada, A.; Rodríguez de Córdoba, S. Complete functional characterization of disease-associated genetic variants in the complement factor H gene. *Kidney Int.* **2018**, *93*, 470–481. [CrossRef]
12. Barbour, T.D.; Ruseva, M.M.; Pickering, M.C. Update on C3 glomerulopathy. *Nephrol. Dial. Transplant.* **2016**, *31*, 717–725. [CrossRef] [PubMed]
13. Spitzer, R.E.; Vallota, E.H.; Forristal, J.; Sudora, E.; Stitzel, A.; Davis, N.C.; West, C.D. Serum C′3 lytic system in patients with glomerulonephritis. *Science* **1969**, *164*, 436–437. [CrossRef] [PubMed]
14. Arroyave, C.M.; Vallota, E.H.; Müller-Eberhard, H.J. Lysis of human erythrocytes due to activation of the alternate complement pathway by nephritic factor (C3NeF). *J. Immunol.* **1974**, *113*, 764–768. [PubMed]
15. Daha, M.R.; Fearon, D.T.; Austen, K.F. Formation in the presence of C3 nephritic factor (C3NeF) of an alternative pathway C3 convertase containing uncleaved B. *Immunology* **1976**, *31*, 789–796. [PubMed]
16. Daha, M.R.; Austen, K.F.; Fearon, D.T. The incorporation of C3 nephritic factor (C3NeF) into a stabilized C3 convertase, C3bBb (C3NeF), and its release after decay of convertase function. *J. Immunol.* **1977**, *119*, 812–817.
17. Williams, D.G.; Bartlett, A.; Duffus, P. Identification of nephritic factor as an immunoglobulin. *Clin. Exp. Immunol.* **1978**, *33*, 425–429.
18. Józsi, M.; Reuter, S.; Nozal, P.; López-Trascasa, M.; Sánchez-Corral, P.; Prohászka, Z.; Uzonyi, B. Autoantibodies to complement components in C3 glomerulopathy and atypical hemolytic uremic syndrome. *Immunol. Lett.* **2014**, *160*, 163–171. [CrossRef]
19. Marinozzi, M.C.; Chauvet, S.; Le Quintrec, M.; Mignotet, M.; Petitprez, F.; Legendre, C.; Cailliez, M.; Deschenes, G.; Fischbach, M.; Karras, A.; et al. C5 nephritic factors drive the biological phenotype of C3 glomerulopathies. *Kidney Int.* **2017**, *92*, 1232–1241. [CrossRef]
20. Halbwachs, L.; Leveillé, M.; Lesavre, P.; Wattel, S.; Leibowitch, J. Nephritic factor of the classical pathway of complement: Immunoglobulin G autoantibody directed against the classical pathway C3 convetase enzyme. *J. Clin. Investig.* **1980**, *65*, 1249–1256. [CrossRef]
21. Tanuma, Y.; Ohi, H.; Hatano, M. Two types of C3 nephritic factor: Properdin-dependent C3NeF and properdin-independent C3NeF. *Clin. Immunol. Immunopathol.* **1990**, *56*, 226–238. [CrossRef]
22. Schena, F.P.; Pertosa, G.; Stanziale, P.; Vox, E.; Pecoraro, C.; Andreucci, V.E. Biological significance of the C3 nephritic factor in membranoproliferative glomerulonephritis. *Clin. Nephrol.* **1982**, *18*, 240–246. [PubMed]
23. Ravindran, A.; Fervenza, F.C.; Smith, R.J.H.; De Vriese, A.S.; Sethi, S. C3 Glomerulopathy: Ten Years' Experience at Mayo Clinic. *Mayo Clin. Proc.* **2018**, *93*, 991–1008. [CrossRef] [PubMed]
24. Donadelli, R.; Pulieri, P.; Piras, R.; Iatropoulos, P.; Valoti, E.; Benigni, A.; Remuzzi, G.; Noris, M. Unraveling the Molecular Mechanisms Underlying Complement Dysregulation by Nephritic Factors in C3G and IC-MPGN. *Front. Immunol.* **2018**, *9*, 2329. [CrossRef] [PubMed]
25. Medjeral-Thomas, N.R.; O'Shaughnessy, M.M.; O'Regan, J.A.; Traynor, C.; Flanagan, M.; Wong, L.; Teoh, C.W.; Awan, A.; Waldron, M.; Cairns, T.; et al. C3 glomerulopathy: Clinicopathologic features and predictors of outcome. *Clin. J. Am. Soc. Nephrol.* **2014**, *9*, 46–53. [CrossRef]

26. Strobel, S.; Zimmering, M.; Papp, K.; Prechl, J.; Józsi, M. Anti-factor B autoantibody in dense deposit disease. *Mol. Immunol.* **2010**, *47*, 1476–1483. [CrossRef]
27. Chen, Q.; Müller, D.; Rudolph, B.; Hartmann, A.; Kuwertz-Bröking, E.; Wu, K.; Kirschfink, M.; Skerka, C.; Zipfel, P.F. Combined C3b and factor B autoantibodies and MPGN type II. *N Engl. J. Med.* **2011**, *365*, 2340–2342. [CrossRef]
28. Smith, R.J.H.; Alexander, J.; Barlow, P.N.; Botto, M.; Cassavant, T.L.; Cook, H.T.; deCórdoba, S.R.; Hageman, G.S.; Jokiranta, T.S.; Kimberling, W.J.; et al. Dense Deposit Disease Focus Group. New approaches to the treatment of dense deposit disease. *J. Am. Soc. Nephrol.* **2007**, *18*, 2447–2456. [CrossRef]
29. Bomback, A.S.; Santoriello, D.; Avasare, R.S.; Regunathan-Shenk, R.; Canetta, P.A.; Ahn, W.; Radhakrishnan, J.; Marasa, M.; Rosenstiel, P.E.; Herlitz, L.C.; et al. C3 glomerulonephritis and dense deposit disease share a similar disease course in a large United States cohort of patients with C3 glomerulopathy. *Kidney Int.* **2018**, *93*, 977–985. [CrossRef]
30. Smith, R.J.H.; Appel, G.B.; Blom, A.M.; Cook, H.T.; D'Agati, V.D.; Fakhouri, F.; Fremeaux-Bacchi, V.; Józsi, M.; Kavanagh, D.; Lambris, J.D.; et al. C3 glomerulopathy—Understanding a rare complement-driven renal disease. *Nat. Rev. Nephrol.* **2019**, *15*, 129–143. [CrossRef]
31. Athanasiou, Y.; Voskarides, K.; Gale, D.P.; Damianou, L.; Patsias, C.; Zavros, M.; Maxwell, P.H.; Cook, H.T.; Demosthenous, P.; Hadjisavvas, A.; et al. Familial C3 glomerulopathy associated with CFHR5 mutations: Clinical characteristics of 91 patients in 16 pedigrees. *Clin. J. Am. Soc. Nephrol.* **2011**, *6*, 1436–1446. [CrossRef]
32. Servais, A.; Noël, L.H.; Roumenina, L.T.; Le Quintrec, M.; Ngo, S.; Dragon-Durey, M.A.; Macher, M.A.; Zuber, J.; Karras, A.; Provot, F.; et al. Acquired and genetic complement abnormalities play a critical role in dense deposit disease and other C3 glomerulopathies. *Kidney Int.* **2012**, *82*, 454–464. [CrossRef] [PubMed]
33. Rabasco, C.; Cavero, T.; Román, E.; Rojas-Rivera, J.; Olea, T.; Espinosa, M.; Cabello, V.; Fernández-Juarez, G.; González, F.; Ávila, A.; et al. Spanish Group for the Study of Glomerular Diseases (GLOSEN). Effectiveness of mycophenolate mofetil in C3 glomerulonephritis. *Kidney Int.* **2015**, *88*, 1153–1160. [CrossRef] [PubMed]
34. Iatropoulos, P.; Noris, M.; Mele, C.; Piras, R.; Valoti, E.; Bresin, E.; Curreri, M.; Mondo, E.; Zito, A.; Gamba, S.; et al. Complement gene variants determine the risk of immunoglobulin-associated MPGN and C3 glomerulopathy and predict long-term renal outcome. *Mol. Immunol.* **2016**, *71*, 131–142. [CrossRef] [PubMed]
35. Caliskan, Y.; Torun, E.S.; Tiryaki, T.O.; Oruc, A.; Ozluk, Y.; Akgul, S.U.; Temurhan, S.; Oztop, N.; Kilicaslan, I.; Sever, M.S. Immunosuppressive Treatment in C3 Glomerulopathy: Is it Really Effective? *Am. J. Nephrol.* **2017**, *46*, 96–107. [CrossRef] [PubMed]
36. Le Quintrec, M.; Lapeyraque, A.L.; Lionet, A.; Sellier-Leclerc, A.L.; Delmas, Y.; Baudouin, V.; Daugas, E.; Decramer, S.; Tricot, L.; Cailliez, M.; et al. Patterns of Clinical Response to Eculizumab in Patients with C3 Glomerulopathy. *Am. J. Kidney Dis.* **2018**, *72*, 84–92. [CrossRef] [PubMed]
37. Gale, D.P.; Goicoechea de Jorge, E.G.; Cook, H.T.; Martinez-Barricate, R.; Hadjisavvas, A.; McLean, A.G. Identification of a mutation in complement factor H-related protein 5 in patients of Cypriot origin with glomerulonephritis. *Lancet* **2010**, *376*, 794–801. [CrossRef]
38. Martínez-Barricarte, R.; Heurich, M.; Valdes-Cañedo, F.; Vazquez-Martul, E.; Torreira, E.; Montes, T.; Tortajada, A.; Pinto, S.; Lopez-Trascasa, M.; Morgan, B.P.; et al. Human C3 mutation reveals a mechanism of dense deposit disease pathogenesis and provides insights into complement activation and regulation. *J. Clin. Investig.* **2010**, *120*, 3702–3712. [CrossRef]
39. Malik, T.H.; Lavin, P.J.; Goicoechea de Jorge, E.; Vernon, K.A.; Rose, K.L.; Patel, M.P.A. A hybrid CFHR3-1 gene causes familial C3 glomerulopathy. *J. Am. Soc. Nephrol.* **2012**, *23*, 1155–1160. [CrossRef]
40. Tortajada, A.; Ye'benes, H.; Abarrategui-Garrido, C.; Anter, J.; García-Fernández, J.M.; Martínez-Barricarte, R.; Alba-Domínguez, M.; Malik, T.H.; Bedoya, R.; Cabrera Pérez, R.; et al. C3 glomerulopathy associated CFHR1 mutation alters FHR oligomerization and complement regulation. *J. Clin. Investig.* **2013**, *123*, 2434–2446. [CrossRef]
41. Medjeral-Thomas, N.R.; Troldborg, A.; Constantinou, N.; Lomax-Browne, H.J.; Hansen, A.G.; Willicombe, M.; Pusey, C.D.; Cook, H.T.; Thiel, S.; Pickering, M.C. Progressive IgA Nephropathy is Associated with low circulating mannan-binding lectin-associated serine protease-3 (MASP-3) and increased glomerular factor H-related protein-5 (FHR5) Deposition. *Kidney Int. Rep.* **2017**, *3*, 426–438. [CrossRef]

42. Hou, J.; Markowitz, G.S.; Bomback, A.S.; Appel, G.B.; Herlitz, L.C.; Barry Stokes, M.; D'Agati, V.D. Toward a working definition of C3 glomerulopathy by immunofluorescence. *Kidney Int.* **2014**, *85*, 450–456. [CrossRef] [PubMed]
43. Sethi, S.; Nasr, S.H.; De Vriese, A.S.; Fervenza, F.C. C4d as a diagnostic tool in proliferative GN. *J. Am. Soc. Nephrol.* **2015**, *26*, 2852–2859. [CrossRef] [PubMed]
44. Singh, G.; Singh, S.K.; Nalwa, A.; Lavleen, S.; Pradeep, I.; Barwad, A.; Sinha, A.; Hari, P.; Bagga, A.; Bagchi, S.; et al. Glomerular C4d staining does not exclude a C3 Glomerulopathy. *Kidney Int. Rep.* **2019**, *4*, 698–709. [CrossRef] [PubMed]
45. Leung, N.; Bridoux, F.; Batuman, V.; Chaidos, A.; Cockwell, P.; D'Agati, V.D.; Dispenzieri, A.; Fervenza, F.C.; Fermand, J.P.; Gibbs, S.; et al. The evaluation of monoclonal gammopathy of renal significance: A consensus report of the International Kidney and Monoclonal Gammopathy Research Group. *Nat. Rev. Nephrol.* **2019**, *15*, 121–135. [CrossRef]
46. Zand, L.; Kattah, A.; Fervenza, F.C.; Smith, R.J.; Nasr, S.H.; Zhang, Y.; Vrana, J.A.; Leung, N.; Cornell, L.D.; Sethi, S. C3 glomerulonephritis associated with monoclonal gammopathy: A case series. *Am. J. Kidney Dis.* **2013**, *62*, 506–514. [CrossRef]
47. Angioi, A.; Fervenza, F.C.; Sethi, S.; Zhang, Y.; Smith, R.J.; Murray, D.; Van Praet, J.; Pani, A.; De Vriese, A.S. Diagnosis of complement alternative pathway disorders. *Kidney Int.* **2016**, *89*, 278–288. [CrossRef]
48. Grumach, A.S.; Kirschfink, M. Are complement deficiencies really rare? Overview on prevalence, clinical importance and modern diagnostic approach. *Mol. Immunol.* **2014**, *61*, 110–117. [CrossRef]
49. Zhang, Y.; Nester, C.M.; Martin, B.; Skjoedt, M.O.; Meyer, N.C.; Shao, D.; Borsa, N.; Palarasah, Y.; Smith, R.J. Defining the complement biomarker profile of C3 glomerulopathy. *Clin. J. Am. Soc. Nephrol.* **2014**, *9*, 1876–1882. [CrossRef]
50. Fervenza, F.C.; Sethi, S. Circulating complement levels and C3 glomerulopathy. *Clin. J. Am. Soc. Nephrol.* **2014**, *9*, 1829–1831. [CrossRef]
51. Corvillo, F.; Okrój, M.; Nozal, P.; Melgosa, M.; Sánchez-Corral, P.; López-Trascasa, M. Nephritic Factors: An Overview of Classification, Diagnostic Tools and Clinical Associations. *Front. Immunol.* **2019**, *10*, 886. [CrossRef]
52. Zhang, Y.; Meyer, N.C.; Wang, K.; Nishimura, C.; Frees, K.; Jones, M.; Katz, L.M.; Sethi, S.; Smith, R.J. Causes of alternative pathway dysregulation in dense deposit disease. *Clin. J. Am. Soc. Nephrol.* **2012**, *7*, 265–274. [CrossRef] [PubMed]
53. Ohi, H.; Yasugi, T. Occurrence of C3 nephritic factor and C4 nephritic factor in membranoproliferative glomerulonephritis (MPGN). *Clin. Exp. Immunol.* **1994**, *95*, 316–321. [CrossRef] [PubMed]
54. Watson, R.; Lindner, S.; Bordereau, P.; Hunze, E.M.; Tak, F.; Ngo, S.; Zipfel, P.F.; Skerka, C.; Dragon-Durey, M.A.; Marchbank, K.J. Standardisation of the factor H autoantibody assay. *Immunobiology* **2014**, *219*, 9–16. [CrossRef] [PubMed]
55. Osborne, A.J.; Breno, M.; Borsa, N.G.; Bu, F.; Frémeaux-Bacchi, V.; Gale, D.P.; van den Heuvel, L.P.; Kavanagh, D.; Noris, M.; Pinto, S.; et al. Statistical Validation of Rare Complement Variants Provides Insights into the Molecular Basis of Atypical Hemolytic Uremic Syndrome and C3 Glomerulopathy. *J. Immunol.* **2018**, *200*, 2464–2478. [CrossRef] [PubMed]
56. Sánchez-Corral, P.; Pouw, R.B.; López-Trascasa, M.; Józsi, M. Self-Damage Caused by Dysregulation of the Complement Alternative Pathway: Relevance of the Factor H Protein Family. *Front. Immunol.* **2018**, *12*, 1607. [CrossRef]
57. Vernon, K.A.; Gale, D.P.; de Jorge, E.G.; McLean, A.G.; Galliford, J.; Pierides, A.; Maxwell, P.H.; Taube, D.; Pickering, M.C.; Cook, H.T. Recurrence of complement factor H-related protein 5 nephropathy in a renal transplant. *Am. J. Transplant.* **2011**, *11*, 152–155. [CrossRef]
58. Cochat, P.; Fargue, S.; Mestrallet, G.; Jungraithmayr, T.; Koch-Nogueira, P.; Ranchin, B.; Zimmerhackl, L.B. Disease recurrence in paediatric renal transplantation. *Pediatr. Nephrol.* **2009**, *11*, 2097–2108. [CrossRef]
59. Wong, L.; Moran, S.; Lavin, P.J.; Dorman, A.M.; Conlon, P.J. Kidney transplant outcomes in familial C3 glomerulopathy. *Clin. Kidney J.* **2016**, *3*, 403–407. [CrossRef]
60. Bomback, A.S.; Smith, R.J.; Barile, G.R.; Zhang, Y.; Heher, E.C.; Herlitz, L.; Stokes, M.B.; Markowitz, G.S.; D'Agati, V.D.; Canetta, P.A.; et al. Eculizumab for dense deposit disease and C3 glomerulonephritis. *Clin. J. Am. Soc. Nephrol.* **2012**, *7*, 748–756. [CrossRef]

61. Abbas, F.; El Kossi, M.; Kim, J.J.; Shaheen, I.S.; Sharma, A.; Halawa, A. Complement-mediated renal diseases after kidney transplantation—Current diagnostic and therapeutic options in de novo and recurrent diseases. *World J. Transplant.* **2018**, *8*, 203–219. [CrossRef]
62. Sánchez-Moreno, A.; De la Cerda, F.; Cabrera, R.; Fijo, J.; López-Trascasa, M.; Bedoya, R.; Rodríguez de Córdoba, S.; Ybot-González, P. Eculizumab in dense-deposit disease after renal transplantation. *Pediatr. Nephrol.* **2014**, *29*, 2055–2059. [CrossRef] [PubMed]
63. Lim, W.H.; Shingde, M.; Wong, G. Recurrent and de novo Glomerulonephritis after Kidney Transplantation. *Front. Immunol.* **2019**, *10*, 1944. [CrossRef] [PubMed]
64. Uffing, A.; Pérez-Sáez, M.J.; La Manna, G.; Comai, G.; Fischman, C.; Farouk, S.; Manfro, R.C.; Bauer, A.C.; Lichtenfels, B.; Mansur, J.B.; et al. A large, international study on post-transplant glomerular diseases: The TANGO project. *BMC Nephrol.* **2018**, *19*, 229. [CrossRef] [PubMed]
65. Legendre, C.M.; Licht, C.; Muus, P.; Greenbaum, L.A.; Babu, S.; Bedrosian, C.; Bingham, C.; Cohen, D.J.; Delmas, Y.; Douglas, K.; et al. Terminal complement inhibitor eculizumab in atypical hemolytic-uremic syndrome. *N. Engl. J. Med.* **2013**, *368*, 2169–2181. [CrossRef]
66. Welte, T.; Arnold, F.; Kappes, J.; Seidl, M.; Häffner, K.; Bergmann, C.; Walz, G.; Neumann-Haefelin, E. Treating C3 glomerulopathy with eculizumab. *BMC Nephrol.* **2018**, *19*, 7. [CrossRef]
67. Von Visger, J.; Cassol, C.; Nori, U.; Franco-Ahumada, G.; Nadasdy, T.; Satoskar, A.A. Complete biopsy-proven resolution of deposits in recurrent proliferative glomerulonephritis with monoclonal IgG deposits (PGNMIGD) following rituximab treatment in renal allograft. *BMC Nephrol.* **2019**, *20*, 53. [CrossRef]
68. McCaughan, J.A.; O'Rourke, D.M.; Courtney, A.E. Recurrent dense deposit disease after renal transplantation: An emerging role for complementary therapies. *Am. J. Transplant.* **2012**, *12*, 1046–1051. [CrossRef]
69. Zand, L.; Lorenz, E.C.; Cosio, F.G.; Fervenza, F.C.; Nasr, S.H.; Gandhi, M.J.; Smith, R.J.; Sethi, S. Clinical findings, pathology, and outcomes of C3GN after kidney transplantation. *J. Am. Soc. Nephrol.* **2014**, *25*, 1110–1117. [CrossRef]
70. Rudnicki, M. Rituximab for Treatment of Membranoproliferative Glomerulonephritis and C3 Glomerulopathies. *BioMed Res. Int.* **2017**, *2017*, 2180508. [CrossRef]
71. Koopman, J.J.E.; Teng, Y.K.O.; Boon, C.J.F.; van den Heuvel, L.P.; Rabelink, T.J.; van Kooten, C.; de Vries, A.P.J. Diagnosis and treatment of C3 glomerulopathy in a center of expertise. *Neth. J. Med.* **2019**, *77*, 10–18.
72. Chauvet, S.; Roumenina, L.T.; Aucouturier, P.; Marinozzi, M.C.; Dragon-Durey, M.A.; Karras, A.; Delmas, Y.; Le Quintrec, M.; Guerrot, D.; Jourde-Chiche, N.; et al. Both Monoclonal and Polyclonal Immunoglobulin Contingents Mediate Complement Activation in Monoclonal Gammopathy Associated-C3 Glomerulopathy. *Front. Immunol.* **2018**, *9*, 2260. [CrossRef] [PubMed]
73. Chauvet, S.; Frémeaux-Bacchi, V.; Petitprez, F.; Karras, A.; Daniel, L.; Burtey, S.; Choukroun, G.; Delmas, Y.; Guerrot, D.; François, A.; et al. Treatment of B-cell disorder improves renal outcome of patients with monoclonal gammopathy-associated C3 glomerulopathy. *Blood* **2017**, *129*, 1437–1447. [CrossRef] [PubMed]
74. Sethi, S.; Sukov, W.R.; Zhang, Y.; Fervenza, F.C.; Lager, D.J.; Miller, D.V.; Cornell, L.D.; Krishnan, S.G.; Smith, R.J. Dense deposit disease associated with monoclonal gammopathy of undetermined significance. *Am. J. Kidney Dis.* **2010**, *56*, 977–982. [CrossRef] [PubMed]
75. Zhang, Y.; Shao, D.; Ricklin, D.; Hilkin, B.M.; Nester, C.M.; Lambris, J.D.; Smith, R.J. Compstatin analog Cp40 inhibits complement dysregulation in vitro in C3 glomerulopathy. *Immunobiology* **2015**, *220*, 993–998. [CrossRef] [PubMed]
76. Paixão-Cavalcante, D.; Torreira, E.; Lindorfer, M.A.; Rodriguez de Cordoba, S.; Morgan, B.P.; Taylor, R.P.; Llorca, O.; Harris, C.L. A humanized antibody that regulates the alternative pathway convertase: Potential for therapy of renal disease associated with nephritic factors. *J. Immunol.* **2014**, *192*, 4844–4851. [CrossRef] [PubMed]
77. Subías, M.; Tortajada, A.; Gastoldi, S.; Galbusera, M.; López-Perrote, A.; Lopez, L.J.; González-Fernández, F.A.; Villegas-Martínez, A.; Dominguez, M.; Llorca, O.; et al. A novel antibody against human factor B that blocks formation of the C3bB proconvertase and inhibits complement activation in disease models. *J. Immunol.* **2014**, *193*, 5567–5575. [CrossRef]
78. Pauly, D.; Nagel, B.M.; Reinders, J.; Killian, T.; Wulf, M.; Ackerman, S.; Ehrenstein, B.; Zipfel, P.F.; Skerka, C.; Weber, B.H. A novel antibody against human properdin inhibits the alternative complement system and specifically detects properdin from blood samples. *PLoS ONE* **2014**, *9*, e96371. [CrossRef]

79. Krmar, R.T.; Holtbäck, U.; Linné, T.; Berg, U.B.; Celsi, G.; Söderberg, M.P.; Wernerson, A.; Szakos, A.; Larsson, S.; Skattum, L.; et al. Acute renal failure in dense deposit disease: Complete recovery after combination therapy with immunosuppressant and plasma exchange. *Clin. Nephrol.* **2011**, *75*, 4–10.
80. Häffner, K.; Michelfelder, S.; Pohl, M. Successful therapy of C3Nef-positive C3 glomerulopathy with plasma therapy and immunosuppression. *Pediatr. Nephrol.* **2015**, *30*, 1951–1959. [CrossRef]
81. Kurtz, K.A.; Schlueter, A.J. Management of membranoproliferative glomerulonephritis type II with plasmapheresis. *J. Clin. Apher.* **2002**, *17*, 135–137. [CrossRef]

13

# Incidence and Cost of Acute Kidney Injury in Hospitalized Patients with Infective Endocarditis

**Victor Ortiz-Soriano [1], Katherine Donaldson [1], Gaixin Du [2], Ye Li [3], Joshua Lambert [3], Mark Rudy [1], Dan Cleland [2], Alice Thornton [4], Laura C. Fanucchi [4], Moises A. Huaman [4,5] and Javier A. Neyra [1,*]**

1 Division of Nephrology, Bone and Mineral Metabolism, Department of Internal Medicine, University of Kentucky Medical Center, Lexington, KY 40506, USA
2 Center for Health Services Research, University of Kentucky, Lexington, KY 40506, USA
3 Department of Statistics, University of Kentucky, Lexington, KY 40506, USA
4 Division of Infectious Diseases, Department of Internal Medicine, University of Kentucky Medical Center, Lexington, KY 40506, USA
5 Division of Infectious Diseases, Department of Internal Medicine, University of Cincinnati, Cincinnati, OH 45221, USA
* Correspondence: javier.neyra@uky.edu

**Abstract:** Acute kidney injury (AKI) is a frequent complication of hospitalized patients with infective endocarditis (IE). Further, AKI in the setting of IE is associated with high morbidity and mortality. We aimed to examine the incidence, clinical parameters, and hospital costs associated with AKI in hospitalized patients with IE in an endemic area with an increasing prevalence of opioid use. This retrospective cohort study included 269 patients admitted to a major referral center in Kentucky with a primary diagnosis of IE from January 2013 to December 2015. Of these, 178 (66.2%) patients had AKI by Kidney Disease Improving Global Outcomes (KDIGO) serum creatinine criteria: 74 (41.6%) had AKI stage 1 and 104 (58.4%) had AKI stage ≥2. In multivariable analysis, higher comorbidity scores and the need for diuretics were independently associated with AKI, while the involvement of the tricuspid valve and the need for vasopressor/inotrope support were independently associated with severe AKI (stage ≥2). The median total direct cost of hospitalization was progressively higher according to each stage of AKI ($17,069 for no AKI; $37,111 for AKI stage 1; and $61,357 for AKI stage ≥2; $p < 0.001$). In conclusion, two-thirds of patients admitted to the hospital due to IE had incident AKI. The occurrence of AKI significantly increased healthcare costs. The higher level of comorbidity, the affection of the tricuspid valve, and the need for diuretics and/or vasoactive drugs were associated with severe AKI in this susceptible population.

**Keywords:** acute kidney injury; infective endocarditis; healthcare costs; opioid use

---

## 1. Introduction

Infective endocarditis (IE) is a severe infectious process that carries high morbidity and mortality [1–3]. Reports indicate that the incidence of IE in the United States has been increasing steadily in recent years [4,5]. The crude incidence has increased from 7.6 to 9.3 cases per 100,000 persons annually from 1998–2013 [5]. Moreover, healthcare costs for patients with IE increased eighteen-fold, from $1.1 million in 2010 to $22.2 million in 2015 [6].

In the United States, some areas such as the Midwest and West have exhibited a steady increase in the incidence of IE in relation to the growing incidence of opioid dependence [7]. According to the National Survey on Drug Use and Health, persons with opioid and other substance use disorder who inject drugs are at higher risk of blood-borne infections and IE [8]. Infectious complications are common and constitute a major cause of hospitalizations [9].

Acute kidney injury (AKI) is a syndrome that occurs in about 20% of hospitalized patients [10,11]. AKI is also associated with high morbidity and mortality and affects hospital resource utilization and healthcare costs [12,13]. Patients with IE can develop distinct forms of acute or subacute kidney disease such as glomerulonephritis, infarction or cortical necrosis [14,15], manifesting as AKI [16]. Prior studies have shown that older age and the degree of thrombocytopenia were associated with an increased risk of AKI in patients with IE [17]. Moreover, some antibiotics commonly used to treat IE (e.g., aminoglycosides, vancomycin, etc.) can exert toxicity to the kidneys under specific circumstances [18].

The main objective of this study was to examine the incidence and clinical parameters associated with AKI in hospitalized patients with IE in Kentucky, a state highly impacted by the opioid epidemic. We also examined hospital costs associated with the occurrence of AKI and major adverse kidney events (MAKE) in this susceptible population.

## 2. Materials and Methods

### 2.1. *Study Design and Participants*

Single-center, retrospective cohort study. The study population included adult patients 18 years or older who were admitted to the University of Kentucky Albert B. Chandler Hospital with IE as the primary diagnosis. Patients were excluded if they had a history of end-stage kidney disease (ESKD), baseline estimated glomerular filtration rate (eGFR) less than 15 mL/min/1.73 $m^2$, were recipients of a kidney transplant, or if they had a prior episode of IE that required hospitalization. The study period was from January 2013–December 2015. The study was approved by the University of Kentucky Institutional Review Board.

### 2.2. *Study Variables and Definitions*

Data were gathered through automated and manual extraction from electronic health records (EHRs) and validated through comprehensive individual review of all records. The presence of comorbidities at the time of index hospitalization was assessed using the Elixhauser score [19], with individual comorbidities identified using ICD-9/10-CM codes. IE as the primary diagnosis was defined by the modified Duke Criteria [20]. IE characteristics including the location, type and number of affected cardiac valves were obtained by individual review of EHRs (consult notes, echocardiography reports, etc.). Baseline eGFR was estimated using the Chronic Kidney Disease Epidemiology Collaboration (CKD-EPI) equation [21], and baseline serum creatinine (SCr) was assessed as follows: (1) Outpatient SCr value closest to index admission within 1 year of hospitalization; if unavailable, (2) last inpatient SCr value from prior hospitalization within 1 year of index admission; if unavailable, (3) lowest SCr value throughout the index hospitalization. We gathered data of substance use disorder specific for opioid and IV drug use with the following ICD-9-CM codes: 292.0–9, 304.00–93, 305.20–93, 648.30–34, 655.50–53, 760.72–75, 779.5, 965.00–09, and V654.2. We extracted medication exposure, procedure data, and total costs related to the index hospitalization from the hospital billing system. The University of Kentucky Albert B. Chandler Hospital utilizes Allscripts Sunrise Clinical Manager™ EHR software (Allscripts, Chicago, IL, USA). Microbiologic data were obtained from blood, valve, abscess fluid, pleural fluid and bone biopsy.

### 2.3. *Study Outcomes*

#### 2.3.1. Clinical Outcomes

The primary outcome was incident in-hospital AKI defined and graded by the Kidney Disease Improving Global Outcomes (KDIGO) SCr-criteria. [22] We grouped AKI stages 2 and 3 due to the low numbers in each category in relation to AKI stage 1 and no AKI. A secondary outcome was MAKE, a composite of all-cause mortality, dependence on renal replacement therapy (RRT), or inability to recover at least 50% (MAKE50) or 25% (MAKE25) of baseline eGFR (if not on RRT) up to 90 days after hospital discharge [23]. Other secondary outcomes included hospital mortality and hospital readmission due to recurrent or a new episode of IE [24,25].

#### 2.3.2. Healthcare Cost Outcomes

The healthcare cost outcome was the median total direct cost of hospitalization in dollars. Other outcomes included hospital length of stay (days) and total days in a telemetry or intensive care unit (ICU) bed.

### *2.4. Statistical Analysis*

Categorical data were reported as number of observations (percentages) and continuous variables as mean ± standard deviation (SD), or median (1st quartile (IQ1)—3rd quartile (IQ3)) as appropriate. Comparisons between groups for categorical variables were made using chi-squared test or Fisher's exact test. Continuous variables were compared using the ANOVA or Kruskal-Wallis test as appropriate.

Multivariable logistic regression modeling was used for AKI stage 1 (vs. no AKI), AKI stage ≥2 (vs. no AKI or AKI stage 1), and MAKE (50% or 25%) as dependent variables and included candidate independent variables that were statistically significant in the bivariate analysis and/or carried clinical significance for the association with the dependent variables. The model section was performed using stepwise regression with a cutoff of 0.1 for variables to enter the model and 0.05 to be removed. All statistical analyses were performed using SAS 9.3 (SAS Institute, Charlotte, NC, USA) with an alpha level set at $p < 0.05$ (two-tailed) for all comparisons.

## 3. Results

### *3.1. Clinical Characteristics*

A total of 269 patients were included in the study. The cohort derivation algorithm is detailed in Figure 1. The mean (SD) age was 45.4 (16.2) years, 59.5% were male, and 95.5% white. The overall incidence of AKI was 66.2%, 74 (41.6%) patients had AKI stage 1 and 104 (58.4%) patients had AKI stage ≥2. The frequency of substance use disorder was not significantly different according to AKI status (54.5% in patients with AKI vs. 50.5% in patients without AKI, $p = 0.540$). Patient's clinical characteristics according to AKI status are detailed in Table 1.

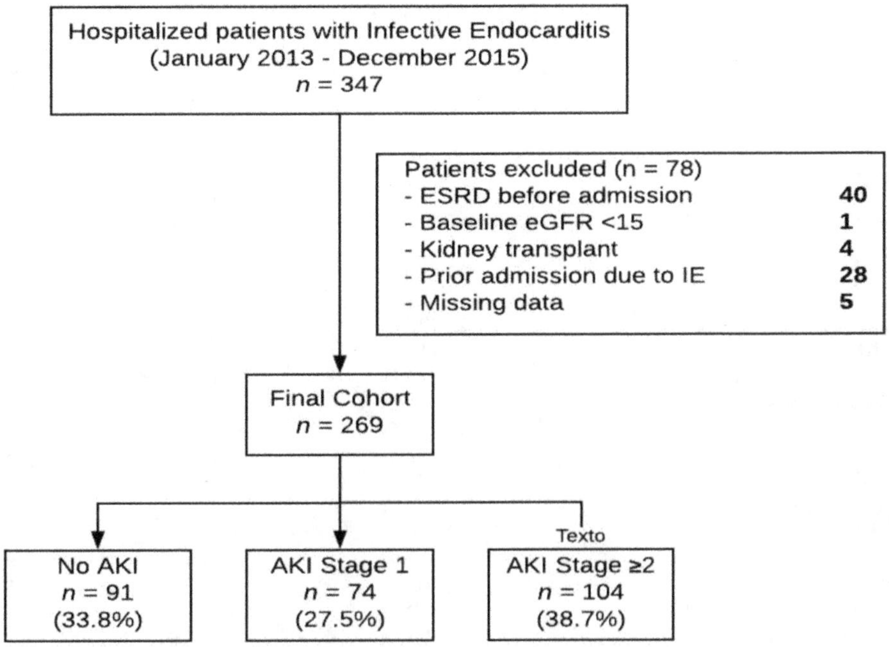


**Figure 1.** Cohort derivation. Abbreviations: AKI (acute kidney injury), eGFR (estimated glomerular filtration rate), ESRD (end-stage renal disease), IE (infective endocarditis).

**Table 1.** Patient characteristics according to acute kidney injury status.

| | No AKI | AKI Stage 1 | AKI Stage ≥2 | *p* |
|---|---|---|---|---|
| | *n* = 91 | *n* = 74 | *n* = 104 | |
| **Demographics** | | | | |
| Age, years, mean ± SD | 44.6 ± 15.6 | 45.5 ± 16.5 | 45.8 ± 16.8 | 0.860 |
| Gender, male, n (%) | 62 (68.1) | 34 (46.0) | 64 (61.5) | 0.013 |
| Ethnic group, white, *n* (%) | 86 (94.5) | 71 (96.0) | 99 (95.2) | 0.939 |
| BMI, kg/m$^2$, mean ± SD | 27.9 ± 10.9 | 29.8 ± 11.0 | 26.9 ± 7.1 | 0.140 |
| **Comorbidity** | | | | |
| Elixhauser Score, median (IQ1-IQ3) | 4.0 (3.0–6.0) | 6.0 (4.0–7.0) | 7.0 (5.0–8.0) | <0.001 |
| Diabetes, *n* (%) | 23 (25.3) | 14 (18.9) | 18 (17.3) | 0.361 |
| Hypertension, *n* (%) | 55 (60.4) | 41 (55.4) | 69 (66.4) | 0.328 |
| Hepatitis B, *n* (%) | 1 (1.1) | 9 (12.2) | 7 (6.7) | 0.011 |
| Hepatitis C, *n* (%) | 27 (29.7) | 38 (51.4) | 51 (49.0) | 0.006 |
| Congenital heart defect, *n* (%) | 6 (6.6) | 8 (10.8) | 9 (8.7) | 0.628 |
| Current substance use disorder, *n* (%) | 46 (50.5) | 42 (56.8) | 55 (52.9) | 0.672 |
| Baseline eGFR, mL/min/1.73 m$^2$, median (IQ1-IQ3) | 105.3 (69.1–127.6) | 96.8 (45.5–123.9) | 103.2 (71.4–122.9) | 0.220 |
| **Medications During Hospitalization** | | | | |
| Opiods, *n* (%) | 3 (3.3) | 6 (8.1) | 9 (8.7) | 0.279 |
| ACEI or ARB, *n* (%) | 36 (39.6) | 12 (16.2) | 21 (20.2) | <0.001 |
| Aminoglycosides, *n* (%) | 36 (39.6) | 31 (41.9) | 52 (50.0) | 0.305 |
| Diuretic, *n* (%) | 38 (41.8) | 51 (68.9) | 83 (79.8) | <0.001 |
| NSAIDs, *n* (%) | 54 (59.3) | 51 (68.9) | 77 (74.0) | 0.088 |
| Pressor or inotrope, *n* (%) | 0 (0.0) | 5 (6.8) | 19 (18.3) | <0.001 |
| Vancomycin, *n* (%) | 76 (83.5) | 69 (93.2) | 89 (85.6) | 0.142 |
| Piperacillin/tazobactam, *n* (%) | 30 (33.0) | 23 (31.1) | 38 (36.5) | 0.733 |
| Cefepime, *n* (%) | 25 (27.5) | 30 (40.5) | 39 (37.5) | 0.169 |
| Vancomycin + Pip/Tazo, *n* (%) | 30 (33.0) | 24 (32.4) | 36 (34.6) | 0.948 |
| Vancomycin + Cefepime, *n* (%) | 26 (28.6) | 32 (43.2) | 37 (35.6) | 0.146 |
| **Infective endocarditis characteristics** | | | | |
| ICU care, *n* (%) | 38 (41.8) | 39 (52.7) | 46 (44.2) | 0.346 |
| Sepsis, *n* (%) | 32 (35.2) | 36 (48.7) | 66 (63.5) | <0.001 |
| Osteomyelitis, *n* (%) | 14 (15.4) | 7 (9.5) | 18 (17.3) | 0.327 |

**Table 1.** *Cont.*

| | No AKI | AKI Stage 1 | AKI Stage ≥2 | *p* |
|---|---|---|---|---|
| | *n* = 91 | *n* = 74 | *n* = 104 | |
| Number of affected cardiac valves, | | | | |
| 0, *n* (%) | 45 (49.5) | 26 (35.1) | 29 (27.9) | 0.006 |
| 1, *n* (%) | 40 (44.0) | 42 (56.8) | 56 (53.8) | |
| ≥2, *n* (%) | 6 (6.5) | 6 (8.1) | 19 (18.3) | |
| Affected valve, | | | | |
| Mitral, *n* (%) | 31 (34.1) | 27 (37.0) | 34 (32.7) | 0.837 |
| Aortic, *n* (%) | 38 (41.8) | 24 (32.9) | 35 (33.7) | 0.395 |
| Tricuspid, *n* (%) | 20 (22.0) | 18 (24.7) | 47 (45.2) | <0.001 |
| Pulmonic, *n* (%) | 1 (1.1) | 2 (2.7) | 2 (1.9) | 0.856 |
| Type of valve, prosthetic, *n* (%) | 23 (25.3) | 20 (27.0) | 33 (31.7) | 0.585 |
| Procedures, | | | | |
| Valve replacement, *n* (%) | 16 (17.6) | 14 (18.9) | 33 (31.7) | 0.037 |
| Valve repair, *n* (%) | 11 (12.1) | 12 (16.2) | 16 (15.4) | 0.716 |
| Other, *n* (%) | 8 (8.8) | 3 (4.1) | 13 (12.5) | 0.165 |
| **Microbiologic data** | | | | |
| MRSA, *n* (%) | 23 (25.3) | 20 (27.0) | 37 (35.6) | 0.286 |
| MSSA, *n* (%) | 16 (17.6) | 12 (16.2) | 27 (26.0) | 0.227 |
| MSSE, *n* (%) | 0 (0.0) | 0 (0.0) | 1 (1.0) | 0.458 |
| Other *Staphylococcus*, *n* (%) | 11 (12.1) | 12 (16.2) | 8 (7.7) | 0.197 |
| *Streptococcus*, *n* (%) | 24 (26.4) | 13 (17.6) | 17 (16.3) | 0.155 |
| *Enterococcus*, *n* (%) | 12 (13.2) | 15 (20.3) | 16 (15.4) | 0.460 |
| Gram-negative rods, *n* (%) | 10 (11.0) | 13 (17.6) | 15 (14.4) | 0.492 |
| *Rothia*, *n* (%) | 2 (2.2) | 2 (2.7) | 1 (1.0) | 0.659 |
| *Candida sp.*, *n* (%) | 1 (1.1) | 5 (6.8) | 9 (8.7) | 0.068 |
| Negative culture, *n* (%) | 4 (4.4) | 4 (5.4) | 2 (1.9) | 0.428 |

Abbreviations: ACEI (angiotensin-converting-enzyme inhibitor), AKI (acute kidney injury), ARB (angiotensin receptor blocker), BMI (body mass index), eGFR (estimated glomerular filtration rate), ICU (intensive care unit), IQ (interquartile), MRSA (methicillin-resistant *Staphylococcus aureus*), MSSA (methicillin-susceptible *Staphylococcus aureus*), MSSE (methicillin-susceptible *Staphylococcus epidermidis*), NSAID (nonsteroidal anti-inflammatory drug), Pip/Tazo (piperacillin/tazobactam), SD (standard deviation).

### *3.2. Clinical Parameters Associated with AKI*

When compared with patients without AKI, patients with AKI had higher Elixhauser comorbidity scores (median (IQ1-IQ3) 4.0 (3.0–6.0) for no AKI, 6.0 (4.0–7.0) for AKI stage 1 and 7.0 (5.0–8.0) for AKI stage ≥2, $p < 0.001$), more likely to have hepatitis B and C coinfection, sepsis, and tricuspid valve involvement (21.9% for no AKI, 24.7% for AKI stage 1 and 45.2% for AKI stage ≥2, $p < 0.001$), and required more frequently diuretics and vasopressor/inotrope support. Patients with AKI more frequently had valve replacement interventions (17.6% for no AKI, 18.9% for AKI stage 1 and 31.7% for AKI stage ≥2, $p = 0.037$) (Table 1). Patients with AKI were less likely to receive angiotensin converting enzyme inhibitors (ACEI) or angiotensin receptor blocker (ARB) (39.6% for no AKI, 16.2% for AKI stage 1 and 20.2% for AKI stage ≥2, $p < 0.001$). There was no difference among the IE causative organisms between patients with and without AKI (Table 1).

In multivariable analysis, higher Elixhauser comorbidity score, more frequent exposure to diuretics and non-steroidal anti-inflammatory drugs (NSAIDs), and less frequent exposure to an ACEI/ARB were independently associated with AKI. Further, requiring vasopressor/inotrope support and having tricuspid valve involvement independently associated with AKI stage ≥2 (adjusted OR of 4.94, 95% CI: 1.52–16.01, $p = 0.008$ and 2.97, 95% CI: 1.59–5.51, $p < 0.001$, respectively) (Table 2).

**Table 2.** Multivariable logistic regression models of AKI stage ≥1 and AKI stage ≥2 as the dependent variables and relevant clinical parameters as the independent variables.

| | AKI Stage ≥1 vs. No AKI | | AKI Stage ≥2 vs. AKI Stage 1 or No AKI | |
|---|---|---|---|---|
| | OR | 95% CI | OR | 95% CI |
| ACEI or ARB, Yes vs. No | 0.28 ** | 0.13–0.57 | 0.66 | 0.33–1.32 |
| Tricuspid valve affected, Yes vs. No | 1.71 | 0.84–3.46 | 2.97 ** | 1.59–5.51 |
| Use of diuretic, Yes Vs. No | 3.18 ** | 1.63–6.23 | 2.04 * | 1.04–4.01 |
| Hepatitis B coinfection, Yes vs. No | 6.57 | 0.78–55.16 | 0.61 | 0.19–1.97 |
| Use of NSAID, Yes vs. No | 1.95 * | 1.01–3.76 | 1.72 | 0.90–3.25 |
| Pressor or Inotrope need, Yes vs. No | - | - | 4.94 * | 1.52–16.01 |
| Diabetes, Yes vs. No | 0.47 | 0.21–1.06 | 0.55 | 0.26–1.19 |
| Elixhauser score, per 1-unit score | 1.35 ** | 1.16–1.56 | 1.35 ** | 1.17–1.55 |

Candidate variables for the multivariable models included age, baseline eGFR, hepatitis B or C coinfection, use of diuretic, use of ACEI or ARB, affection of the tricuspid valve, use of NSAID, need of pressor or inotrope, Elixhauser comorbidity score, history of diabetes, and zip code with the highest percentage of population below poverty level. C-statistic: 0.830, 0.788 for AKI stage ≥1 vs. no AKI and AKI stage ≥2 vs. AKI stage 1 or no AKI, respectively. * $p < 0.05$; ** $p < 0.01$. Abbreviations: ACEI (angiotensin-converting enzyme inhibitor), ARB (angiotensin-receptor blocker), NSAID (nonstereoidal anti-inflammatory drug).

### 3.3. Clinical Outcomes Associated with AKI

Patients with AKI stage ≥2 had slightly higher hospital mortality rates than those without AKI or AKI stage 1 (19.2% vs. 13.3%, $p = 0.194$). The frequency of MAKE50 was significantly higher in patients with AKI vs. those without AKI (38.5% for no AKI, 54.1% for AKI Stage 1, and 59.6% for AKI Stage ≥2, $p = 0.011$) (Table 3). Patients with AKI had also a slightly higher frequency of MAKE25 than those without AKI (71.9% vs. 60.4%, $p = 0.125$). There was no difference in hospital readmission rates due to IE according to AKI classification (Table 3).

**Table 3.** Study outcomes in hospitalized patients with infective endocarditis according to acute kidney injury status.

| | No AKI $n = 91$ | AKI Stage 1 $n = 74$ | AKI Stage ≥2 $n = 104$ | $p$ Value |
|---|---|---|---|---|
| **Clinical outcomes** | | | | |
| Hospital mortality, $n$ (%) | 14 (15.4) | 8 (10.8) | 20 (19.2) | 0.312 |
| Readmission due to IE, (%) | 4 (4.4) | 4 (5.4) | 3 (2.9) | 0.687 |
| MAKE50 *, $n$ (%) | 35 (38.5) | 40 (54.1) | 62 (59.6) | 0.011 |
| MAKE25 #, $n$ (%) | 55 (60.4) | 51 (68.9) | 77 (74.0) | 0.125 |
| **Healthcare cost outcomes** | | | | |
| Total direct hospitalization cost, dollars, median (IQ1-IQ3) | 17,069 (6722–31,910) | 37,111 (20,100–58,258) | 61,357 (34,164–88,495) | <0.001 |
| Hospital length of stay, days, median (IQ1-IQ3) | 9.0 (5.0–17.5) | 23.0 (12.0–43.8) | 34.5 (16.8–48.0) | <0.001 |
| Telemetry bed days, median (IQ1-IQ3) | 3.0 (0.0–10.0) | 8.0 (2.0–17.0) | 9.5 (1.0–20.0) | <0.001 |
| ICU length of stay, median (IQ1-IQ3) | 0.0 (0.0–2.0) | 1.5 (0.0–5.0) | 6.0 (1.5–14.5) | <0.001 |

* MAKE50 = Major Adverse Kidney Event, which includes mortality at or within 90 days of hospital discharge, continued RRT-dependence at 90 days after hospital discharge, or recovery of at least 50% of baseline eGFR within 90 days of discharge.# MAKE25 = Major Adverse Kidney Event, which includes mortality at or within 90 days of hospital discharge, continued RRT-dependence at 90 days after hospital discharge, or recovery of at least 25% of baseline eGFR within 90 days of discharge. Abbreviations: AKI (acute kidney injury), ICU (intensive care unit), IQ (interquartile range), MAKE (major adverse kidney event).

In multivariable analysis, the occurrence of sepsis as a complication of IE was independently associated with MAKE50 (adjusted OR 2.03, 95% CI: 1.23–3.36, $p = 0.006$). Further, AKI stage ≥2 had a borderline significant association with MAKE50 (adjusted OR 1.97, 95% CI: 1.09–3.58, $p = 0.126$) (Table 4).

**Table 4.** Multivariable logistic regression models of major adverse kidney events as the dependent variable and relevant clinical parameters as the independent variables.

| | MAKE50 | | MAKE25 | |
|---|---|---|---|---|
| | OR | 95% CI | OR | 95% CI |
| Sepsis, Yes vs. No | 2.03 ** | 1.23–3.36 | 1.56 | 0.91–2.66 |
| AKI Severity | | | | |
| Stage ≥2 vs. No AKI | 1.97 | 1.09–3.58 | 1.66 | 0.89–3.10 |
| Stage 1 vs. No AKI | 1.74 | 0.92–3.28 | 1.37 | 0.71–2.64 |

Candidate variables for the multivariable models included age, gender, history of hypertension, sepsis during indexed admission, affection of tricuspid valve, use of NSAID, use of ACEI or ARB, and AKI severity. C-statistic: 0.641, 0.590 for MAKE50 and MAKE25 respectively. ** $p < 0.01$. MAKE50 = Major Adverse Kidney Event, which includes mortality at or within 90 days of hospital discharge, continued RRT-dependence at 90 days after hospital discharge, or no recovery of at least 50% of baseline eGFR within 90 days of discharge. MAKE25 = Major Adverse Kidney Event, which includes mortality at or within 90 days of hospital discharge, continued RRT-dependence at 90 days after hospital discharge, or no recovery of at least 25% of baseline eGFR within 90 days of discharge. Abbreviations: AKI (acute kidney injury), KDIGO (kidney disease improving global outcomes), MAKE (major adverse kidney event).

### *3.4. Healthcare Costs Outcomes*

The median cost of hospitalization was $35,552. The median cost of hospitalization in the AKI group was three times higher than in the no AKI group ($52,654 (25,846–73,946) vs. 17,069 (6722–31,910), $p < 0.001$) and increased accordingly to AKI severity (Figure 2 and Table 3). Patients with AKI had a longer length of hospital stay (median (IQ1–IQ3) 9.0 (5.0–17.5) days for no AKI, 23.0 (12.0–43.8) for AKI stage 1 and 34.5 (16.8–48.0) for AKI stage ≥2, $p < 0.001$). Similarly, patients with AKI had a longer length of ICU stay and more days on telemetry beds when compared with those without AKI (Table 3).

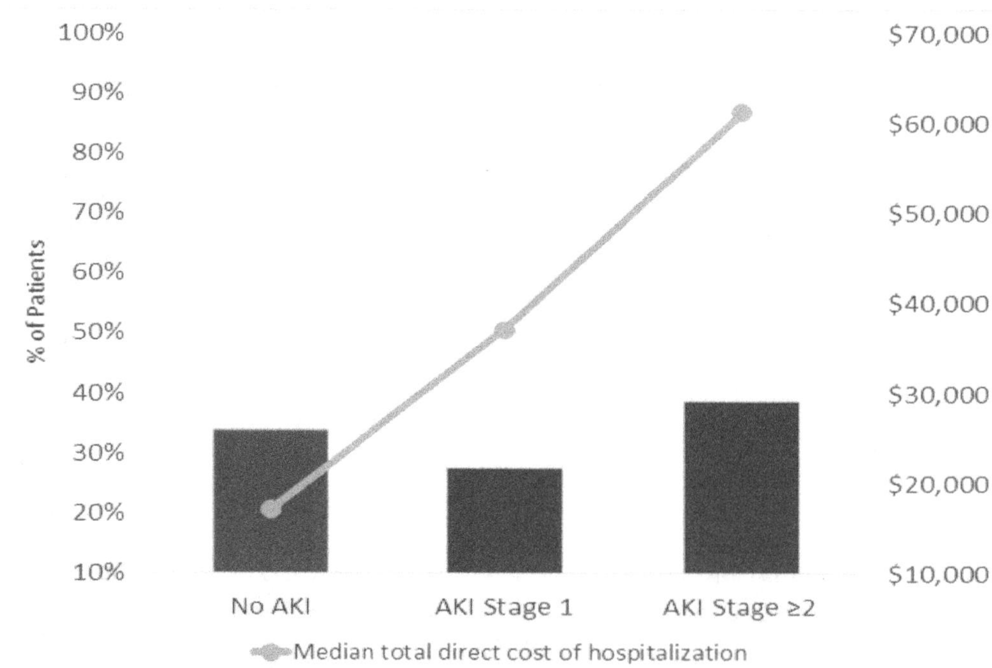


**Figure 2.** Incidence of acute kidney injury and median total hospitalization direct cost in hospitalized patients with a primary diagnosis of infective endocarditis.

## 4. Discussion

The main finding of our study is the high incidence of AKI in a large cohort of hospitalized patients with IE. About 2 out of 3 patients (66.2%) suffered from an episode of AKI while in the hospital, which translated into higher resource utilization and healthcare costs. The median cost of hospitalization was 3.6 times higher in patients with severe AKI (stage ≥2) vs. those without AKI. We also found that tricuspid valve involvement, the need for vasopressor/inotrope support and diuretics, and a higher level of comorbidity were associated with severe AKI (stage ≥2).

Other studies have also reported the incidence of AKI in patients with IE. Ritchie et al., [18] studied a cohort of 211 patients diagnosed with bacterial endocarditis at the Brigham and Women's Hospital between January 2009 and October 2013. They reported a lower incidence of AKI of 38.9% (only 15.2% of patients in their cohort had substance use disorder vs. 53.2% in our cohort). In contrast, our study used the KDIGO SCr-criteria to define AKI, while they used the Acute Kidney Injury Network's (AKIN) SCr and urine output criteria [26]. Furthermore, in our cohort, patients had overall higher comorbidity scores in comparison to the referred study. In addition, Boils et al., [16] reported a biopsy-based pathologic series of 49 patients who had kidney function impairment in the setting of IE. The most common presentation of kidney disease in this population was AKI (79% of the cases) and the most common kidney biopsy findings were necrotizing and crescentic glomerulonephritis (53%) and endocapillary proliferative glomerulonephritis (37%). In addition, acute tubular injury was present in 86% of the cases.

Patients with severe AKI (stage ≥2) had slightly higher hospital mortality rates than those without AKI or AKI stage 1. Further, patients with severe AKI (stage ≥2) had significantly higher rates of major adverse kidney events than patients without AKI. Emerging evidence suggests that not only those patients with clinical evidence of AKI but also approximately 20% of patients that do not meet SCr-criteria of AKI still have increased risk of developing acute kidney disease (persistent alterations in kidney function or structure within the next 3 months following an episode of AKI), which is associated with incident or progression of CKD, ESKD, and death [27,28]. It is possible that some patients in the no AKI group may have had subclinical AKI [29] not detected by SCr changes precluding a more pronounced differentiation in clinical outcomes among those with vs. without AKI. In addition, the observed absence of mortality differentiation according to incident AKI or AKI severity stages may be due to the low event rate and lack of power. Overall rates of hospital mortality in patients with IE reported in other studies range between 18% and 24% [30–32], similar to the hospital mortality rate reported in our study (15.6%). Further, Wallace et al., [32] studied a cohort of 208 patients with IE and reported that mortality at discharge was 18% and at 6 months post-discharge was 27%, demonstrating that after discharge these patients are still at high risk of death.

Our study showed that higher comorbidity scores, exposure to NSAIDs, and the need for diuretics were associated with AKI. Diuretics are commonly used in patients with AKI since fluid overload is one of the major complications of decreased kidney function, and diuretics are also used for risk-stratification of AKI progression (furosemide stress test) [33]. Therefore, the association of diuretic use with AKI may be a reflection of more severe forms of AKI (e.g., oliguric/anuric AKI) and not necessarily thought to be contributory to the development or progression of AKI. Few studies have reported clinical parameters associated with AKI in the setting of IE. In multivariable analysis, Ritchie et al., [18] identified independent clinical parameters associated with AKI such as CKD, treatment with nafcillin or oxacillin, treatment with aminoglycoside and vancomycin, and similarly to our study, need of or exposure to loop diuretics. In contrast, we did not find major differences in relation to antibiotic exposure in those with vs. without AKI.

Our study also found that patients with severe AKI (stage ≥2) were more likely to have tricuspid valve involvement and required vasopressor/inotrope support more frequently than patients without AKI. Right-side IE (RSIE) occurs more commonly in persons with substance use disorder, especially persons who inject drugs [34]. In our cohort, patients with tricuspid valve affection (vs. other valves) had more substance use disorder, hepatitis C coinfection and sepsis (74.1% vs. 44.3%; 61.2% vs. 35%; 70.6% vs. 40.4%, respectively, $p < 0.001$ for all), which may have influenced the higher frequency of severe AKI. Lemaire et al., [35] studied 6264 patients with IE who underwent valvular surgery, 809 (12.9%) with a diagnosis of substance use disorder. They found that patients with a substance use disorder were more likely to have post-operative complications, especially infectious complications such as pneumonia (OR 1.4, 95% CI 1.14–1.74), sepsis (OR 1.4, 95% CI 1.16–1.63), and renal complications (OR 1.5, 95% CI 1.23–1.77), defined based on ICD-9-CM diagnosis codes.

We also found that healthcare resource utilization and costs were higher in IE patients with AKI vs. those without AKI. In a different cohort study of 25,495 hospitalized patients who had AKI, Collister et al., reported that AKI was associated with longer length of hospital stay and increased hospital total cost [36]. They also found that incident AKI Stage 1 and 2 resulted in 1.2–1.3 times higher hospital total cost than no AKI while AKI Stage 3 and the need of dialysis were associated with 1.8–2.5 times higher cost. Fleischauer et al., [6] gathered data from 128 hospitals in North Carolina ($n$ = 505 patients) and reported healthcare costs related to IE. They found that hospital admissions for drug dependence-associated IE increased twelve-fold from 2010 to 2015 (0.2 to 2.7 cases per 100,000 persons per year). Similarly, the total cost of hospitalization of IE patients increased eighteen-fold in the same period of time (from 1.1 to ~22.2 million). The major limitation of this study is that they only included hospitalizations with drug dependence-related IE listed as an ICD-9/10 CM diagnosis.

Our study has limitations. First, our study is a retrospective, single-center, cohort study of relatively small sample size and therefore the results may not be generalizable to other populations, particularly those with a low prevalence of substance use disorder or more diverse racial backgrounds (>90% of our study population was white). Second, we did not use urine output criteria as part of the AKI definition or examined the clinical etiology of AKI due to lack of data availability. Third, the time point at which antibiotics or other drugs were administered during the course of AKI was not characterized. Therefore, exposure to these drugs may have occurred before, during or after AKI, which can introduce confounding by indication to the interpretation of the results (e.g., more or less exposure in the context of clinically evident AKI rather than a drug-related attributable risk for the AKI event).

Our study has several strengths. First, we examined a large cohort of hospitalized patients with a primary diagnosis of IE compared to other studies examining AKI in the setting of IE [16,18]. Second, we examined distinct clinical parameters (patient-specific, IE-specific and medication exposure) associated with AKI as well as resource utilization and healthcare cost associated with the occurrence of AKI. Our study therefore further contributes to identifying patients with IE at high risk of AKI. Third, our cohort is unique in that is from an area with a high prevalence of opioid use disorder. Finally, our study highlights the need to identify clinical parameters that may inform risk-stratification of AKI and adverse outcomes in this susceptible population.

## 5. Conclusions

Two out of three patients admitted to the hospital with a primary diagnosis of IE had AKI. A higher level of comorbidity was independently associated with AKI. Patients with AKI more frequently received diuretics and patients with severe AKI (stage ≥2) more frequently required pressor/inotrope support. The affection of the tricuspid valve was independently associated with severe AKI (stage ≥2). Patients with severe AKI (stage ≥2) had more frequently major adverse kidney events up to 90 days post-discharge. Further, resource utilization and healthcare cost were significantly higher in patients with AKI vs. those without AKI. Future studies should aim to develop risk-stratification tools for AKI and adverse outcomes in hospitalized patients with IE and therefore guide preventive strategies that ameliorate the burden of complications in this susceptible population.

**Author Contributions:** V.O.-S.: Project design, manuscript writing, revision and submission; K.D.: Project design, manuscript revision; G.D.: Statistical analysis, manuscript revision; Y.L.: Statistical analysis, manuscript revision; J.L.: Statistical analysis, manuscript revision; M.R.: Data gathering and validation, manuscript revision; D.C.: Data gathering, data extraction and validation, manuscript revision; A.T.: Project design, manuscript revision; L.C.F.: Project design, regulatory procedures, manuscript revision; M.A.H.: Project design, manuscript revision; J.A.N.: Project and analysis design and supervision, manuscript writing and revision.

**Acknowledgments:** Neyra is currently supported by an Early Career Pilot Grant from the National Center for Advancing Translational Sciences (NCATS), National Institutes of Health (NIH), through Grant UL1 TR001998. Huaman is currently supported by NCATS, NIH through grant KL2 TR001426.

## References


1. Murdoch, D.R.; Corey, G.R.; Hoen, B.; Miro, J.M.; Fowler, V.G., Jr.; Bayer, A.S.; Karchmer, A.W.; Olaison, L.; Pappas, P.A.; Moreillon, P.; et al. Clinical presentation, etiology, and outcome of infective endocarditis in the 21st century: The International Collaboration on Endocarditis-Prospective Cohort Study. *Arch. Intern. Med.* **2009**, *169*, 463–473. [CrossRef] [PubMed]
2. Thuny, F.; Grisoli, D.; Cautela, J.; Riberi, A.; Raoult, D.; Habib, G. Infective endocarditis: Prevention, diagnosis, and management. *Can. J. Cardiol.* **2014**, *30*, 1046–1057. [CrossRef] [PubMed]
3. Baddour, L.M.; Wilson, W.R.; Bayer, A.S.; Fowler, V.G., Jr.; Bolger, A.F.; Levison, M.E.; Ferrieri, P.; Gerber, M.A.; Tani, L.Y.; Gewitz, M.H.; et al. Infective endocarditis: Diagnosis, antimicrobial therapy, and management of complications: A statement for healthcare professionals from the Committee on Rheumatic Fever, Endocarditis, and Kawasaki Disease, Council on Cardiovascular Disease in the Young, and the Councils on Clinical Cardiology, Stroke, and Cardiovascular Surgery and Anesthesia, American Heart Association: Endorsed by the Infectious Diseases Society of America. *Circulation* **2005**, *111*, e394–e434. [CrossRef] [PubMed]
4. Pant, S.; Patel, N.J.; Deshmukh, A.; Golwala, H.; Patel, N.; Badheka, A.; Hirsch, G.A.; Mehta, J.L. Trends in infective endocarditis incidence, microbiology, and valve replacement in the United States from 2000 to 2011. *J. Am. Coll. Cardiol.* **2015**, *65*, 2070–2076. [CrossRef] [PubMed]
5. Toyoda, N.; Chikwe, J.; Itagaki, S.; Gelijns, A.C.; Adams, D.H.; Egorova, N.N. Trends in Infective Endocarditis in California and New York State, 1998–2013. *JAMA* **2017**, *317*, 1652–1660. [CrossRef] [PubMed]
6. Fleischauer, A.T.; Ruhl, L.; Rhea, S.; Barnes, E. Hospitalizations for Endocarditis and Associated Health Care Costs Among Persons with Diagnosed Drug Dependence—North Carolina, 2010–2015. *MMWR Morb. Mortal. Wkly. Rep.* **2017**, *66*, 569–573. [CrossRef]
7. Vivolo-Kantor, A.M.; Seth, P.; Gladden, R.M.; Mattson, C.L.; Baldwin, G.T.; Kite-Powell, A.; Coletta, M.A. Vital Signs: Trends in Emergency Department Visits for Suspected Opioid Overdoses—United States, July 2016–September 2017. *MMWR Morb. Mortal. Wkly. Rep.* **2018**, *67*, 279–285. [CrossRef]
8. Jones, C.M. Heroin use and heroin use risk behaviors among nonmedical users of prescription opioid pain relievers—United States, 2002–2004 and 2008–2010. *Drug Alcohol Depend.* **2013**, *132*, 95–100. [CrossRef]
9. Scheidegger, C.; Zimmerli, W. Incidence and spectrum of severe medical complications among hospitalized HIV-seronegative and HIV-seropositive narcotic drug users. *AIDS* **1996**, *10*, 1407–1414. [CrossRef]
10. Susantitaphong, P.; Cruz, D.N.; Cerda, J.; Abulfaraj, M.; Alqahtani, F.; Koulouridis, I.; Jaber, B.L. World incidence of AKI: A meta-analysis. *Clin. J. Am. Soc. Nephrol.* **2013**, *8*, 1482–1493. [CrossRef]
11. Szczech, L.A.; Harmon, W.; Hostetter, T.H.; Klotman, P.E.; Powe, N.R.; Sedor, J.R.; Smedberg, P.; Himmelfarb, J. World Kidney Day 2009: Problems and challenges in the emerging epidemic of kidney disease. *J. Am. Soc. Nephrol.* **2009**, *20*, 453–455. [CrossRef] [PubMed]
12. Silver, S.A.; Long, J.; Zheng, Y.; Chertow, G.M. Cost of Acute Kidney Injury in Hospitalized Patients. *J. Hosp. Med.* **2017**, *12*, 70–76. [CrossRef] [PubMed]
13. Rewa, O.; Bagshaw, S.M. Acute kidney injury—Epidemiology, outcomes and economics. *Nat. Rev. Nephrol.* **2014**, *10*, 193–207. [CrossRef] [PubMed]
14. Neugarten, J.; Gallo, G.R.; Baldwin, D.S. Glomerulonephritis in bacterial endocarditis. *Am. J. Kidney. Dis.* **1984**, *3*, 371–379. [CrossRef]
15. Majumdar, A.; Chowdhary, S.; Ferreira, M.A.; Hammond, L.A.; Howie, A.J.; Lipkin, G.W.; Littler, W.A. Renal pathological findings in infective endocarditis. *Nephrol. Dial. Transplant.* **2000**, *15*, 1782–1787. [CrossRef]
16. Boils, C.L.; Nasr, S.H.; Walker, P.D.; Couser, W.G.; Larsen, C.P. Update on endocarditis-associated glomerulonephritis. *Kidney Int.* **2015**, *87*, 1241–1249. [CrossRef]
17. Conlon, P.J.; Jefferies, F.; Krigman, H.R.; Corey, G.R.; Sexton, D.J.; Abramson, M.A. Predictors of prognosis and risk of acute renal failure in bacterial endocarditis. *Clin. Nephrol.* **1998**, *49*, 96–101.
18. Ritchie, B.M.; Hirning, B.A.; Stevens, C.A.; Cohen, S.A.; DeGrado, J.R. Risk factors for acute kidney injury associated with the treatment of bacterial endocarditis at a tertiary academic medical center. *J. Chemother.* **2017**, *29*, 292–298. [CrossRef]
19. Elixhauser, A.; Steiner, C.; Harris, D.R.; Coffey, R.M. Comorbidity measures for use with administrative data. *Med. Care* **1998**, *36*, 8–27. [CrossRef]
20. Durack, D.T.; Lukes, A.S.; Bright, D.K. New criteria for diagnosis of infective endocarditis: Utilization of

specific echocardiographic findings. Duke Endocarditis Service. *Am. J. Med.* **1994**, *96*, 200–209. [CrossRef]

21. Levey, A.S.; Stevens, L.A.; Schmid, C.H.; Zhang, Y.L.; Castro, A.F., 3rd; Feldman, H.I.; Kusek, J.W.; Eggers, P.; Van Lente, F.; Greene, T.; et al. A new equation to estimate glomerular filtration rate. *Ann. Intern. Med.* **2009**, *150*, 604–612. [CrossRef] [PubMed]
22. Keslin, M.H.; Messner, R.P.; Williams, R.C., Jr. Glomerulonephritis with subacute bacterial endocarditis. Immunofluorescent studies. *Arch. Intern. Med.* **1973**, *132*, 578–581. [CrossRef] [PubMed]
23. Kellum, J.A.; Zarbock, A.; Nadim, M.K. What endpoints should be used for clinical studies in acute kidney injury? *Intensive Care Med.* **2017**, *43*, 901–903. [CrossRef] [PubMed]
24. Leaf, D.E.; Jacob, K.A.; Srivastava, A.; Chen, M.E.; Christov, M.; Juppner, H.; Sabbisetti, V.S.; Martin, A.; Wolf, M.; Waikar, S.S. Fibroblast Growth Factor 23 Levels Associate with AKI and Death in Critical Illness. *J. Am. Soc. Nephrol.* **2017**, *28*, 1877–1885. [CrossRef] [PubMed]
25. Rubenfeld, G.D.; Angus, D.C.; Pinsky, M.R.; Curtis, J.R.; Connors, A.F., Jr.; Bernard, G.R. Outcomes research in critical care: Results of the American Thoracic Society Critical Care Assembly Workshop on Outcomes Research. The Members of the Outcomes Research Workshop. *Am. J. Resp. Crit. Care.* **1999**, *160*, 358–367. [CrossRef] [PubMed]
26. Mehta, R.L.; Kellum, J.A.; Shah, S.V.; Molitoris, B.A.; Ronco, C.; Warnock, D.G.; Levin, A. Acute Kidney Injury Network: Report of an initiative to improve outcomes in acute kidney injury. *Crit. Care* **2007**, *11*, R31. [CrossRef] [PubMed]
27. James, M.T.; Levey, A.S.; Tonelli, M.; Tan, Z.; Barry, R.; Pannu, N.; Ravani, P.; Klarenbach, S.W.; Manns, B.J.; Hemmelgarn, B.R. Incidence and Prognosis of Acute Kidney Diseases and Disorders Using an Integrated Approach to Laboratory Measurements in a Universal Health Care. *JAMA Netw. Open* **2019**, *2*, e191795. [CrossRef] [PubMed]
28. Haase, M.; Kellum, J.A.; Ronco, C. Subclinical AKI—An emerging syndrome with important consequences. *Nat. Rev. Nephrol.* **2012**, *8*, 735–739. [CrossRef]
29. Ronco, C.; Kellum, J.A.; Haase, M. Subclinical AKI is still AKI. *Crit. Care* **2012**, *16*, 313. [CrossRef]
30. Cresti, A.; Chiavarelli, M.; Scalese, M.; Nencioni, C.; Valentini, S.; Guerrini, F.; D'Aiello, I.; Picchi, A.; De Sensi, F.; Habib, G. Epidemiological and mortality trends in infective endocarditis, a 17-year population-based prospective study. *Cardiovasc. Diagn. Ther.* **2017**, *7*, 27–35. [CrossRef]
31. Alkhawam, H.; Sogomonian, R.; Zaiem, F.; Vyas, N.; El-Hunjul, M.; Jolly, J.; Al-Khazraji, A.; Ashraf, A. Morbidity and mortality of infective endocarditis in a hospital system in New York City serving a diverse urban population. *J. Invest. Med.* **2016**, *64*, 1118–1123. [CrossRef] [PubMed]
32. Wallace, S.M.; Walton, B.I.; Kharbanda, R.K.; Hardy, R.; Wilson, A.P.; Swanton, R.H. Mortality from infective endocarditis: Clinical predictors of outcome. *Heart* **2002**, *88*, 53–60. [CrossRef]
33. Koyner, J.L.; Davison, D.L.; Brasha-Mitchell, E.; Chalikonda, D.M.; Arthur, J.M.; Shaw, A.D.; Tumlin, J.A.; Trevino, S.A.; Bennett, M.R.; Kimmel, P.L.; et al. Furosemide Stress Test and Biomarkers for the Prediction of AKI Severity. *J. Am. Soc. Nephrol.* **2015**, *26*, 2023–2031. [CrossRef] [PubMed]
34. Hussain, S.T.; Witten, J.; Shrestha, N.K.; Blackstone, E.H.; Pettersson, G.B. Tricuspid valve endocarditis. *Ann. Cardiothorac. Surg.* **2017**, *6*, 255–261. [CrossRef] [PubMed]
35. Lemaire, A.; Dombrovskiy, V.; Saadat, S.; Batsides, G.; Ghaly, A.; Spotnitz, A.; Lee, L.Y. Patients with Infectious Endocarditis and Drug Dependence Have Worse Clinical Outcomes after Valvular Surgery. *Surg. Infect.* **2017**, *18*, 299–302. [CrossRef] [PubMed]
36. Collister, D.; Pannu, N.; Ye, F.; James, M.; Hemmelgarn, B.; Chui, B.; Manns, B.; Klarenbach, S.; Alberta Kidney Disease Network. Health Care Costs Associated with AKI. *Clin. J. Am. Soc. Nephrol.* **2017**, *12*, 1733–1743. [CrossRef]

# 14

# Secretory Leukocyte Protease Inhibitor (SLPI)—A Novel Predictive Biomarker of Acute Kidney Injury after Cardiac Surgery

**Luisa Averdunk [1,2], Christina Fitzner [1], Tatjana Levkovich [1], David E. Leaf [3,4], Michael Sobotta [1], Jil Vieten [1], Akinobu Ochi [5], Gilbert Moeckel [5], Gernot Marx [1] and Christian Stoppe [1,*]**

1 Department of Intensive Care Medicine, RWTH Aachen University Hospital, 52074 Aachen, Germany; luisa.aver@gmail.com (L.A.); cfitzner@ukaachen.de (C.F.); tlevkovich@ukaachen.de (T.L.); msobotta@ukaachen.de (M.S.); jil.vieten@rwth-aachen.de (J.V.); gmarx@ukaachen.de (G.M.)
2 Institute of Human Genetics, Medical Faculty, Heinrich Heine University, 40225 Düsseldorf, Germany
3 Division of Renal Medicine, Brigham and Women's Hospital, Boston, MA 02115, USA; deleaf@bwh.harvard.edu
4 Department of Medicine, Harvard Medical School, Boston, MA 02115, USA
5 Department of Nephropathology, Yale University School of Medicine, New Haven, CT 06510, USA; akiaki5733@med.osaka-cu.ac.jp (A.O.); gilbert.moeckel@yale.edu (G.M.)
* Correspondence: christian.stoppe@gmail.com

**Abstract:** Acute kidney injury (AKI) is one of the most frequent complications after cardiac surgery and is associated with poor outcomes. Biomarkers of AKI are crucial for the early diagnosis of this condition. Secretory leukocyte protease inhibitor (SLPI) is an alarm anti-protease that has been implicated in the pathogenesis of AKI but has not yet been studied as a diagnostic biomarker of AKI. Using two independent cohorts (development cohort (DC), $n = 60$; validation cohort (VC), $n = 148$), we investigated the performance of SLPI as a diagnostic marker of AKI after cardiac surgery. Serum and urinary levels of SLPI were quantified by ELISA. SLPI was significantly elevated in AKI patients compared with non-AKI patients (6 h, DC: 102.1 vs. 64.9 ng/mL, $p < 0.001$). The area under the receiver operating characteristic curve of serum SLPI 6 h after surgery was 0.87 ((0.76–0.97); DC). The addition of SLPI to standard clinical predictors significantly improved the predictive accuracy of AKI (24 h, VC: odds ratio (OR) = 3.91 (1.44–12.13)). In a subgroup, the increase in serum SLPI was evident before AKI was diagnosed on the basis of serum creatinine or urine output (24 h, VC: OR = 4.89 (1.54–19.92)). In this study, SLPI was identified as a novel candidate biomarker for the early diagnosis of AKI after cardiac surgery.

**Keywords:** acute kidney injury; cardiovascular surgery; ICU; complications; biomarkers

## 1. Introduction

Acute kidney injury (AKI) is one of the most common complications after major surgery, especially after cardiac surgery [1,2]. Despite substantial improvement in intraoperative management and perioperative care, the incidence of AKI in patients in the intensive care unit (ICU) remains high and ranges between 20% and 67% [3]. AKI necessitates a prolonged ICU stay and is an important prognostic factor of poor mid- to long-term outcomes: it is associated with increased postoperative infections and cardiovascular complications, as well as markedly increased morbidity and mortality rates, even years after surgery [4–8]. Although distinct consensus criteria for the early detection of AKI have been defined by the Kidney Disease Improving Global Outcomes (KDIGO) clinical practice guidelines, AKI continues to be underdiagnosed [9]. To date, the treatment options for AKI are limited, and renal replacement therapy is the standard approach to treating severe cases of AKI. The early identification of patients at risk could enable the timely initiation of preventive measures to reduce the sequelae of AKI [10]. In this context, the currently established and routinely used AKI indicators, such as serum creatinine and urine output, have been repeatedly demonstrated to be insufficient for the early detection of AKI because changes in serum creatinine indicative of altered kidney function are evident only after more than 50% of the baseline renal function has been compromised [11]. Moreover, serum creatinine only serves as a surrogate parameter to estimate the excretory function of the kidney. Thus, serum creatinine does not provide information about the underlying renal pathology and is unable to discriminate between reversible and irreversible injuries [12]. For a better approximation of the extent of injury and the early diagnosis, differential diagnosis, and prognosis of AKI, the international KDIGO board has called for the identification of appropriate AKI markers, analogous to serum troponin or liver enzymes used to identify organ injury [13].

Accordingly, studies have investigated several new biomarkers of AKI, and urinary tissue inhibitor of metalloproteinase-2 (TIMP-2) and insulin-like growth factor-binding protein 7 (IGFBP7) ([TIMP-2]·[IGFBP7]) have been deemed promising markers [14]. The assessment of whole-genome mRNA profiles in human kidney biopsies from post-transplant AKI revealed that the most upregulated mRNA (15-fold) was that of secretory leukocyte protease inhibitor (SLPI) [15]. Despite these promising findings, to date, observational studies have not been conducted to evaluate circulating concentrations of SLPI as a biomarker of AKI. Therefore, in a cardiac surgery setting, we tested the predictive value of SLPI as a novel AKI biomarker in two independent prospective observational studies: one development cohort and one validation cohort.

## 2. Materials and Methods

### 2.1. Study Design and Patients

The aim of the study was to investigate the association between serum SLPI levels and the incidence of postoperative AKI after cardiac surgery. The studies, registered at clinicaltrials.gov (NCT 02488876, April 2009), were approved by the institutional review board (Ethics committee, RWTH Aachen University, Aachen, Germany) and performed in adherence to the Declaration of Helsinki. All patients were scheduled for elective cardiac surgery involving aortic cross-clamping, cardioplegic myocardial arrest, and cardiopulmonary bypass. Exclusion criteria were emergency operations, pregnancy, lack of informed consent, an age of less than 18 years, and end-stage renal disease requiring dialysis.

First, an explorative development study was conducted between September 2015 and March 2016. Second, the results of the development study were used as the basis for a prospective observational validation study, which was conducted from January to June 2017.

Serum creatinine was measured daily. The serum creatinine level on the day before cardiac surgery was used as the reference value. Urine output was quantified hourly by Foley catheter drainage while the patient remained in the intensive care unit.

In both the development and validation studies, serum samples for enzyme-linked immunosorbent assays (ELISA) were drawn one day prior to surgery and immediately (0 h) and 24 h after surgery. In the development study, additional samples were drawn 6 and 12 h after surgery, and, in the validation study, an additional sample was collected 48 h after surgery (Figure 1B).

After blood collection, the samples were centrifuged (3000 rpm for 10 min), and the supernatants were transferred to cryotubes for storage at −80 °C until further analysis. Urine samples were collected preoperatively, immediately postoperatively, and 24 h after surgery and transferred to cryotubes for storage at −80 °C.

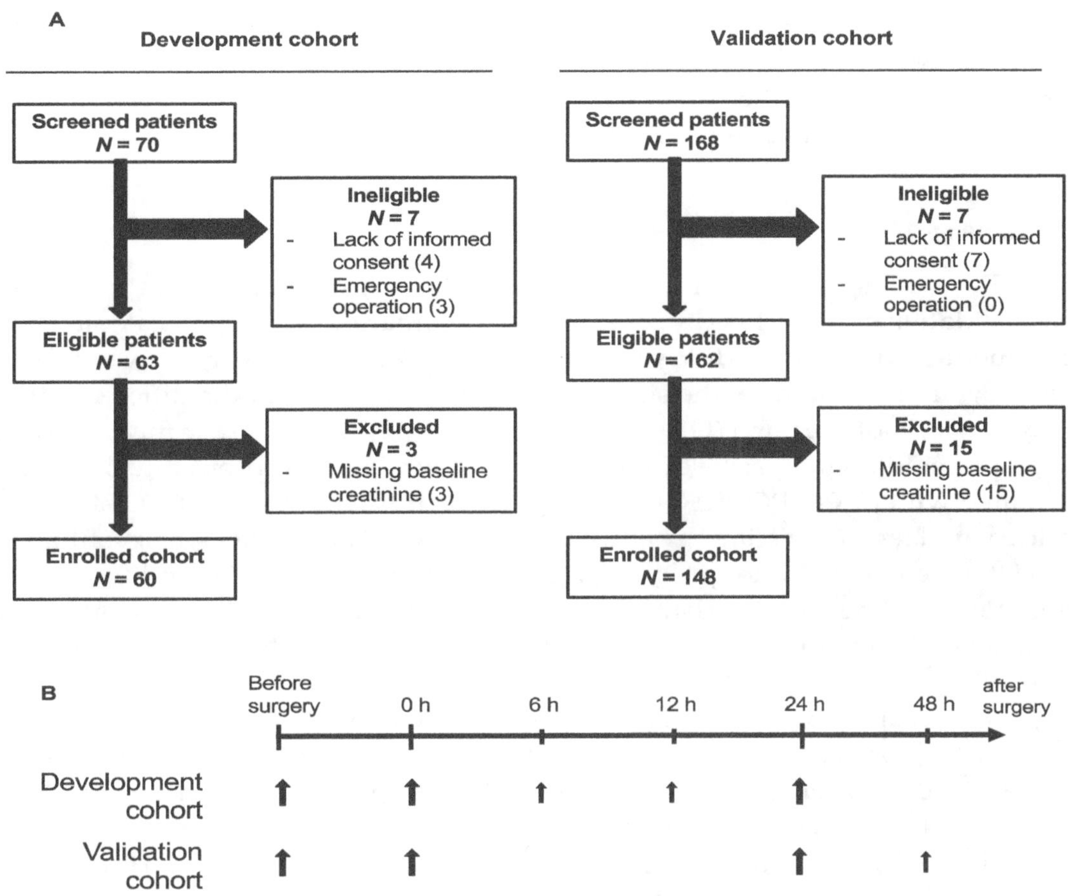


**Figure 1.** (**A**) Flowcharts of the two independent observational studies investigating SLPI as a biomarker of AKI after cardiac surgery. (**B**) The time points of sample collection for analysis. Larger arrows represent the collection of blood and urine, and smaller arrows represent the collection of blood only. SLPI, secretory leukocyte protease inhibitor; AKI, acute kidney injury.

### 2.2. Study Endpoints

The primary endpoint of both studies was the development of AKI within 72 h after cardiac surgery. AKI was diagnosed according to the KDIGO clinical practice guidelines by (1) an increase in serum creatinine of at least 0.3 mg/dL or a 50% increase from baseline and/or (2) a decline in urine output to below 0.5 mL/kg/h for at least 6 h [16].

The following patients' baseline characteristics are known to affect the risk of AKI and were thus determined: age, sex, body mass index (BMI), intake of heart medication, arterial hypertension, pulmonary hypertension, congestive heart disease, reduced left ventricular ejection fraction (LVEF) <35%, chronic kidney disease, chronic obstructive pulmonary disease (COPD), diabetes, and previous cardiac surgery. On the basis of these data, we calculated the Cleveland Clinic Foundation Score—a clinical score used to estimate the risk of developing AKI after cardiac surgery [17]. We recorded the operational characteristics, including the type and duration of surgery, and the postoperative Sequential Organ Failure Score (SOFA) on the first day after surgery (POD1).

### 2.3. Biomarkers

Serum and urine levels of SLPI were measured by ELISA as previously described and according to the manufacturer's instructions (R&D Systems, Minneapolis, MN, USA) [18]. For the urine samples taken from patients in the development study, we additionally quantified urine neutrophil gelatinase-associated lipocalin (NGAL)—a previously described biomarker of AKI—using a commercially available ELISA kit (R&D Systems, Minneapolis, MN, USA) [19,20]. Before analysis, the serum samples were diluted 1:200 for SLPI ELISA, and urine samples were diluted 1:10 for SLPI ELISA and 1:100 for NGAL ELISA. In a subgroup of 25 patients (the first 25 patients of the validation cohort), we normalized SLPI to the creatinine concentration in the urine. The average coefficient of variation (CV) between duplicates was 9.7% (intra-assay CV) and the average inter-assay cooefficient was 11.9%.

### 2.4. Statistical Methods

Because SLPI serum levels ranged widely in the first study (development study), we performed an additional validation study. The sample size of the validation study was calculated on the basis of the development study. The median of the SLPI levels 24 h after surgery was used as a cut-off. We assumed a power of 90% and set the significance level to 0.05. From the difference in proportions of the "AKI events" in both groups (G1 (≤median SLPI) = 10.7% and G2 (>median SLPI) = 34.5%), we calculated a preferable sample size of 168 patients, assuming a drop-out rate of 25%. The sample size was calculated with PROC POWER, SAS 9.4 (SAS Institute Inc., Cary, NC, USA).

Categorical variables are described by absolute numbers and percentages, and continuous variables are reported as the median and interquartile range (IQR) with the first (Q1) and third (Q3) quartiles.

Differences in baseline characteristics between the two outcome groups were analyzed using univariable logistic regression. Correlations between SLPI and NGAL were calculated using Spearman's correlation.

The diagnostic accuracy of the biomarkers was calculated by the receiver operating characteristic (ROC) curve and the corresponding area under the curve (AUC). $p$-values were calculated for a hypothesis of AUC > 0.5. Optimal cut-offs were calculated using the Youden index, and 95% confidence intervals, sensitivities, and specificities are reported.

A univariable logistic regression model was used to investigate the performance of SLPI as a predictor of AKI. Given a nonlinear relationship between SLPI and the incidence of AKI, SLPI was considered a binary variable and categorized by the corresponding median to avoid biased estimates [21].

Using multivariable logistic regression models, we adjusted SLPI for the Cleveland Clinic Foundation Score (including sex, congestive heart disease, left ventricular ejection fraction, use of intra-aortic balloon-pump, chronic obstructive pulmonary disease, insulin-requiring diabetes, previous heart surgery, emergency surgery, type of surgery, and preoperative creatinine level) [17]. We applied Firths' bias reduction implemented in SAS-Macro %fl (SAS Institute Inc., Cary, NC, USA); the odds ratios (OR) with 95% confidence intervals (CI) and $P$-values are reported. To evaluate whether serum SLPI is able to predict AKI before an increase in serum creatinine is evident, we analyzed the time point at which a rise in serum creatinine was detected [22]. Then, in a subgroup analysis, we only considered the patients who received an AKI diagnosis after the time point of SLPI measurement. For example, when analyzing serum SLPI 24 h after surgery, all patients whose serum creatinine had already increased at 24 h after surgery or later were excluded.

In all cases, two-sided testing was used, and $p$ <0.05 was considered statistically significant. If not otherwise stated, statistical analyses were performed using SAS Software, version 9.4 (SAS Institute Inc., Cary, NC, USA) and SPSS 25 (IBM SPSS Statistics for Windows, version 21.0. IBM Corp., Armonk, NY, USA).

## 3. Results

### 3.1. Baseline Characteristics and Outcomes of Patients

Of the 70 cardiac surgery patients initially screened for the development study, 60 patients were successfully enrolled. For the validation study, 148 of the 168 screened patients were enrolled (Figure 1A). The incidence of AKI during the first 72 h after cardiac surgery was 25% in the development cohort (DC; 14 of 60 patients) and 15% in the validation cohort (VC; 22 of 148 patients) (Table 1).

In both cohorts and for all cases, the diagnostic criterion "increased creatine" was met before oliguria occurred. Oliguria was detected in 21% of AKI cases in the DC and in 23% of AKI cases in the VC (Table 1). In most cases, AKI was diagnosed 48 h after surgery (DC, 50% of cases; VC, 41% of cases) (Table 1). In both cohorts, the overall proportion of AKI patients affected by persistent AKI (>48 h) was approximately 40% (Table 1).

**Table 1.** Incidence, diagnostic criteria, and time point of diagnosis of AKI by cohort. Categorical data are presented as the absolute number and percentage. Diagnosis of AKI was based on Kidney Disease Improving Global Outcomes (KDIGO) clinical practice guidelines ((1) an increase in serum creatinine of at least 0.3 mg/dL or an increase of 50% above baseline and/or (2) a decline in urine output to below 0.5 mL/kg/h for at least 6 h) [16]. Most patients diagnosed with AKI were affected by AKI stage 1 and were diagnosed 48 h after surgery. All patients suffering from AKI showed an increase in serum creatinine. Approximately 40% of AKI patients had persistent AKI lasting >48 h. AKI, acute kidney injury.

| Acute Kidney Injury within 72 h after Cardiac Surgery | Development Cohort ($n$ = 60) | | Persistent AKI > 48 h | Validation Cohort ($n$ = 148) | | Persistent AKI > 48 h |
|---|---|---|---|---|---|---|
| AKI according to KDIGO diagnostic criteria | 14 | (25%) | 6 (43%) | 22 | (15%) | 9 (41%) |
| KDIGO Stage 1 | 8 | (57%) | | 12 | (54%) | |
| KDIGO Stage 2 | 5 | (36%) | | 8 | (36%) | |
| KDIGO Stage 3 | 1 | (7%) | | 2 | (9%) | |
| Diagnostic criteria met | | | | | | |
| Increased creatinine | 14 | (100%) | | 22 | (100%) | |
| Oliguria (<0.5 mL/kg/h for ≥6 h) | 3 | (21%) | | 5 | (23%) | |
| Time point of diagnosis | | | | | | |
| 24 h after surgery | 3 | (21%) | 1 (33%) | 6 | (27%) | 2 (33%) |
| 48 h after surgery | 7 | (50%) | 3 (42%) | 9 | (41%) | 6 (67%) |
| 72 h after surgery | 4 | (29%) | 2 (50%) | 7 | (32%) | 1 (14%) |

The majority of patients who developed AKI had significantly elevated baseline creatinine levels before surgery (DC: 0.93 mg/dL vs. 1.22 mg/dL, $p = 0.011$; VC: 0.99 mg/dL vs. 1.08 mg/dL, $p = 0.018$) (Table 2). In the development study, AKI was significantly associated with older age ($p = 0.047$), diabetes mellitus ($p = 0.012$), the intake of calcium channel blockers ($p = 0.037$), and an increased Cleveland Clinic Foundation Score ($p = 0.005$). In the VC, AKI was associated with a longer duration of cardiopulmonary bypass ($p = 0.046$, Table 2). No sex-based differences were observed.

### 3.2. AKI Was Associated with Higher Serum SLPI in Cardiac Surgery Patients

After cardiac surgery, serum SLPI significantly increased in both cohorts and peaked at 24 h after surgery (DC and VC: $p < 0.001$). Compared with patients not diagnosed with AKI, those diagnosed with AKI had significantly elevated SLPI serum levels 6, 12, 24, and 48 h after surgery (e.g., 24 h, DC: $p = 0.001$; 24 h, VC: $p = 0.008$; Table 3, Figure 2A,B). Serum SLPI did not differ significantly between transient (<48 h) and persistent (>48 h) AKI cases (Figure S1). Patients with high serum SLPI (higher the median value) 24 h after surgery had a significantly higher incidence of AKI (DC: 10% vs. 38%, $p = 0.03$; VC: 7% vs. 24%, $p = 0.01$; Figure 3). Similar to serum SLPI, urinary SLPI levels were significantly increased 24 h after cardiac surgery (Figure 2C,D). Compared with serum SLPI, urinary levels of SLPI were low overall (approximately 5–10 times lower). After surgery, urinary SLPI levels did not significantly differ between patients with and without AKI (Table 3, Figure 2C,D). When normalized to urinary creatinine, patients with AKI showed significantly higher SLPI levels 24 h after surgery (subgroup of VC, $n = 25$, $p = 0.01$; Figure 2F).

**Table 2.** Baseline and operative characteristics by cohort and AKI. Data are expressed as the median (Q1–Q3) or number (percentage). ACE, angiotensin-converting enzyme; AKI, acute kidney injury; BMI, body mass index; CABG, coronary artery bypass graft; COPD, chronic obstructive pulmonary disease; LVEF, left ventricular ejection fraction; POD1, first postoperative day; Q1, Q3, first and third quartile, respectively; and SOFA, Sequential Organ Failure Score. The influence of baseline characteristics on AKI was analyzed by univariable logistic regression. Bold fonts indicate $p$-values < 0.05.

| Characteristic | Development Cohort | | | | | Validation Cohort | | | | |
|---|---|---|---|---|---|---|---|---|---|---|
| | No AKI ($n$ = 46) | | AKI ($n$ = 14) | | $p$-Value | No AKI ($n$ = 126) | | AKI (n = 22) | | $p$-Value |
| Demographics | | | | | | | | | | |
| Age (years) | 67 | (59–75) | 69 | (68–78) | **0.047** | 67 | (59–75) | 69 | (68–78) | 0.171 |
| Sex (female) | 11 | (24) | 4 | (29) | 0.678 | 33 | (26) | 6 | (27) | 0.869 |
| BMI (kg/m$^2$) | 27.4 | (25.0–29.9) | 26.5 | (23.8–33.2) | 0.767 | 27.1 | (24.8–30.3) | 28.5 | (22.9–30.4) | 0.876 |
| Medication, No (%) | | | | | | | | | | |
| Beta blockers | 40 | (87) | 9 | (75) | 0.292 | 91 | (73) | 17 | (77) | 0.733 |
| ACE Inhibitors | 35 | (76) | 8 | (67) | 0.478 | 69 | (55) | 12 | (55) | 0.943 |
| Sartans | 6 | (13) | 1 | (8) | 0.840 | 27 | (22) | 7 | (32) | 0.271 |
| Calcium channel blockers | 6 | (13) | 5 | (42) | **0.037** | 35 | (28) | 6 | (27) | 0.993 |
| Diuretics | 36 | (78) | 11 | (92) | 0.456 | 52 | (42) | 13 | (59) | 0.138 |
| Statins | 45 | (98) | 12 | (100) | 0.929 | 106 | (85) | 19 | (86) | 0.975 |
| Acetylsalicylic acid | 44 | (96) | 12 | (100) | 0.860 | 103 | (82) | 18 | (82) | 0.848 |
| Comorbidities, No (%) | | | | | | | | | | |
| Arterial hypertension | 28 | (61) | 11 | (85) | 0.159 | 89 | (71) | 18 | (82) | 0.362 |
| Pulmonary hypertension | 3 | (7) | 1 | (8) | 0.741 | 6 | (5) | 2 | (9) | 0.328 |
| Congestive heart disease | 7 | (15) | 4 | (29) | 0.255 | 16 | (13) | 0 | (0) | 0.201 |
| LVEF < 35% | 10 | (22) | 2 | (14) | 0.651 | 6 | (5) | 2 | (9) | 0.328 |
| Chronic kidney disease | 3 | (7) | 2 | (14) | 0.345 | 9 | (7) | 4 | (18) | 0.090 |
| COPD | 3 | (7) | 2 | (14) | 0.345 | 15 | (12) | 3 | (14) | 0.707 |
| Diabetes, insulin | 3 | (7) | 5 | (38) | **0.012** | 13 | (10) | 3 | (14) | 0.545 |
| Previous cardiac surgery | 3 | (7) | 0 | (0) | 0.632 | 8 | (6) | 1 | (5) | 0.970 |
| Serum creatinine at baseline (mg/dL) | 0.93 | (0.78–1.04) | 1.22 | (0.83–1.36) | **0.011** | 0.99 | (0.80–1.10) | 1.08 | (0.94–1.28) | **0.018** |
| Type of Surgery | | | | | | | | | | |
| Isolated CABG | 24 | (52) | 3 | (21) | 0.064 | 78 | (62) | 11 | (50) | 0.274 |
| Isolated valvular surgery | 8 | (17) | 4 | (29) | 0.344 | 16 | (13) | 4 | (18) | 0.425 |
| Combined procedure | 14 | (30) | 7 | (50) | 0.191 | 30 | (24) | 7 | (32) | 0.403 |
| other | | | | | | 5 | (4) | 1 | (5) | |
| Risk of AKI | | | | | | | | | | |
| Cleveland Clinic Foundation Score | 3 | (2–3) | 4 | (3–5) | **0.005** | 3 | (2–4) | 3 | (2–4) | 0.636 |
| Duration of Surgery | | | | | | | | | | |
| Aortic cross clamp | 74.5 | (57.5–99) | 78.5 | (47–105) | 0.934 | 73 | (55–89) | 78 | (60–101) | 0.232 |
| Cardiopulmonary bypass | 115 | (91–144) | 118.5 | (89.5–148.5) | 0.769 | 109 | (87–133) | 139 | (97–150) | **0.046** |
| SOFA on POD 1 | 10 | (7.5–12) | 9 | (7–10) | 0.674 | 8 | (6–9) | 9 | (7–12) | **0.044** |

**Table 3.** SLPI measured at different time points. Serum and urinary SLPI concentrations quantified by ELISA and compared between patients with and without AKI. Bold fonts indicate $p$-values < 0.05.

| Serum SLPI | | | | | | | | | | |
|---|---|---|---|---|---|---|---|---|---|---|
| **SLPI (ng/mL)** | **Development Cohort ($n$ = 60)** | | | | | **Validation Cohort ($n$ = 148)** | | | | |
| | **No AKI ($n$ = 46)** | | **AKI ($n$ = 14)** | | ***p*-Value** | **No AKI ($n$ = 226)** | | **AKI ($n$ = 22)** | | ***p*-Value** |
| Pre-OP | 67.3 | (57.2–82.1) | 87.6 | (65.3–98.5) | **0.14** | 40.1 | (31.6 –48.5) | 43.7 | (36.6–52.4) | 0.280 |
| 0 h after surgery | 66.3 | (52.8–81.15) | 102.7 | (83.2–128.2) | **0.06** | 29.7 | (22.4–39.9) | 37.9 | (25.4–45.3) | 0.127 |
| 6 h after surgery | 64.9 | (53.9–84.7) | 102.1 | (93.2–131.5) | **<0.001** | | | | | |
| 12 h after surgery | 74.7 | (52.0–88.1) | 114.5 | (95.0–134.5) | **<0.001** | | | | | |
| 24 h after surgery | 86.1 | (69.0–113.5) | 117.9 | (105.6–145.2) | **0.001** | 80.4 | (64.7–111.7) | 106.6 | (83.0–135.3) | **0.008** |
| 48 h after surgery | | | | | | 58.5 | (58.5–90.0) | 98.8 | (76.0–110.4) | **0.000** |
| **Urinary SLPI** | | | | | | | | | | |
| **SLPI (ng/mL)** | **Development Cohort ($n$ = 60)** | | | | | **Validation Cohort ($n$ = 148)** | | | | |
| | **No AKI ($n$ = 46)** | | **AKI ($n$ = 14)** | | ***p*-Value** | **No AKI ($n$ = 226)** | | **AKI ($n$ = 22)** | | ***p*-Value** |
| Pre-OP | 1.10 | (0.40–2.09) | 0.40 | (0.17–0.96) | 0.022 | 0.51 | (0.15–1.53) | 0.8 | (0.20–1.36) | 0.520 |
| 0 h after surgery | 0.23 | (0.07–1.09) | 0.58 | (0.31–2.02) | 0.056 | 0.13 | (0.025–0.35) | 0.98 | (0.98–1.40) | 0.073 |
| 24 h after surgery | 2.20 | (0.74–5.05) | 2.38 | (0.33–9.23) | 0.942 | 1.15 | (0.71–1.92) | 1.08 | (0.90–1.62) | 0.575 |

Patients with AKI showed significantly elevated serum SLPI after surgery. AKI, acute kidney injury; Pre-OP, before surgery; SLPI, secretory leukocyte protease inhibitor. Data are reported as median (Q1–Q3). $p$-values were analyzed using the Mann–Whitney U test.

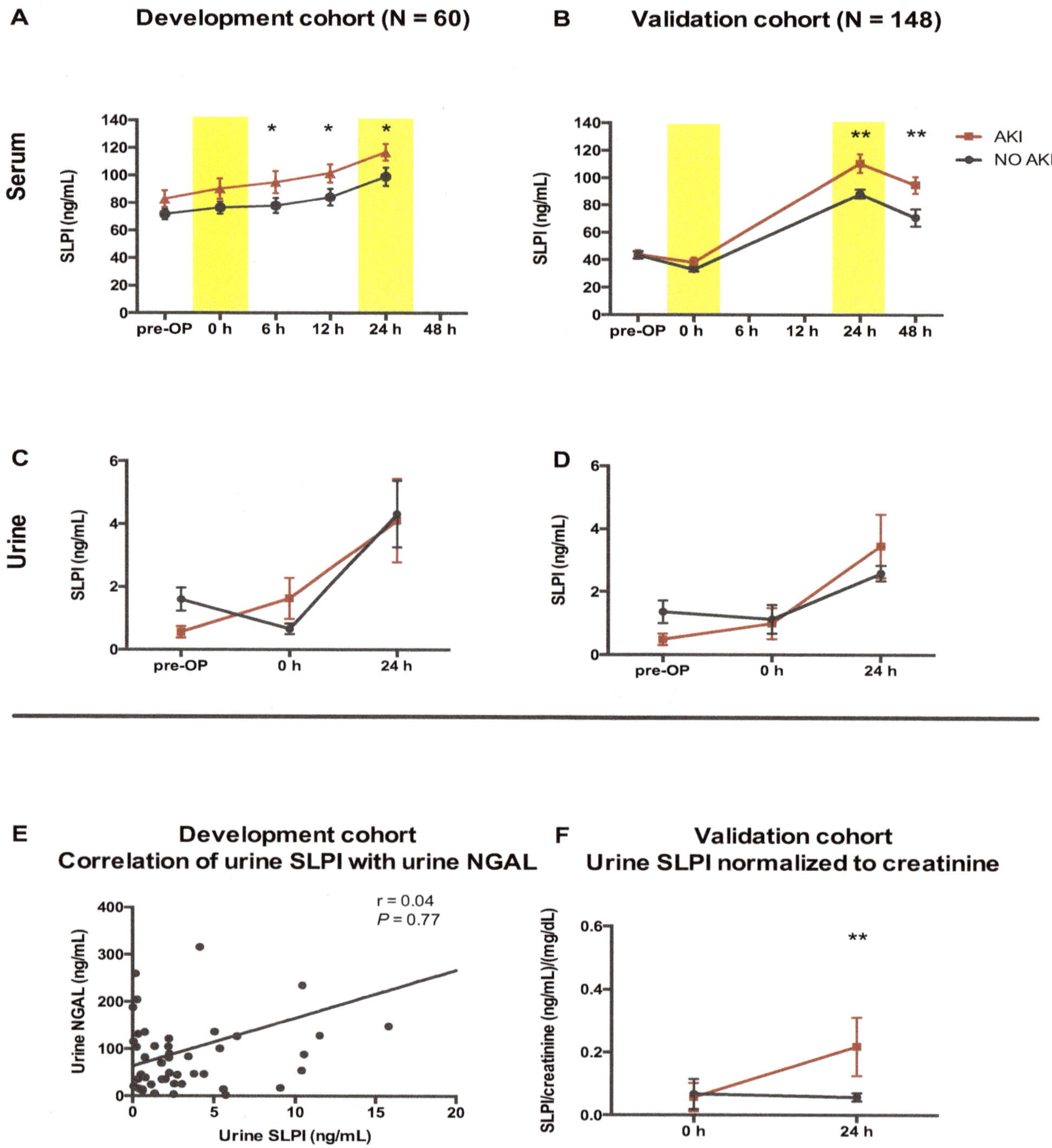


**Figure 2.** Higher serum SLPI levels were associated with a greater risk of AKI. (**A**,**B**) Perioperative kinetics of serum SLPI in patients without postoperative AKI compared with patients with AKI. (**C**,**D**) Perioperative kinetics of urinary SLPI. (**E**) Correlation between postoperative urinary SLPI and postoperative urinary NGAL 24 h after cardiac surgery. (**F**) Postoperative kinetics of urinary SLPI normalized to urinary creatinine. AKI, acute kidney injury; NGAL, neutrophil gelatinase-associated lipocalin; Pre-OP, before surgery; SLPI, secretory leukocyte protease inhibitor. Data are means ± SEM; *r*, Spearman's coefficient. (**A**,**B**) * $p < 0.05$, ** $p < 0.01$ versus other groups at the corresponding time point (difference between groups).

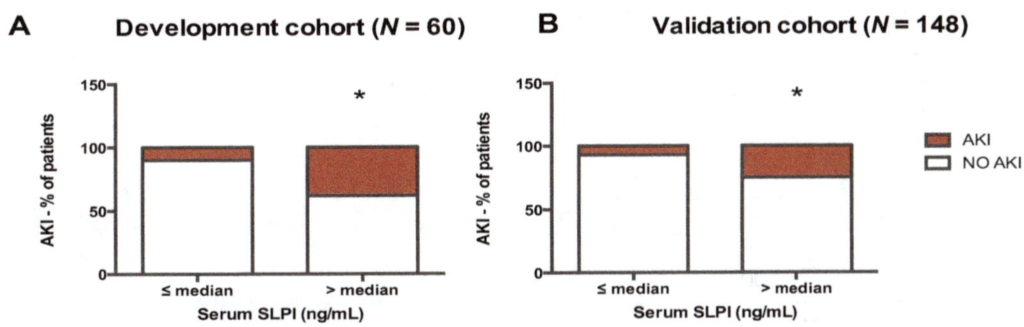


**Figure 3.** Percentage of patients with AKI within 72 h after cardiac surgery, stratified by median serum SLPI concentration 24 h after surgery (**A**) in the development cohort and (**B**) validation cohort. AKI, acute kidney injury; SLPI, secretory leukocyte protease inhibitor. * $p < 0.05$ analyzed by Fisher's exact test.

### 3.3. Accuracy of SLPI for Diagnosis of AKI

We assessed the predictive accuracy of SLPI for AKI by the ROC curve and the corresponding AUC. At 24 h after surgery, the area under the ROC curve of serum SLPI was 0.81 (95% CI 0.69–0.92) in the development cohort and 0.69 (95% CI 0.58–0.80) in the validation cohort (Figure 4). The additional earlier time points in the development cohort yielded AUCs of 0.87 (95% CI 0.76–0.97) 6 h after surgery and 0.85 (95% CI 0.74–0.95) 12 h after surgery. When only patients with a Cleveland Clinic Foundation Score ≥3 ("at risk for AKI") were selected, the diagnostic accuracy did not improve significantly (Figure S2). The AUCs of the absolute increase of SLPI from baseline before surgery (delta from pre-OP) were not superior to absolute SLPI (Figure S3). Compared with urinary NGAL, with an AUC of 0.52 (95% CI 0.31–0.73) 24 h after surgery, serum SLPI was more accurate in diagnosing AKI 24 h after surgery (Figure 4, Figure S4). However, urinary SLPI, even when normalized to urine creatinine, did not demonstrate significant results (AUC = 0.71, 95% CI 0.44–1.0). Table 4 lists the optimal cut-off concentrations calculated using the Youden index and the related sensitivities and specificities.

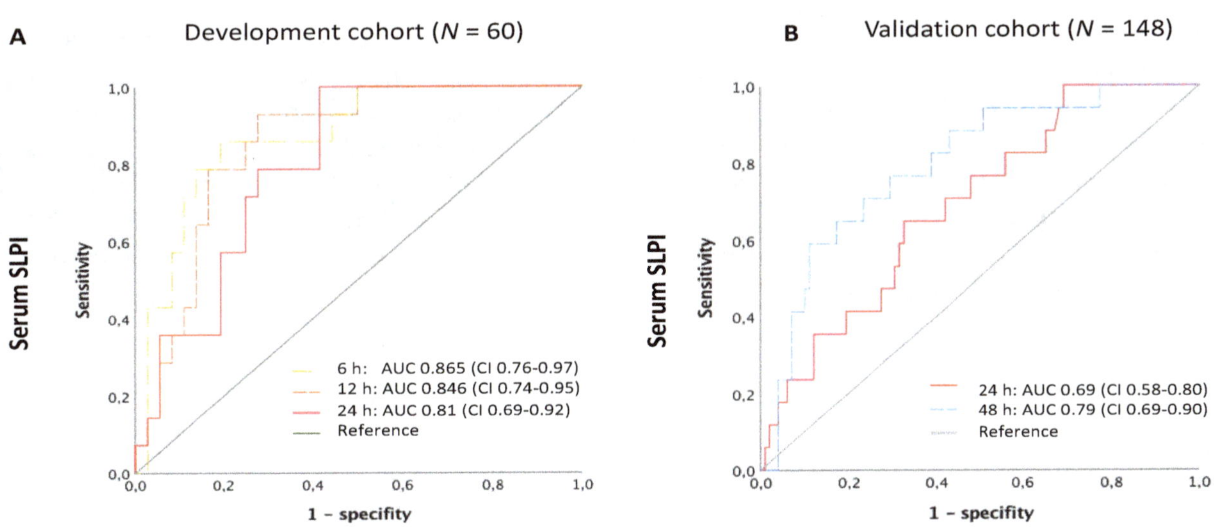


**Figure 4.** Receiver operating characteristic (ROC) curves of SLPI and NGAL for the diagnosis of AKI at different time points after surgery. (**A**) ROC of serum SLPI in the development study and (**B**) in the validation study. AKI, acute kidney injury; AUC, area under the curve; CI, 95% confidence interval; SLPI, secretory leukocyte protease inhibitor.

**Table 4.** Sensitivity and specificity of SLPI as a biomarker for AKI at optimal cut-off values.

| Time Point after Surgery | Optimal Cut-off (ng/mL) | Sensitivity (%) | 95% CI | Specificity (%) | 95% CI | Likelihood Ratio | Youden Index |
|---|---|---|---|---|---|---|---|
| Development cohort, Serum SLPI | | | | | | | |
| 6 h | >85.20 | 64.3 | 35.1–87.2 | 68.29 | 51.9–81.9 | 2.027 | 0.32 |
| 12 h | >92.72 | 66.7 | 34.9–90.1 | 73.17 | 57.1–85.8 | 2.485 | 0.39 |
| 24 h | >87.93 | 100.0 | 75.3–100.0 | 54.55 | 38.9–69.6 | 2.200 | 0.54 |
| Validation cohort, Serum SLPI | | | | | | | |
| 24 h | >101.8 | 70.0 | 45.7–88.1 | 67.6 | 57.8–76.4 | 2.162 | 0.38 |
| 48 h | >78.45 | 77.8 | 52.4–93.6 | 71.2 | 61.4–79.9 | 2.709 | 0.49 |

Optimal cut-off concentrations were calculated with the help of the Youden index; CI, confidence interval; Pre-OP, before surgery; SLPI, secretory leukocyte protease inhibitor.

### 3.4. SLPI as a Predictor of AKI in Univariate and Multivariate Analyses

As calculated in a univariate analysis, patients with higher postoperative serum SLPI (>median) had a significantly higher risk of AKI (e.g., validation cohort, 24 h, OR = 3.89, 95% CI 1.44–12.08, $p = 0.007$; 48 h, OR = 9.24, 95% CI 2.69–48.30, $p < 0.001$; Table 4).

Because the Cleveland Clinic Foundation Score is a clinical score for risk stratification of AKI after open cardiac surgery, this score was included in the multivariable analysis as the reference model (independent variable). The Cleveland Clinic Foundation Score includes the variables sex, congestive heart disease, left ventricular ejection fraction, use of intra-aortic balloon-pump, chronic obstructive pulmonary disease, insulin-requiring diabetes, previous heart surgery, emergency surgery, type of surgery, and preoperative serum creatinine. When adjusted for the Cleveland Clinic Foundation Score, serum SLPI remained a significant predictor of AKI at 6, 12, and 24 h after surgery in the development cohort and 24 and 48 h in the validation cohort (e.g., 6 h, DC: OR = 1.74; 95% CI 1.18–2.84, $p = 0.004$; 24 h, VC: OR = 3.91 95% CI, 1.44–12.13, $p = 0.007$; Table 5).

To determine whether SLPI can be regarded as a predictive biomarker, we performed a subgroup analysis in which we only considered AKI cases that were diagnosed after the respective SLPI measurement. Thus, for SLPI measured at 24 h, we only considered cases of AKI that were diagnosed at 48 or 72 h ($n = 11$ in the development and $n = 16$ in the validation study), and for SLPI measured at 48 h, we only considered cases of AKI that were diagnosed at 72 h after surgery. In addition to the early time points (6 and 12 h after surgery), in these univariable and multivariable analyses, SLPI was significantly predictive of AKI 24 h (multivariable: OR = 4.89; 95% CI, 1.54–19.92; $p = 0.006$) and 48 h (multivariable: OR = 15.24; 95% CI, 1.63–2025.31; $p = 0.013$) after surgery (Table 5).

**Table 5.** SLPI as a predictor of AKI. **(A)** Univariable logistic regression. Serum SLPI was a significant predictor of AKI 12, 24, and 48 h after surgery. Multivariable logistic regression adjusted for Cleveland Clinic Foundation Score (including the variables sex, congestive heart disease, left ventricular ejection fraction, use of intra-aortic balloon-pump, chronic obstructive pulmonary disease, insulin-requiring diabetes, previous heart surgery, emergency surgery, type of surgery, and preoperative serum creatinine). After adjustment for the Cleveland Clinic Foundation Score, serum SLPI remained a significant predictor of AKI. **(B)** Subgroup analysis of cases of AKI that were diagnosed after the respective SLPI measurement. For SLPI measured at 24 h, only the cases of AKI that were diagnosed at 48 or 72 h ($n = 11$ in the DC and $n = 16$ in the VC) were considered. For SLPI measured at 48 h, only the cases of AKI that were diagnosed at 72 h after surgery were considered. SLPI was categorized by the corresponding median; CI, confidence interval; OR, odds ratio; Pre-OP, before surgery; SLPI, secretory leukocyte protease inhibitor; bold fonts indicate $p$-values < 0.05.

| **(A) AKI, Time Point not Considered** | | | | | | | | | |
|---|---|---|---|---|---|---|---|---|---|
| | | **Univariable Logistic Regression (Median)** | | | | **Multivariable Logistic Regression (Median)** | | | |
| **Time Point after Surgery** | **Median** | **OR** | **95% CI** | | ***p*-value** | **OR** | **adj. 95% CI** | | ***p*-value** |
| Development Cohort | | | | | | | | | |
| Pre-OP | 71.3 | 1.37 | 0.42 | 4.57 | 0.601 | 1.12 | 0.30 | 4.16 | 0.868 |
| 0 h after surgery | 77.2 | 2.06 | 0.63 | 7.28 | 0.230 | 1.69 | 0.46 | 6.61 | 0.431 |
| 6 h after surgery | 69.6 | 2.19 | 0.67 | 7.82 | 0.197 | **1.74** | 1.18 | 2.84 | **0.004** |
| 12 h after surgery | 79.9 | **3.80** | 1.03 | 17.09 | **0.045** | **1.72** | 1.15 | 2.83 | **0.008** |
| 24 h after surgery | 95 | **3.92** | 1.10 | 17.31 | **0.035** | **1.76** | 1.16 | 2.98 | **0.007** |
| Validation Cohort | | | | | | | | | |
| Pre-OP | 41.00 | 1.46 | 0.58 | 3.75 | 0.417 | 1.47 | 0.59 | 3.76 | 0.412 |
| 0 h after surgery | 13.00 | 1.029 | 0.41 | 2.59 | 0.945 | 1.01 | 0.38 | 2.66 | 0.19 |
| 24 h after surgery | 88.3 | **3.89** | 1.44 | 12.08 | **0.007** | **3.91** | 1.44 | 12.13 | **0.007** |
| 48 h after surgery | 65.3 | **9.24** | 2.69 | 48.30 | **<0.001** | **9.45** | 2.74 | 49.55 | **<0.001** |
| **(B) AKI, Time Point Considered** | | | | | | | | | |
| | | **Univariable logistic regression (median)** | | | | **Multivariable Logistic Regression (Median)** | | | |
| **Time Point** | **Median** | **OR** | **95% CI** | | ***p*-value** | **OR** | **adj. 95% CI** | | ***p*-value** |
| Development Cohort | | | | | | | | | |
| SLPI measured at 24 h for AKI diagnosed later: 48 or 72 h after surgery (11 of 14 cases of AKI) | 95 | **4.45** | 1.07 | 25.61 | **0.039** | 2.48 | 0.50 | 15.35 | 0.268 |
| Validation Cohort | | | | | | | | | |
| SLPI measured at 24 h for AKI diagnosed later: 48 or 72 h after surgery (16 of 22 AKI cases) | 88.3 | **4.94** | 1.55 | 20.15 | **0.006** | **4.89** | 1.54 | 19.92 | **0.006** |
| SLPI measured at 48 h for AKI diagnosed later: 72 h after surgery (7 of 22 cases of AKI) | 65.3 | **15.4** | 1.67 | 2042 | **0.011** | **15.24** | 1.63 | 2025.31 | **0.013** |

## 4. Discussion

SLPI is a 12 kDa (107 amino acids) non-glycosylated single-chain protein that is broadly expressed in myeloid and other epithelial cells [23–25]. SLPI functions as a non-redundant alarm anti-protease and is considered important in the defense against proteolytic attack from liberated granulocyte proteases [26]. Apart from its anti-protease activity, SLPI has antibacterial, antiviral, and anti-inflammatory properties and promotes wound healing [27].

Cardiac surgery patients with AKI, even those who achieve complete renal recovery, have a significantly increased risk of death and adverse long-term consequences compared with patients without AKI [8]. Over time, 10%–20% of patients with AKI develop chronic kidney disease [28,29]. The KDIGO clinical practice guideline recommends the early identification of patients at risk and suggests a bundle of preventive measures for the early treatment of kidney injury. Because serum creatinine and urine output show changes in renal function only after the occurrence of significant kidney injury, new biomarkers are needed to earlier identify patients who will later benefit from therapeutic measures [9]. In the 2006 Clinical Path Opportunities List, the Food and Drug Administration declared the identification of new biomarkers as a key area for improving clinical trials and medical therapies [30]. A major limitation in the identification of suitable biomarkers of AKI is the limited availability of human biopsies from kidneys with AKI; therefore, relevant tissue analyses have not yet been conducted in large-scale studies. In post-transplant kidney graft dysfunction, however, the retrieval of kidney biopsies is part of the routine diagnostic panel. The assessment of whole-genome mRNA profiles in eight injured kidney allografts with AKI revealed not only the upregulated expression of established biomarkers such as NGAL but also the significantly enhanced expression of *SLPI* mRNA [15]. The increase in *SLPI* gene expression is correlated with the protein levels of SLPI in the plasma and urine, which indicates a link between elevated SLPI in the urine and blood and the status of the kidney. In fact, immunohistochemical staining and in situ hybridization detected local SLPI protein expression in the kidney tubular epithelial cells, suggesting that the tubule epithelial cells are a source of elevated serum SLPI in patients suffering from post-transplant AKI [31]. Despite the striking baseline-adjusted increase in mRNA expression (15-fold change) that first implicated SLPI as a promising biomarker of AKI, to the best of our knowledge, SLPI has been exclusively tested in the post-transplant AKI setting and has not been examined in AKI after cardiac surgery.

In this prospective observational study, we investigated the possibility of using SLPI to diagnose and predict AKI in patients undergoing cardiac surgery. The incidence of AKI ranged between 15% (in the validation cohort) and 25% (in the development cohort), which is within the normal range of incidence of AKI observed after cardiac surgery [3]. Only a minority of patients met the KDIGO diagnostic criterion of oliguria lasting at least 6 h, which might be attributed to strict counteractive measures, including diuretics and fluid management, undertaken in the ICU setting.

The levels of serum and urinary SLPI considerably increased in the postoperative course and peaked 24 h after the surgical intervention. Compared with healthy blood donors with an average serum SLPI of 49 ng/mL, the serum concentrations of SLPI were approximately twice as high 24 h after cardiac surgery [32]. Contrasting the perioperative values of serum SLPI in the development and validation cohorts, we detected different baseline SLPI levels, whereas the relative changes were comparable. Whether these differences arose from different patient characteristics could not be reliably established.

Patients affected by AKI during the first 72 h after surgery had significantly higher serum SLPI 6, 12, 24, and 48 h after surgery compared with non-AKI patients. SLPI levels exceeding the median 24 h after surgery were associated with a markedly increased risk of AKI. Serum SLPI showed promising accuracy in the diagnosis of AKI, with an AUC of over 0.85 six hours after surgery in the development cohort. However, samples from later time points only yielded moderate results for the AUC and the corresponding sensitivity or specificity of cut-off values. Considering the optimal cut-off values calculated using the Youden index for the different time points, the overall cut-off value of serum SLPI to predict AKI might ranges from around 85 to 90 ng/mL. Compared with patient characteristics that were prognostic for AKI, the addition of SLPI to the risk assessment models significantly improved the prediction of AKI. SLPI was found to detect AKI before a rise in serum creatinine or before decreased urine output became evident. These findings suggest that SLPI is a novel predictive marker of AKI, which may be of particular clinical significance after cardiac surgery but also in a broader intensive care setting associated with AKI.

To date, the functional role of SLPI in the pathogenesis of AKI after cardiac surgery is unknown and requires further examination in experimental studies. In animal models, SLPI has been shown to be an important protective mediator during ischemia–reperfusion injury in the liver and brain, as well as after cardiac transplantation [27,33–35]. In a renal ischemia–reperfusion injury mouse model, SLPI was suggested to contribute to tubular cell regeneration via Cyclin-D1 upregulation [36]. Cardiac surgery patients are exposed to a high risk of developing a systemic inflammatory response, which is a substantial factor in the pathogenesis of postoperative AKI [37,38]. After cardiac surgery, SLPI was significantly upregulated and might play a role as a counter-regulatory factor against the detrimental inflammatory response by modulating nuclear factor κ-light-chain-enhancer of activated B cells (NF-κB) and promoting organ repair, such as proximal tubular cell regeneration [35,36,39–41]. The sufficient degradation of SLPI in the tubular cells of healthy individuals can be assumed [42,43]. The elevation of serum SLPI levels in acute kidney injury might be a multifactorial and multidirectional resulting from (1) SLPI release from injured kidney tissue, (2) impaired renal elimination, and (3) acute and chronic inflammatory conditions.

One strength of this study is the robust results obtained from two independent and heterogeneous cohorts with significant comorbidities related to AKI, including patients with chronic kidney disease. Compared with some other recently discovered biomarkers, SLPI seems to function accurately as an AKI marker in these unselected study cohorts, which might increase the generalizability of the received findings [44].

Some study limitations exist, and the presented findings need to be interpreted cautiously. Long-term data for the prediction of chronic kidney disease and long-term mortality were not captured in our database and therefore could not be analyzed. Another limitation to our trial is that, for the validation study, only postoperative samples taken 24 and 48 h after surgery were available; thus, the results obtained at 6 and 12 h in the development study could not be compared. However, the results obtained from the development study at 24 h after surgery were successfully confirmed in the validation cohort. Additionally, the appearance that serum SLPI is superior to urinary SLPI as a predictor of AKI should be approached carefully. If a tubular source of SLPI is assumed, then the concentration of SLPI in the urine should be robustly elevated, although we only detected elevated urinary SLPI levels when they were normalized to serum creatinine. As leukocytes are the best-established source of SLPI, elevated SLPI during AKI might, in part, result from a systemic inflammatory response. However, urine concentrations are subject to fluctuations caused by dilution effects (e.g., by diuretics). This might explain why we only observed a significant elevation of urinary SLPI after its normalization to creatinine.

Among the newly identified biomarkers of AKI, urine neutrophil gelatinase-associated lipocalin (NGAL) and [TIMP-2]·[IGFBP7] have provided promising results [14,19,45]. The combined measurement of [TIMP-2]·[IGFBP7] reflects the idea that biomarker panels might better depict the heterogeneous etiology of AKI than single markers. The combination of these identified markers with new biomarkers, such as SLPI, might further improve diagnostic accuracy [46–49].

## 5. Conclusions

In conclusion, we identified SLPI as a novel biomarker for the early detection of AKI after cardiac surgery. Our findings may lead to future perspectives of biomarker-based risk stratification and may identify patients who would benefit from the early initiation of preventive and treatment strategies.

**Supplementary Materials:**
Figure S1. Comparison of serum SLPI in patients affected by transient AKI (<48 h) versus persistent AKI (>48 h).

Figure S2. Diagnostic accuracy of serum SLPI in patients "at risk" as identified by Cleveland Clinic Foundation Score. Figure S3. Association of absolute increase of serum SLPI from baseline (pre-OP, before surgery) with AKI. Figure S4. Receiver operating characteristic (ROC) curves of urine NGAL for the diagnosis of AKI. Figure S5. Association of perioperative serum SLPI with postoperative death and ICU length of stay.

**Author Contributions:** L.A., C.S., A.O., and G.M. (Gilbert Moeckel) substantially contributed to the design of the clinical studies; L.A., T.L., M.S., and J.V. acquired the clinical data and performed the experimental analyses; L.A., C.F., and C.S. performed the statistical analyses and contributed to the interpretation of presented findings; L.A. drafted the manuscript. C.S., D.E.L., and G.M. (Gernot Marx) substantially revised the manuscript. All authors read and approved the final manuscript.

**Acknowledgments:** We are thankful for the technical support and assistance of C. Beckers, M. Tatarek-Nossol, and S. Brömler.

## References

1. Kheterpal, S.; Tremper, K.K.; Heung, M.; Rosenberg, A.L.; Englesbe, M.; Shanks, A.M.; Campbell, D.A., Jr. Development and validation of an acute kidney injury risk index for patients undergoing general surgery: Results from a national data set. *Anesthesiology* **2009**, *110*, 505–515. [CrossRef] [PubMed]
2. Thiele, R.H.; Isbell, J.M.; Rosner, M.H. AKI associated with cardiac surgery. *Clin. J. Am. Soc. Nephrol.* **2015**, *10*, 500–514. [CrossRef] [PubMed]
3. Grams, M.E.; Sang, Y.; Coresh, J.; Ballew, S.; Matsushita, K.; Molnar, M.Z.; Szabo, Z.; Kalantar-Zadeh, K.; Kovesdy, C.P. Acute Kidney Injury After Major Surgery: A Retrospective Analysis of Veterans Health Administration Data. *Am. J. Kidney Dis.* **2016**, *67*, 872–880. [CrossRef] [PubMed]
4. Thakar, C.V.; Yared, J.P.; Worley, S.; Cotman, K.; Paganini, E.P. Renal dysfunction and serious infections after open-heart surgery. *Kidney Int.* **2003**, *64*, 239–246. [CrossRef] [PubMed]
5. Go, A.S.; Chertow, G.M.; Fan, D.; McCulloch, C.E.; Hsu, C.Y. Chronic kidney disease and the risks of death, cardiovascular events, and hospitalization. *N. Engl. J. Med.* **2004**, *351*, 1296–1305. [CrossRef] [PubMed]
6. Chertow, G.M.; Burdick, E.; Honour, M.; Bonventre, J.V.; Bates, D.W. Acute kidney injury, mortality, length of stay, and costs in hospitalized patients. *J. Am. Soc. Nephrol.* **2005**, *16*, 3365–3370. [CrossRef] [PubMed]
7. Bihorac, A.; Yavas, S.; Subbiah, S.; Hobson, C.E.; Schold, J.D.; Gabrielli, A.; Layon, A.J.; Segal, M.S. Long-term risk of mortality and acute kidney injury during hospitalization after major surgery. *Ann. Surg.* **2009**, *249*, 851–858. [CrossRef]
8. Hobson, C.E.; Yavas, S.; Segal, M.S.; Schold, J.D.; Tribble, C.G.; Layon, A.J.; Bihorac, A. Acute kidney injury is associated with increased long-term mortality after cardiothoracic surgery. *Circulation* **2009**, *119*, 2444–2453. [CrossRef]
9. Meersch, M.; Volmering, S.; Zarbock, A. Prevention of acute kidney injury. *Best Pract. Res. Clin. Anaesthesiol.* **2017**, *31*, 361–370. [CrossRef]
10. Zarbock, A.; Kellum, J.A.; Schmidt, C.; Van Aken, H.; Wempe, C.; Pavenstadt, H.; Boanta, A.; Gerss, J.; Meersch, M. Effect of Early vs. Delayed Initiation of Renal Replacement Therapy on Mortality in Critically Ill Patients with Acute Kidney Injury: The ELAIN Randomized Clinical Trial. *JAMA* **2016**, *315*, 2190–2199. [CrossRef]
11. Moran, S.M.; Myers, B.D. Course of acute renal failure studied by a model of creatinine kinetics. *Kidney Int.* **1985**, *27*, 928–937. [CrossRef] [PubMed]
12. Kellum, J.A.; Prowle, J.R. Paradigms of acute kidney injury in the intensive care setting. *Nat. Rev. Nephrol.* **2018**, *14*, 217–230. [CrossRef] [PubMed]
13. James, M.; Bouchard, J.; Ho, J.; Klarenbach, S.; LaFrance, J.P.; Rigatto, C.; Wald, R.; Zappitelli, M.; Pannu, N. Canadian Society of Nephrology commentary on the 2012 KDIGO clinical practice guideline for acute kidney injury. *Am. J. Kidney Dis.* **2013**, *61*, 673–685. [CrossRef] [PubMed]
14. Kashani, K.; Al-Khafaji, A.; Ardiles, T.; Artigas, A.; Bagshaw, S.M.; Bell, M.; Bihorac, A.; Birkhahn, R.; Cely, C.M.; Chawla, L.S.; et al. Discovery and validation of cell cycle arrest biomarkers in human acute kidney injury. *Crit. Care* **2013**, *17*, R25. [CrossRef]
15. Wilflingseder, J.; Sunzenauer, J.; Toronyi, E.; Heinzel, A.; Kainz, A.; Mayer, B.; Perco, P.; Telkes, G.; Langer, R.M.; Oberbauer, R. Molecular pathogenesis of post-transplant acute kidney injury: Assessment of whole-genome mRNA and miRNA profiles. *PLoS ONE* **2014**, *9*, e104164. [CrossRef]
16. Palevsky, P.M.; Liu, K.D.; Brophy, P.D.; Chawla, L.S.; Parikh, C.R.; Thakar, C.V.; Tolwani, A.J.; Waikar, S.S.; Weisbord, S.D. KDOQI US commentary on the 2012 KDIGO clinical practice guideline for acute kidney injury. *Am. J. Kidney Dis.* **2013** *61*, 649–672. [CrossRef]

17. Thakar, C.V.; Arrigain, S.; Worley, S.; Yared, J.P.; Paganini, E.P. A clinical score to predict acute renal failure after cardiac surgery. *J. Am. Soc. Nephrol.* **2005**, *16*, 162–168. [CrossRef]
18. Stoppe, C.; Rex, S.; Goetzenich, A.; Kraemer, S.; Emontzpohl, C.; Soppert, J.; Averdunk, L.; Sun, Y.; Rossaint, R.; Lue, H.; et al. Interaction of MIF family proteins in myocardial ischemia/reperfusion damage and their influence on clinical outcome of cardiac surgery patients. *Antioxid. Redox Signal.* **2015**, *23*, 865–879. [CrossRef]
19. Haase, M.; Bellomo, R.; Devarajan, P.; Schlattmann, P.; Haase-Fielitz, A.; NGAL Meta-analysis Investigator Group. Accuracy of neutrophil gelatinase-associated lipocalin (NGAL) in diagnosis and prognosis in acute kidney injury: A systematic review and meta-analysis. *Am. J. Kidney Dis.* **2009**, *54*, 1012–1024. [CrossRef]
20. Ho, J.; Tangri, N.; Komenda, P.; Kaushal, A.; Sood, M.; Brar, R.; Gill, K.; Walker, S.; MacDonald, K.; Hiebert, B.M.; et al. Urinary, Plasma, and Serum Biomarkers' Utility for Predicting Acute Kidney Injury Associated With Cardiac Surgery in Adults: A Meta-analysis. *Am. J. Kidney Dis.* **2015**, *66*, 993–1005. [CrossRef]
21. Altman, D.G.; McShane, L.M.; Sauerbrei, W.; Taube, S.E. Reporting recommendations for tumor marker prognostic studies (REMARK): Explanation and elaboration. *BMC Med.* **2012**, *10*, 51. [CrossRef] [PubMed]
22. Heinze, G.; Schemper, M. A solution to the problem of separation in logistic regression. *Stat. Med.* **2002**, *21*, 2409–2419. [CrossRef] [PubMed]
23. King, A.E.; Critchley, H.O.; Kelly, R.W. Presence of secretory leukocyte protease inhibitor in human endometrium and first trimester decidua suggests an antibacterial protective role. *Mol. Hum. Reprod.* **2000**, *6*, 191–196. [CrossRef] [PubMed]
24. Ohlsson, K.; Bjartell, A.; Lilja, H. Secretory leucocyte protease inhibitor in the male genital tract: PSA-induced proteolytic processing in human semen and tissue localization. *J. Androl.* **1995**, *16*, 64–74. [PubMed]
25. Bergenfeldt, M.; Nystrom, M.; Bohe, M.; Lindstrom, C.; Polling, A.; Ohlsson, K. Localization of immunoreactive secretory leukocyte protease inhibitor (SLPI) in intestinal mucosa. *J. Gastroenterol.* **1996**, *31*, 18–23. [CrossRef] [PubMed]
26. Thompson, R.C.; Ohlsson, K. Isolation, properties, and complete amino acid sequence of human secretory leukocyte protease inhibitor, a potent inhibitor of leukocyte elastase. *Proc. Natl. Acad. Sci. USA* **1986**, *83*, 6692–6696. [CrossRef]
27. Hannila, S.S. Secretory Leukocyte Protease Inhibitor (SLPI): Emerging Roles in CNS Trauma and Repair. *Neuroscientist* **2015**, *21*, 630–636. [CrossRef]
28. Basile, D.P.; Bonventre, J.V.; Mehta, R.; Nangaku, M.; Unwin, R.; Rosner, M.H.; Kellum, J.A.; Ronco, C.; Group, A.X.W. Progression after AKI: Understanding Maladaptive Repair Processes to Predict and Identify Therapeutic Treatments. *J. Am. Soc. Nephrol.* **2016**, *27*, 687–697. [CrossRef]
29. Coca, S.G.; Singanamala, S.; Parikh, C.R. Chronic kidney disease after acute kidney injury: A systematic review and meta-analysis. *Kidney Int.* **2012**, *81*, 442–448. [CrossRef]
30. Mahajan, R.; Gupta, K. Food and drug administration's critical path initiative and innovations in drug development paradigm: Challenges, progress, and controversies. *J. Pharm. Bioall. Sci.* **2010**, *2*, 307–313. [CrossRef]
31. Ohlsson, S.; Ljungkrantz, I.; Ohlsson, K.; Segelmark, M.; Wieslander, J. Novel distribution of the secretory leucocyte proteinase inhibitor in kidney. *Mediat. Inflamm.* **2001**, *10*, 347–350. [CrossRef] [PubMed]
32. Bergenfeldt, M.; Bjork, P.; Ohlsson, K. The elimination of secretory leukocyte protease inhibitor (SLPI) after intravenous injection in dog and man. *Scand. J. Clin. Lab. Investig.* **1990**, *50*, 729–737. [CrossRef] [PubMed]
33. Schneeberger, S.; Hautz, T.; Wahl, S.M.; Brandacher, G.; Sucher, R.; Steinmassl, O.; Steinmassl, P.; Wright, C.D.; Obrist, P.; Werner, E.R.; et al. The effect of secretory leukocyte protease inhibitor (SLPI) on ischemia/reperfusion injury in cardiac transplantation. *Am. J. Transplant.* **2008**, *8*, 773–782. [CrossRef] [PubMed]
34. Lentsch, A.B.; Yoshidome, H.; Warner, R.L.; Ward, P.A.; Edwards, M.J. Secretory leukocyte protease inhibitor in mice regulates local and remote organ inflammatory injury induced by hepatic ischemia/reperfusion. *Gastroenterology* **1999**, *117*, 953–961. [CrossRef]
35. Grobmyer, S.R.; Barie, P.S.; Nathan, C.F.; Fuortes, M.; Lin, E.; Lowry, S.F.; Wright, C.D.; Weyant, M.J.; Hydo, L.; Reeves, F.; et al. Secretory leukocyte protease inhibitor, an inhibitor of neutrophil activation, is elevated in serum in human sepsis and experimental endotoxemia. *Crit. Care Med.* **2000**, *28*, 1276–1282. [CrossRef]
36. Ochi, A.; Chen, D.; Schulte, W.; Leng, L.; Moeckel, N.; Piecychna, M.; Averdunk, L.; Stoppe, C.; Bucala, R.; Moeckel, G. MIF-2/D-DT enhances proximal tubular cell regeneration through SLPI- and ATF4-dependent mechanisms. *Am. J. Physiol.* **2017** *313*, F767–F780. [CrossRef]

37. Billings, F.T.t.; Pretorius, M.; Schildcrout, J.S.; Mercaldo, N.D.; Byrne, J.G.; Ikizler, T.A.; Brown, N.J. Obesity and oxidative stress predict AKI after cardiac surgery. *J. Am. Soc. Nephrol.* **2012**, *23*, 1221–1228. [CrossRef]
38. Sureshbabu, A.; Ryter, S.W.; Choi, M.E. Oxidative stress and autophagy: Crucial modulators of kidney injury. *Redox Biol.* **2015**, *4*, 208–214. [CrossRef]
39. Lopez-Bermejo, A.; Ortega, F.J.; Castro, A.; Ricart, W.; Fernandez-Real, J.M. The alarm secretory leukocyte protease inhibitor increases with progressive metabolic dysfunction. *Clin. Chim. Acta* **2011**, *412*, 1122–1126. [CrossRef]
40. Taggart, C.C.; Cryan, S.A.; Weldon, S.; Gibbons, A.; Greene, C.M.; Kelly, E.; Low, T.B.; O'Neill, S.J.; McElvaney, N.G. Secretory leucoprotease inhibitor binds to NF-kappaB binding sites in monocytes and inhibits p65 binding. *J. Exp. Med.* **2005**, *202*, 1659–1668. [CrossRef]
41. Taggart, C.C.; Greene, C.M.; McElvaney, N.G.; O'Neill, S. Secretory leucoprotease inhibitor prevents lipopolysaccharide-induced IkappaBalpha degradation without affecting phosphorylation or ubiquitination. *J. Biol. Chem.* **2002**, *277*, 33648–33653. [CrossRef] [PubMed]
42. Nystrom, M.; Bergenfeldt, M.; Ohlsson, K. The elimination of secretory leukocyte protease inhibitor (SLPI) from the gastrointestinal tract in man. *Scand. J. Clin. Lab. Investig.* **1997**, *57*, 119–125. [CrossRef] [PubMed]
43. Strober, W.; Waldmann, T.A. The role of the kidney in the metabolism of plasma proteins. *Nephron* **1974**, *13*, 35–66. [CrossRef] [PubMed]
44. Smertka, M.; Chudek, J. Using NGAL as an early diagnostic test of acute kidney injury. *Ren. Fail.* **2012**, *34*, 130–133. [CrossRef] [PubMed]
45. Zhou, F.; Luo, Q.; Wang, L.; Han, L. Diagnostic value of neutrophil gelatinase-associated lipocalin for early diagnosis of cardiac surgery-associated acute kidney injury: A meta-analysis. *Eur. J. Cardiothorac. Surg.* **2016**, *49*, 746–755. [CrossRef] [PubMed]
46. Hall, P.S.; Mitchell, E.D.; Smith, A.F.; Cairns, D.A.; Messenger, M.; Hutchinson, M.; Wright, J.; Vinall-Collier, K.; Corps, C.; Hamilton, P.; et al. The future for diagnostic tests of acute kidney injury in critical care: Evidence synthesis, care pathway analysis and research prioritisation. *Health Technol. Assess.* **2018**, *22*, 1–274. [CrossRef]
47. Nisula, S.; Yang, R.; Kaukonen, K.M.; Vaara, S.T.; Kuitunen, A.; Tenhunen, J.; Pettila, V.; Korhonen, A.M.; Group, F.S. The urine protein NGAL predicts renal replacement therapy, but not acute kidney injury or 90-day mortality in critically ill adult patients. *Anesth. Analg.* **2014**, *119*, 95–102. [CrossRef] [PubMed]
48. Bihorac, A.; Chawla, L.S.; Shaw, A.D.; Al-Khafaji, A.; Davison, D.L.; Demuth, G.E.; Fitzgerald, R.; Gong, M.N.; Graham, D.D.; Gunnerson, K.; et al. Validation of cell-cycle arrest biomarkers for acute kidney injury using clinical adjudication. *Am. J. Respir. Crit. Care Med.* **2014**, *189*, 932–939. [CrossRef]
49. Honore, P.M.; Nguyen, H.B.; Gong, M.; Chawla, L.S.; Bagshaw, S.M.; Artigas, A.; Shi, J.; Joannes-Boyau, O.; Vincent, J.L.; Kellum, J.A.; et al. Urinary Tissue Inhibitor of Metalloproteinase-2 and Insulin-Like Growth Factor-Binding Protein 7 for Risk Stratification of Acute Kidney Injury in Patients With Sepsis. *Crit. Care Med.* **2016**, *44*, 1851–1860. [CrossRef]

# 15

# Pseudoxanthoma Elasticum, Kidney Stones and Pyrophosphate: From a Rare Disease to Urolithiasis and Vascular Calcifications

**Emmanuel Letavernier [1,*], Elise Bouderlique [1], Jeremy Zaworski [1], Ludovic Martin [2] and Michel Daudon [1]**

1 UMR S 1155 and Physiology Unit, AP-HP, Hôpital Tenon, Sorbonne Université and INSERM, F-75020 Paris, France; eliseboud@aol.com (E.B.); jyzaworski@gmail.com (J.Z.); michel.daudon@aphp.fr (M.D.)

2 PXE Consultation Center, MAGEC Reference Center for Rare Skin Diseases, Angers University Hospital, MITOVASC Institute, UMR CNRS 6015 INSERM U1083 Angers University, 49000 Angers, France; lumartin@chu-angers.fr

* Correspondence: emmanuel.letavernier@aphp.fr

**Abstract:** Pseudoxanthoma elasticum is a rare disease mainly due to *ABCC6* gene mutations and characterized by ectopic biomineralization and fragmentation of elastic fibers resulting in skin, cardiovascular and retinal calcifications. It has been recently described that pyrophosphate (a calcification inhibitor) deficiency could be the main cause of ectopic calcifications in this disease and in other genetic disorders associated to mutations of *ENPP1* or *CD73*. Patients affected by Pseudoxanthoma Elasticum seem also prone to develop kidney stones originating from papillary calcifications named Randall's plaque, and to a lesser extent may be affected by nephrocalcinosis. In this narrative review, we summarize some recent discoveries relative to the pathophysiology of this mendelian disease responsible for both cardiovascular and renal papillary calcifications, and we discuss the potential implications of pyrophosphate deficiency as a promoter of vascular calcifications in kidney stone formers and in patients affected by chronic kidney disease.

**Keywords:** pseudoxanthoma elasticum; pyrophosphate; kidney; Randall's plaque

---

## 1. Introduction: Pseudoxanthoma Elasticum and Related Diseases

### 1.1. Clinical Manifestations

Pseudoxanthoma elasticum (PXE; OMIM #264800, prevalence 1/25,000 to 1/50,000) is an autosomal recessive disease resulting mainly from mutations in *ABCC6* gene [1,2]. PXE is characterized by the fragmentation of elastin fibers, elastorrhexis, and calcifications of soft tissues involving mainly skin, arteries and retina [3,4]. The 2/3 female to 1/3 male ratio in patients diagnosed with PXE remains unexplained to date.

The disease may present during infancy but is classically discovered in teenagers or young adults, because of cutaneous manifestations [3–6].

Xanthoma-like papules may be sparse or form coalescent plaques and folds of esthetic concern. They give the name to the disease and predominate in flexion zones and neck. Skin biopsy and histopathological examination reveal calcifications with destruction of the elastic fibers [7]. It remains uncertain whether elastorrhexis precedes calcifications or whether calcified elastin fibers are broken in a second step.

PXE also affects retina, inducing fragmentation and rupture of calcified elastin fibers of the Bruch's membrane. The examination of the fundus of the eye reveals a typical "peau d'orange" aspect in

PXE patients, with angioid streaks and choroidal neovascularization leading to hemorrhages [8,9]. When affecting the macula, these lesions lead to the loss of central vision.

Cardiovascular calcifications are a hallmark of PXE but clinical manifestations are relatively delayed, predominating after the fourth decade of life, and their severity is extremely variable among PXE patients [5]. Peripheral arterial disease is frequent and there is a significantly increased risk of stroke [10,11]. Coronary calcifications are also frequent but the risk of cardiac infarction seems only mildly increased (if any) in comparison to the general population [5,12]. The earliest arterial calcifications observed in PXE affect elastic fibers of the medial layer, and predominate in medium and small-sized musculo-elastic arteries. Cardiovascular remodeling in large and medium sized musculo-elastic arteries is characterized by an increased intima-media thickening [13,14]. The arterial lesions affecting PXE peripheral arteries differ from those due to aging, hypertension or classic atherosclerosis and share similarities with calcifications and remodeling observed in chronic kidney disease [5,15].

To date, there is no specific curative or preventive therapy for PXE patients. Bisphosphonates such as Etidronate seem promising to prevent cardiovascular calcifications and anti-Vascular Endothelial Growth Factor (VEGF) intraocular injections limit neoangiogenesis [9,16,17].

Two other autosomal recessive mendelian diseases share phenotypic similarities with PXE: the generalized arterial calcifications of infancy (GACI), caused by mutations of the ectonucleotide pyrophosphatase phosphodiesterase NPP1 encoded by the *ENPP1* gene (OMIM 208000) and Arterial calcification due to deficiency of CD73 (ACDC, OMIM 211800), due to mutation of the *NT5E* gene encoding CD73, an ecto 5′-nucleotidase adenosine (ADO)-generating enzyme [18–21] GACI is an extremely severe but fortunately rare disorder characterized by extensive arterial calcification and stenosis affecting young children leading to heart failure. In some cases, the disease is less severe and patients with *ENPP1* mutations may present with the PXE phenotype. ACDC has been discovered more recently in a few families and is also characterized by cardiovascular calcifications and stenosis [19,20].

In addition to phenotypic resemblances, these three diseases share a common pathophysiological link: pyrophosphate (PPi) deficiency.

### 1.2. Pathophysiology of PXE, GACI and ACDC: Pyrophosphate Deficiency

During decades, the mechanism responsible for ectopic calcifications in PXE patients remained a mystery. *ABCC6* mutations are responsible for most of the PXE syndromes diagnosed. *ABCC6* encodes an adenosine triphosphate (ATP)-binding cassette transporter mainly expressed in the liver and to a lesser extent in kidney proximal tubular cells [1,22,23]. This specific expression raised the hypothesis that PXE would be a metabolic disease responsible for distant manifestations, i.e., connective tissue calcifications [24]. Due to its structure, close to other ABC-type transporters, ABCC6 could promote the efflux of calcification inhibitors from hepatocytes and tubular cells toward the systemic circulation [24].

A role for vitamin K has been suggested by several observations [25]. First, antivitamin K therapy is associated with vascular calcifications and sometimes calciphylaxis in hemodialyzed patients [26]. Second, *GGCX* mutations cause a PXE-like calcification phenotype and are associated with deficiency in vitamin K clotting factors [25]. The *GGCX* gene encodes a gamma-glutamyl carboxylase which catalyzes the conversion of glutamate residues to gamma-carboxyglutamate residues (gamma-carboxylation). This posttranslational modification process uses vitamin K as an essential cofactor. Gamma-carboxylation is necessary to activate multiple vitamin K-dependent proteins including coagulation factors (Factors II, VII, IX and X) and proteins such as Matrix Gla Protein (MGP). Third, PXE patients have lower serum levels of vitamin K in comparison with a control population [25]. Finally, MGP is a vitamin K-dependent mineralization inhibitor. *MGP* homozygous mutations are responsible for Keutel syndrome, characterized by cartilage calcification and pulmonary artery stenoses [27]. Nevertheless, administration of vitamin K was not efficient to reduce clinical manifestations in patients or to improve significantly the ectopic calcification which also occur in *Abcc6*$^{-/-}$ mice [28,29].

A major breakthrough in the field of calcifying diseases has been the identification that the hepatic (and probably tubular) ABCC6 transporter promotes the release of extracellular adenosine triphosphate (ATP), which serves as a substrate for NPP1 in the vasculature to generate adenosine monophosphate (AMP) and PPi, a potent anticalcifying molecule [30,31]. This process is the main source of circulating PPi, that counteracts the formation of calcium phosphate ectopic calcifications. PPi inhibits the crystallization and the growth of calcium phosphate crystalline phases such as hydroxyapatite [32]. Patients with PXE and GACI as well as *Abcc6*$^{-/-}$ and *Enpp1* mutant (tiptoe walking: ttw/ttw) mice have a reduced plasma PPi level, explaining, at least in part, their mineralization disorder [22]. Of note, PPi treatment is sufficient to prevent ectopic mineralization in both *Abcc6*$^{-/-}$ and *Enpp1*$^{ttw/ttw}$ murine models [33–35].

Moreover, ABCC6 and NPP1 combined activity generates AMP in addition to PPi. AMP is rapidly converted into adenosine by CD73, which exerts a tonic inhibition on tissue non-specific alkaline enzyme (TNAP). In ACDC, mutations in *NT5E/CD73* lead to insufficient adenosine levels, increasing TNAP activity: TNAP degrades PPi to generate inorganic phosphate and eventually promotes hydroxyapatite precipitation in ectopic tissues [22,33,35].

Thus, ABCC6, NPP1 and CD73 increase PPi systemic synthesis and decrease endogenous PPi degradation through TNAP inhibition (Figure 1).

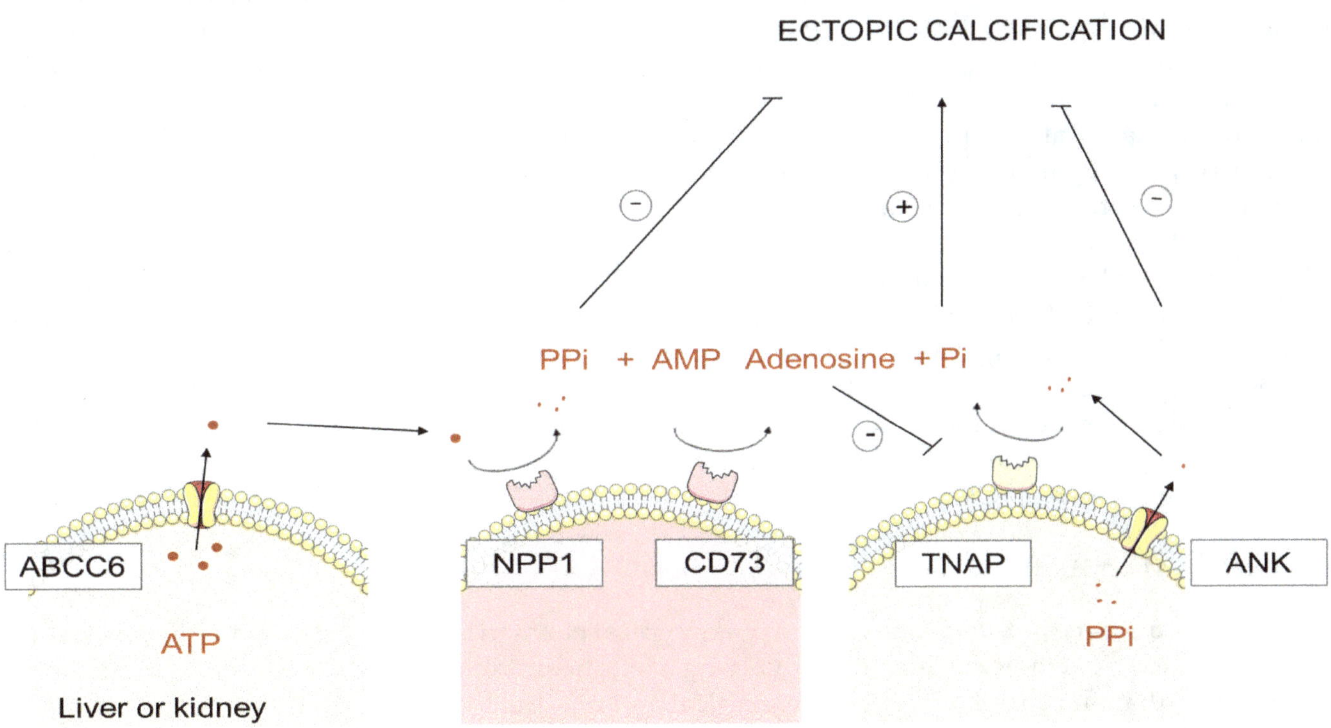


**Figure 1.** Systemic Pyrophosphate (PPi) synthesis. ABCC6 (expressed in hepatocytes and proximal tubular cells) and NPP1 (in arteries and capillaries) combined activity generates AMP in addition to PPi. AMP is rapidly converted into adenosine by CD73, which exerts a tonic inhibition on tissue non-specific alkaline enzyme (TNAP). TNAP degrades PPi to generate inorganic phosphate and promotes hydroxyapatite precipitation in ectopic tissues. ANK allows PPi externalization from cells, its role in ectopic calcifications is unclear.

## 2. Pseudoxanthoma Elasticum and Kidney Calcifications

### 2.1. *Nephrocalcinosis and Kidney Stones: Preliminary Reports*

A few preliminary and sparse reports have suggested that PXE patients may be affected by kidney stones [36]. In addition to kidney stones, the presence of typical nephrocalcinosis has been reported in a few patients affected by PXE [37–39]. When exposed to a procalcifying diet (high phosphate, vitamin D and low magnesium), *Abcc6*$^{-/-}$ and *Enpp1*$^{-/-}$ mice develop rapidly a nephrocalcinosis consisting in multiple calcium phosphate tubular plugs [40].

### 2.2. High Prevalence of Kidney Stones in PXE Patients

In a recent PXE cohort study that was not specifically designed to record kidney stone prevalence, observations suggested that nephrolithiasis was an unrecognized but a prevalent feature of PXE, affecting at least 10% of patients [11]. To better characterize the prevalence of kidney stones among patients with PXE, we conducted a retrospective study in 170 patients participating in the Angers PXE cohort [41]. Among the 164 patients who received the survey, 113 fulfilled the questionaire (33 men and 80 women). Among these patients, 45 (39.8%) declared they had a past medical history of kidney stones (asymptomatic stones in four patients or renal colic in 41 patients). Although this type of study may be biased, as patients affected by kidney stones may be more prone to fulfill the survey, the prevalence of kidney stones and renal colic in PXE patients appears to be extremely high. As a matter of comparison, the lifetime expected incidence of kidney stones is nearing 10% in the general population. Usually, urolithiasis is more frequent in males than females but in PXE patients approximately two thirds of the patients are women. This is consistent with the higher prevalence of PXE in women.

The analysis of six computed tomography (CT)-scans from PXE patients revealed the presence of papillary calcifications, Randall's plaques, the first step of kidney stone formation in five of them [41]. This is remarkable as only the presence of massive plaques can be determined by imaging. These calcifications affected rather the tip of the renal papilla than the renal medulla. One patient had both papillary calcifications and medullary calcifications, i.e., nephrocalcinosis. CT scans had been performed in patients with a past medical history of kidney stones, but one may hypothesize that patients with PXE and without a past medical history of urolithiasis may also be affected by asymptomatic papillary calcifications. We examined a limited number of CT-scans so that we cannot estimate the prevalence of papillary calcifications/Randall's plaque and nephrocalcinosis in PXE patients. A few stones from PXE patients have been analyzed and presented Randall's plaque fragments made of carbonated apatite, suggesting that stone formation in these individuals was initiated by these plaques. No specific study dedicated to the biological risk factors of kidney stone formation in PXE has been performed to date. In the same way, chronic kidney disease (CKD) is not a classic feature of PXE and we still ignore whether some PXE patients affected by kidney stones and papillary calcifications may be at risk to develop CKD.

### 2.3. *Abcc6*$^{-/-}$ Mice: A Murine Model of Randall's Plaque

*Abcc6*$^{-/-}$ mice recapitulate many of the phenotypical characteristics of the human PXE disease [42]. Mice are affected by ectopic calcifications involving aorta, heart, retina and vibrissae and their PPi serum level is lower than in control mice. As renal cortical and medullary calcifications had been described in these animals, especially after an "acceleration diet", we hypothesized that papillary calcification could develop in this model [40]. Aging *Abcc6*$^{-/-}$ mice actually developed kidney calcifications electively at the tip of the papilla, mainly in the interstitial tissue, round shaped and surrounding the loops of Henle and the vasa recta: they differed from the tubular plugs observed after an acceleration diet. These calcifications were made of carbonated apatite spheres as evidenced by scanning electron microscopy and Fourier transform infrared microspectroscopy [41]. At the nanometer scale, by using transmission electron microscopy coupled to electron energy loss spectroscopy, we evidenced that incipient calcifications were made of concentric layers containing calcium and phosphate alternating with organic compounds, as described in incipient human calcifications forming the Randall's plaque. Remarkably, the renal calcification observed in aging *Abcc6*$^{-/-}$ mice met the four essential criteria of Randall's plaque: (i) interstitial deposits surrounding tubules and vasa recta, (ii) electively located at the tip of the renal papilla, (iii) made of carbonated apatite, and (iv) forming nanometer-scale elementary structures made of minerals and organic compounds.

*Abcc6*$^{-/-}$ mice had also a lower urinary excretion of PPi than control mice, and as previously described lower serum levels of PPi [41]. *Abcc6*$^{-/-}$ mice expressing a functional human ABCC6 protein in the liver had an increase in serum PPi circulating levels and were protected against kidney calcifications at 18 months of age [33]. It seems therefore very likely that the systemic PPi deficiency in these mice was at the origin of calcium phosphate supersaturation at the tip of the papilla, leading to papillary calcification.

## 3. The Mystery of Randall's Plaque Formation: A Role for Calcification Inhibitors and Pyrophosphate?

### *3.1. Randall's Plaque: the Origin of Renal Calculi*

Randall's plaque is the first step of calcium oxalate stone formation in many cases. Alexander Randall proposed its original theory in 1936 when he claimed the identification of the origin of renal calculi [43]. He performed extensive forensic studies and observed, at the tip of the renal papilla, whitish deposits made of calcium phosphate and carbonate, originating from the renal interstitium. In some cases, these lesions disrupted the urothelium cellular barrier and brown calcium oxalate stones were attached to these "Randall's" plaques, forming a heterogeneous nucleation process. He identified that the calcium oxalate stones had an umbilication due the shape of the papilla and that calcium phosphate remnants, fragments of Randall's plaque, were present in this umbilication once the stone was passed, identifying the origin of the stone. Other authors performed similar studies during this period [44]. It has been postulated early that the high concentration in calcium in renal papilla could be at the origin of the plaque. The interest in Randall's plaque has grown during the last decades, as the development of endourology evidenced the presence of stones attached to Randall's plaque in situ. Randall's plaque was found in stone formers in 57%–99% of patients when reno-ureterocopy was performed. The prevalence seems lower in France than in North American studies [45–49]. Although Randall's plaques seem to be very frequent, common papillary calcifications are usually too small to be evidenced by CT-scan (unlike PXE patients).

### *3.2. Determinants of Randall's Plaque Formation*

The main risk factors responsible for calcium oxalate supersaturation and crystals or stone formation are relatively well identified: low diuresis, hypercalciuria, hyperoxaluria and/or hypocitraturia [47,50]. However, the origin of the Randall's plaque itself is less understood. The prevalence of calcium oxalate stones is increasing worldwide [47,51]. As there is no longitudinal study taking into account stone morphology or papillary plaque coverage, the role of Randall's plaque in this epidemic is difficult to assess. However, we identified that the proportion of stones with a papillary umbilication and typical plaque remnants was three times more frequent in recent years than three decades ago, especially in young adults [52]. In 2003, Evan et al. analyzed papilla biopsies and identified that incipient Randall's plaque at the tip of the renal papillae were made of subepithelial apatite deposits surrounding the loop of Henle [53]. These observations suggested that apatite droplets formed in around the loop of Henle in contact with basement membrane could spread in the interstitium and form plaques. It has been suggested that calcium phosphate supersaturation in the thin limb of the loop of Henle could promote calcium phosphate particle precipitation and that some of these particles attached to epithelial cells could migrate by endocytosis to the interstitial tissue and form plaques [54,55]. We performed analyses of incipient Randall's plaque in dozens of healthy papillae and identified that early calcifications could also appear around vasa recta at the tip of renal papilla, as previously highlighted by Stoller et al. [56,57]. This suggests that calcium phosphate supersaturation should be extremely high in this environment. Kuo et al. have identified that hypercalciuria, low diuresis and low urine pH correlated with the surface of Randall's plaque in kidney stone formers [58]. More than seven decades ago, Vermooten had performed forensic studies in South Africa and identified Randall's plaque in 17% of whites and only in 4% of the local native Bantus, known to have low calciuria and to be rarely affected by calcium-related stones [44,59]. Hypercalciuria could therefore be involved first in Randall's plaque formation and several years or decades later in calcium oxalate stone formation, once plaque has developed and eroded urothelium locally.

### 3.3. *Randall's Plaque and Calcification Inhibitors*

Calcium concentration is predicted to be extremely high at the tip of the renal papilla, especially around vasa recta [60,61]. Considering (i) that phosphate concentration is certainly significant, although reabsorbed partly in the proximal tubule, and (ii) that papillary pH should stand within physiological range (7.4), calcium phosphate supersaturation should be extremely high at the tip of the papilla. This suggests that calcification inhibitors play a key role to prevent Randall's plaque formation. A very large number of low-weight and macromolecular calcification inhibitors have been studied in the field of urolithiasis [62]. Currently, there is no monogenic mendelian disease responsible for calcification inhibitor deficiency and kidney stone formation, maybe with the exception of distal renal tubular acidosis, which is responsible for hypocitraturia and nephrocalcinosis [63]. Interestingly, *ABCC6* mutation in PXE patients and *Abcc6* knock-out murine models are sufficient to induce papillary calcification [41]. This monogenic defect responsible for PPi deficiency is clearly not compensated by other calcification inhibitors. This observation is remarkable as the development of kidney tissue calcifications is extremely difficult to achieve in rodent models. We previously tried to induce Randall's plaque in Sprague Dawley rats exposed to vitamin D and calcium supplementation for 6 months. These animals developed tubular plugs and stones but none of them developed papillary interstitial calcifications [64]. Similar observations have been performed in the genetic hypercalciuric stone forming rat extensively studied by Bushinsky et al. [65]. These data confirm that calcification inhibitors, especially PPi, play a major role to prevent Randall's plaque formation.

Further studies are required to assess whether kidney stone formers affected by Randall's plaque have lower urine (or serum) PPi levels than kidney stone formers without Randall's plaque or than general population. Of note, seminal studies had previously highlighted that kidney stone formers may have lower urinary PPi excretion than matched subjects [66]. However, this field of research has probably been limited during the last decades by the lack of reliable methods to measure PPi, due to pre-analytic pitfalls and to the very low concentration of PPi in biological fluids.

### 3.4. *The Abcc6$^{-/-}$ Murine Model: A Tool to Identify Randall's Plaque Determinants and New Therapeutics*

*Abcc6$^{-/-}$* mice expressing a functional human ABCC6 protein in the liver or supplemented with PPi were protected against kidney calcification [33,34]. It has been shown that oral PPi is partly absorbed in human subjects and increases serum PPi circulating levels. Taken together, these data suggest that PPi or drugs increasing PPi synthesis could potentially be used as a treatment against kidney calcifications and Randall's plaque.

*Abcc6$^{-/-}$* mice can also be used to test whether drugs or dietary factors could influence Randall's plaque formation. We hypothesized that the increased proportion of stones grown on Randall's plaque during the past decades could, at least partly, be explained by the widespread use of vitamin D supplementation in the general population [52]. Although the question is extremely controversial, some studies highlighted a relationship between vitamin D intakes, especially in addition with calcium supplementation, and stone formation [67]. *Abcc6$^{-/-}$* and wild-type mice were exposed to vitamin D supplementation, with or without a calcium-rich diet, to promote the formation of Randall's plaque. The combined administration of vitamin D and calcium accelerated significantly Randall's plaque formation in *Abcc6$^{-/-}$* mice, although the animal did not develop hypercalcemia or even a significant increase in urine calcium excretion [68]. This model raises some concerns regarding the potential role of long-term vitamin D supplementation and calcium intakes in predisposed individuals.

## 4. Pyrophosphate Deficiency, the Common Link between Vascular Calcifications, Kidney Stones and Chronic Kidney Disease?

Epidemiological studies have highlighted an association between nephrolithiasis and systemic conditions including cardiovascular diseases but the underlying mechanisms remain unidentified [69]. Vascular calcifications are highly associated with cardiovascular mortality. Kidney stone formers, even young patients, have an increased carotid intima-media wall thickness and an increased arterial stiffness in comparison with matched populations [70,71]. Kidney stone formers have a higher degree of aortic calcification than age- and sex-matched non-stone formers and more severe coronary artery calcification, suggesting that vascular calcifications and kidney stones may have a common underlying mechanism [72].

The potential implication of PPi in vascular calcification is not a novel hypothesis, as Schibler et al. have reported in 1968 that PPi and polyphosphate can inhibit the induction of aortic calcifications by vitamin D, but the recent evidence that PXE patients are affected by both cardiovascular calcifications and kidney stones and Randall's plaque suggests that PPi deficiency could be involved in the development of vascular calcifications in kidney stone formers [41,73]. Here again, further studies based upon a reliable assay of serum PPi levels would be necessary to assess whether PPi deficiency is the missing link between kidney stone/Randall's plaque and vascular calcifications.

Moreover, a relative deficiency in PPi could be involved in the vascular calcifications observed in patients affected by CKD, responsible for an increased cardiovascular morbidity and mortality [74]. TNAP activity is increased in uremic rats, reducing PPi/inorganic phosphate ratio and ABCC6 expression is reduced in uremic mice and rats [75,76]. Exogenous PPi could in theory be of help to protect against vascular calcifications in CKD.

## 5. Conclusions

An increased prevalence of kidney stones has been reported recently in patients affected by PXE, a disease characterized by low circulating PPi levels and vascular calcifications. These patients are affected by massive Randall's plaques and in some cases by nephrocalcinosis. In clinical practice, patients affected by PXE should be aware that they are at high risk to form kidney stones, and preventive measures should be considered, as for any kidney stone former (increased diuresis, decreased urine calcium excretion, etc.). These observations from a rare monogenic disease evidence that PPi probably prevents the development of Randall's plaque and, in the long term, the formation of kidney stones, a disease with a lifetime incidence nearing 10% of the population. Further studies are required to assess whether PPi deficiency is involved in Randall's plaque and kidney stone formation in the general population, but also whether administration of PPi could be protective in that setting. *Abcc6*$^{-/-}$ mice can also be used as a model of Randall's plaque to test new drugs or identify potential determinants of plaque formation or worsening. In addition, PPi could be a missing link between kidney stones and the high prevalence of cardiovascular calcifications observed in kidney stone formers, a deficiency in PPi and potentially in other calcification inhibitors could promote both papillary and vascular mineralization.

**Acknowledgments:** The authors thank Georges Leftheriotis (Nice, France) and Olivier Le Saux (Hawai'i, USA), all the colleagues that participated in the studies dedicated to the role of Abcc6 in kidney stone formation, the COST action CA16115 EuroSoftCalcNet and Patients associations.

## Abbreviations

| | |
|---|---|
| PXE | Pseudoxanthoma elasticum |
| VEGF | Vascular Endothelial Growth Factor |
| GACI | Generalized arterial calcification of infancy |
| (E)NPP1 | ectonucleotide pyrophosphatase phosphodiesterase |

| | |
|---|---|
| ACDC | Arterial calcification due to deficiency of CD73 |
| PPi | Pyrophosphate |
| CT | Computed Tomography |
| CKD | Chronic kidney disease |
| TNAP | Tissue nonspecific alkaline phosphatase |

## References

1. Le Saux, O.; Urban, Z.; Tschuch, C.; Csiszar, K.; Bacchelli, B.; Quaglino, D.; Pasquali-Ronchetti, I.; Pope, F.M.; Richards, A.; Terry, S.; et al. Mutations in a gene encoding an ABC transporter cause pseudoxanthoma elasticum. *Nat. Genet.* **2000**, *25*, 223–227. [CrossRef] [PubMed]
2. Le Saux, O.; Beck, K.; Sachsinger, C.; Silvestri, C.; Treiber, C.; Göring, H.H.; Johnson, E.W.; De Paepe, A.; Pope, F.M.; Pasquali-Ronchetti, I.; et al. A spectrum of ABCC6 mutations is responsible for pseudoxanthoma elasticum. *Am. J. Hum. Genet.* **2001**, *69*, 749–764. [CrossRef]
3. Neidner, K.H. History. *Clin. Dermatol.* **1988**, *6*, 1–4. [CrossRef]
4. Uitto, J.; Li, Q.; Jiang, Q. Pseudoxanthoma Elasticum: Molecular Genetics and Putative Pathomechanisms. *J. Investig. Dermatol.* **2010**, *130*, 661–670. [CrossRef] [PubMed]
5. Leftheriotis, G.; Omarjee, L.; Le Saux, O.; Henrion, D.; Abraham, P.; Prunier, F.; Willoteaux, S.; Martin, L. The vascular phenotype in Pseudoxanthoma elasticum and related disorders: Contribution of a genetic disease to the understanding of vascular calcification. *Front. Genet.* **2013**, *4*, 4. [CrossRef] [PubMed]
6. Naouri, M.; Boisseau, C.; Bonicel, P.; Daudon, P.; Bonneau, D.; Chassaing, N.; Martin, L. Manifestations of pseudoxanthoma elasticum in childhood. *Br. J. Dermatol.* **2009**, *161*, 635–639. [CrossRef]
7. Hosen, M.J.; Lamoen, A.; De Paepe, A.; Vanakker, O.M. Histopathology of Pseudoxanthoma Elasticum and Related Disorders: Histological Hallmarks and Diagnostic Clues. *Scientifica* **2012**, *2012*, 598262. [CrossRef]
8. Audo, I.; Vanakker, O.M.; Smith, A.; Leroy, B.P.; Robson, A.G.; Jenkins, S.A.; Coucke, P.J.; Bird, A.C.; Paepe, A.D.; Holder, G.E.; et al. Pseudoxanthoma Elasticum with Generalized Retinal Dysfunction, a Common Finding? *Investig. Ophthalmol. Vis. Sci.* **2007**, *48*, 4250–4256. [CrossRef]
9. Ebran, J.-M.; Milea, D.; Trelohan, A.; Bonicel, P.; Hamel, J.-F.; Leftheriotis, G.; Martin, L. New insights into the visual prognosis of pseudoxanthoma elasticum. *Br. J. Ophthalmol.* **2014**, *98*, 142–143. [CrossRef]
10. De Vilder, E.Y.G.; Cardoen, S.; Hosen, M.J.; Le Saux, O.; De Zaeytijd, J.; Leroy, B.P.; De Reuck, J.; Coucke, P.J.; De Paepe, A.; Hemelsoet, D.; et al. Pathogenic variants in the ABCC6 gene are associated with an increased risk for ischemic stroke. *Brain Pathol. Zurich Switz.* **2018**, *28*, 822–831. [CrossRef]
11. Legrand, A.; Cornez, L.; Samkari, W.; Mazzella, J.-M.; Venisse, A.; Boccio, V.; Auribault, K.; Keren, B.; Benistan, K.; Germain, D.P.; et al. Mutation spectrum in the ABCC6 gene and genotype-phenotype correlations in a French cohort with pseudoxanthoma elasticum. *Genet. Med. Off. J. Am. Coll. Med. Genet.* **2017**, *19*, 909–917. [CrossRef] [PubMed]
12. Prunier, F.; Terrien, G.; Le Corre, Y.; Apana, A.L.Y.; Bière, L.; Kauffenstein, G.; Furber, A.; Bergen, A.A.B.; Gorgels, T.G.M.F.; Le Saux, O.; et al. Pseudoxanthoma elasticum: Cardiac findings in patients and Abcc6-deficient mouse model. *PLoS ONE* **2013**, *8*, e68700. [CrossRef] [PubMed]
13. Germain, D.P.; Boutouyrie, P.; Laloux, B.; Laurent, S. Arterial Remodeling and Stiffness in Patients With Pseudoxanthoma Elasticum. *Arterioscler. Thromb. Vasc. Biol.* **2003**, *23*, 836–841. [CrossRef] [PubMed]
14. Germain, D.P. Pseudoxanthoma elasticum. *Orphanet J. Rare Dis.* **2017**, *12*, 85. [CrossRef] [PubMed]
15. Leftheriotis, G.; Kauffenstein, G.; Hamel, J.F.; Abraham, P.; Le Saux, O.; Willoteaux, S.; Henrion, D.; Martin, L. The contribution of arterial calcification to peripheral arterial disease in pseudoxanthoma elasticum. *PLoS ONE* **2014**, *9*, e96003. [CrossRef] [PubMed]
16. Kranenburg, G.; de Jong, P.A.; Bartstra, J.W.; Lagerweij, S.J.; Lam, M.G.; Ossewaarde-van Norel, J.; Risseeuw, S.; van Leeuwen, R.; Imhof, S.M.; Verhaar, H.J.; et al. Etidronate for Prevention of Ectopic Mineralization in Patients With Pseudoxanthoma Elasticum. *J. Am. Coll. Cardiol.* **2018**, *71*, 1117–1126. [CrossRef] [PubMed]
17. Bauer, C.; le Saux, O.; Pomozi, V.; Aherrahrou, R.; Kriesen, R.; Stölting, S.; Liebers, A.; Kessler, T.; Schunkert, H.; Erdmann, J.; et al. Etidronate prevents dystrophic cardiac calcification by inhibiting macrophage aggregation. *Sci. Rep.* **2018**, *8*, 5812. [CrossRef]
18. Ruf, N.; Uhlenberg, B.; Terkeltaub, R.; Nürnberg, P.; Rutsch, F. The mutational spectrum of ENPP1 as arising after the analysis of 23 unrelated patients with generalized arterial calcification of infancy (GACI). *Hum. Mutat.* **2005** *25*, 98. [CrossRef]

19. Nitschke, Y.; Baujat, G.; Botschen, U.; Wittkampf, T.; du Moulin, M.; Stella, J.; Le Merrer, M.; Guest, G.; Lambot, K.; Tazarourte-Pinturier, M.-F.; et al. Generalized arterial calcification of infancy and pseudoxanthoma elasticum can be caused by mutations in either ENPP1 or ABCC6. *Am. J. Hum. Genet.* **2012**, *90*, 25–39. [CrossRef]
20. St Hilaire, C.; Ziegler, S.G.; Markello, T.C.; Brusco, A.; Groden, C.; Gill, F.; Carlson-Donohoe, H.; Lederman, R.J.; Chen, M.Y.; Yang„ D.; et al. NT5E mutations and arterial calcifications. *N. Engl. J. Med.* **2011**, *364*, 432–442. [CrossRef]
21. Nitschke, Y.; Rutsch, F. Inherited Arterial Calcification Syndromes: Etiologies and Treatment Concepts. *Curr. Osteoporos. Rep.* **2017**, *15*, 255–270. [CrossRef] [PubMed]
22. Favre, G.; Laurain, A.; Aranyi, T.; Szeri, F.; Fulop, K.; Le Saux, O.; Duranton, C.; Kauffenstein, G.; Martin, L.; Lefthériotis, G. The ABCC6 Transporter: A New Player in Biomineralization. *Int. J. Mol. Sci.* **2017**, *18*, 1941. [CrossRef] [PubMed]
23. Pomozi, V.; Le Saux, O.; Brampton, C.; Apana, A.; Iliás, A.; Szeri, F.; Martin, L.; Monostory, K.; Paku, S.; Sarkadi, B.; et al. ABCC6 is a basolateral plasma membrane protein. *Circ. Res.* **2013**, *112*, e148–e151. [CrossRef] [PubMed]
24. Le Saux, O.; Bunda, S.; VanWart, C.M.; Douet, V.; Got, L.; Martin, L.; Hinek, A. Serum factors from pseudoxanthoma elasticum patients alter elastic fiber formation in vitro. *J. Investig. Dermatol.* **2006**, *126*, 1497–1505. [CrossRef] [PubMed]
25. Vanakker, O.M.; Martin, L.; Schurgers, L.J.; Quaglino, D.; Costrop, L.; Vermeer, C.; Pasquali-Ronchetti, I.; Coucke, P.J.; De Paepe, A. Low serum vitamin K in PXE results in defective carboxylation of mineralization inhibitors similar to the GGCX mutations in the PXE-like syndrome. *Lab. Investig. J. Tech. Methods Pathol.* **2010**, *90*, 895–905. [CrossRef] [PubMed]
26. Nigwekar, S.U.; Bloch, D.B.; Nazarian, R.M.; Vermeer, C.; Booth, S.L.; Xu, D.; Thadhani, R.I.; Malhotra, R. Vitamin K-Dependent Carboxylation of Matrix Gla Protein Influences the Risk of Calciphylaxis. *J. Am. Soc. Nephrol. JASN* **2017**, *28*, 1717–1722. [CrossRef] [PubMed]
27. Munroe, P.B.; Olgunturk, R.O.; Fryns, J.P.; Van Maldergem, L.; Ziereisen, F.; Yuksel, B.; Gardiner, R.M.; Chung, E. Mutations in the gene encoding the human matrix Gla protein cause Keutel syndrome. *Nat. Genet.* **1999**, *21*, 142–144. [CrossRef]
28. Brampton, C.; Yamaguchi, Y.; Vanakker, O.; Van Laer, L.; Chen, L.-H.; Thakore, M.; De Paepe, A.; Pomozi, V.; Szabó, P.T.; Martin, L.; et al. Vitamin K does not prevent soft tissue mineralization in a mouse model of pseudoxanthoma elasticum. *Cell Cycle Georget. Tex* **2011**, *10*, 1810–1820. [CrossRef]
29. Gorgels, T.G.M.F.; Waarsing, J.H.; Herfs, M.; Versteeg, D.; Schoensiegel, F.; Sato, T.; Schlingemann, R.O.; Ivandic, B.T.; Vermeer, C.; Schurgers, L.J.; et al. Vitamin K supplementation increases vitamin K tissue levels but fails to counteract ectopic calcification in a mouse model for pseudoxanthoma elasticum. *J. Mol. Med.* **2011**, *89*, 1125–1135. [CrossRef]
30. Jansen, R.S.; Küçükosmanoglu, A.; de Haas, M.; Sapthu, S.; Otero, J.A.; Hegman, I.E.M.; Bergen, A.A.B.; Gorgels, T.G.M.F.; Borst, P.; van de Wetering, K. ABCC6 prevents ectopic mineralization seen in pseudoxanthoma elasticum by inducing cellular nucleotide release. *Proc. Natl. Acad. Sci. USA* **2013**, *110*, 20206–20211. [CrossRef]
31. Jansen, R.S.; Duijst, S.; Mahakena, S.; Sommer, D.; Szeri, F.; Váradi, A.; Plomp, A.; Bergen, A.A.; Oude Elferink, R.P.J.; Borst, P.; et al. ABCC6-mediated ATP secretion by the liver is the main source of the mineralization inhibitor inorganic pyrophosphate in the systemic circulation-brief report. *Arterioscler. Thromb. Vasc. Biol.* **2014**, *34*, 1985–1989. [CrossRef] [PubMed]
32. Fleisch, H.; Bisaz, S. Mechanism of calcification: Inhibitory role of pyrophosphate. *Nature* **1962**, *195*, 911. [CrossRef] [PubMed]
33. Pomozi, V.; Brampton, C.; van de Wetering, K.; Zoll, J.; Calio, B.; Pham, K.; Owens, J.B.; Marh, J.; Moisyadi, S.; Váradi, A.; et al. Pyrophosphate Supplementation Prevents Chronic and Acute Calcification in ABCC6-Deficient Mice. *Am. J. Pathol.* **2017**, *187*, 1258–1272. [CrossRef] [PubMed]
34. Pomozi, V.; Julian, C.B.; Zoll, J.; Pham, K.; Kuo, S.; Tőkési, N.; Martin, L.; Váradi, A.; Le Saux, O. Dietary Pyrophosphate Modulates Calcification in a Mouse Model of Pseudoxanthoma Elasticum: Implication for Treatment of Patients. *J. Investig. Dermatol.* **2019** *139*, 1082–1088. [CrossRef] [PubMed]
35. Dedinszki, D.; Szeri, F.; Kozák, E.; Pomozi, V.; Tőkési, N.; Mezei, T.R.; Merczel, K.; Letavernier, E.; Tang, E.; Le Saux, O.; et al. Oral administration of pyrophosphate inhibits connective tissue calcification. *EMBO Mol.*

*Med.* **2017**, *9*, 1463–1470. [CrossRef] [PubMed]

36. Fabre, B.; Bayle, P.; Bazex, J.; Durand, D.; Lamant, L.; Chassaing, N. Pseudoxanthoma elasticum and nephrolithiasis. *J. Eur. Acad. Dermatol. Venereol.* **2005**, *19*, 212–215. [CrossRef] [PubMed]
37. Chraïbi, R.; Ismaili, N.; Belgnaoui, F.; Akallal, N.; Bouhllab, J.; Senouci, K.; Hassam, B. Pseudoxanthoma elasticum and nephrocalcinosis. *Ann. Dermatol. Venereol.* **2007**, *134*, 764–766. [CrossRef]
38. Gayen, T.; Das, A.; Roy, S.; Biswas, S.; Shome, K.; Chowdhury, S.N. Pseudoxanthoma elasticum and nephrocalcinosis: Incidental finding or an infrequent manifestation? *Indian Dermatol. Online J.* **2014**, *5*, 176–178.
39. Seeger, H.; Mohebbi, N. Pseudoxanthoma elasticum and nephrocalcinosis. *Kidney Int.* **2016**, *89*, 1407. [CrossRef]
40. Li, Q.; Chou, D.W.; Price, T.P.; Sundberg, J.P.; Uitto, J. Genetic modulation of nephrocalcinosis in mouse models of ectopic mineralization: The Abcc6(tm1Jfk) and Enpp1(asj) mutant mice. *Lab. Investig. J. Tech. Methods Pathol.* **2014**, *94*, 623–632. [CrossRef]
41. Letavernier, E.; Kauffenstein, G.; Huguet, L.; Navasiolava, N.; Bouderlique, E.; Tang, E.; Delaitre, L.; Bazin, D.; de Frutos, M.; Gay, C.; et al. ABCC6 Deficiency Promotes Development of Randall Plaque. *J. Am. Soc. Nephrol.* **2018**, *29*, 2337–2347. [CrossRef] [PubMed]
42. Gorgels, T.G.M.F.; Hu, X.; Scheffer, G.L.; van der Wal, A.C.; Toonstra, J.; de Jong, P.T.V.M.; van Kuppevelt, T.H.; Levelt, C.N.; de Wolf, A.; Loves, W.J.P.; et al. Disruption of Abcc6 in the mouse: Novel insight in the pathogenesis of pseudoxanthoma elasticum. *Hum. Mol. Genet.* **2005**, *14*, 1763–1773. [CrossRef] [PubMed]
43. Randall, A. THE ORIGIN AND GROWTH OF RENAL CALCULI. *Ann. Surg.* **1937**, *105*, 1009–1027. [CrossRef] [PubMed]
44. Vermooten, V. The incidence and significance of the deposition of calcium plaques in the renal papilla as observed in the Caucasian and Bantu population in South Africa. *J. Urol.* **1941**, 193–196. [CrossRef]
45. Low, R.K.; Stoller, M.L. Endoscopic mapping of renal papillae for Randall's plaques in patients with urinary stone disease. *J. Urol.* **1997**, *158*, 2062–2064. [CrossRef]
46. Matlaga, B.R.; Williams, J.C.; Kim, S.C.; Kuo, R.L.; Evan, A.P.; Bledsoe, S.B.; Coe, F.L.; Worcester, E.M.; Munch, L.C.; Lingeman, J.E. Endoscopic evidence of calculus attachment to Randall's plaque. *J. Urol.* **2006**, *175*, 1720–1724. [CrossRef]
47. Khan, S.R.; Pearle, M.S.; Robertson, W.G.; Gambaro, G.; Canales, B.K.; Doizi, S.; Traxer, O.; Tiselius, H.-G. Kidney stones. *Nat. Rev. Dis. Primer* **2016**, *2*, 16008. [CrossRef]
48. Daudon, M.; Bazin, D.; Letavernier, E. Randall's plaque as the origin of calcium oxalate kidney stones. *Urolithiasis* **2015**, *43*, 5–11. [CrossRef]
49. Letavernier, E.; Bazin, D.; Daudon, M. Randall's plaque and kidney stones: Recent advances and future challenges. *Comptes Rendus Chim.* **2016**, *19*, 1456–1460. [CrossRef]
50. Daudon, M.; Letavernier, E.; Frochot, V.; Haymann, J.-P.; Bazin, D.; Jungers, P. Respective influence of calcium and oxalate urine concentration on the formation of calcium oxalate monohydrate or dihydrate crystals. *Comptes Rendus Chim.* **2016**, *19*, 1504–1513. [CrossRef]
51. Ziemba, J.B.; Matlaga, B.R. Epidemiology and economics of nephrolithiasis. *Investig. Clin. Urol.* **2017**, *58*, 299–306. [CrossRef] [PubMed]
52. Letavernier, E.; Vandermeersch, S.; Traxer, O.; Tligui, M.; Baud, L.; Ronco, P.; Haymann, J.-P.; Daudon, M. Demographics and characterization of 10,282 Randall plaque-related kidney stones: A new epidemic? *Medicine (Baltimore)* **2015**, *94*, e566. [CrossRef]
53. Evan, A.P.; Lingeman, J.E.; Coe, F.L.; Parks, J.H.; Bledsoe, S.B.; Shao, Y.; Sommer, A.J.; Paterson, R.F.; Kuo, R.L.; Grynpas, M. Randall's plaque of patients with nephrolithiasis begins in basement membranes of thin loops of Henle. *J. Clin. Investig.* **2003**, *111*, 607–616. [CrossRef]
54. Asplin, J.R.; Mandel, N.S.; Coe, F.L. Evidence of calcium phosphate supersaturation in the loop of Henle. *Am. J. Physiol.* **1996**, *270*, F604–F613. [CrossRef]
55. Lieske, J.C.; Norris, R.; Swift, H.; Toback, F.G. Adhesion, internalization and metabolism of calcium oxalate monohydrate crystals by renal epithelial cells. *Kidney Int.* **1997**, *52*, 1291–1301. [CrossRef]
56. Verrier, C.; Bazin, D.; Huguet, L.; Stéphan, O.; Gloter, A.; Verpont, M.-C.; Frochot, V.; Haymann, J.-P.; Brocheriou, I.; Traxer, O.; et al. Topography, Composition and Structure of Incipient Randall Plaque at the Nanoscale Level. *J. Urol.* **2016** *196*, 1566–1574. [CrossRef]

57. Stoller, M.L.; Low, R.K.; Shami, G.S.; McCormick, V.D.; Kerschmann, R.L. High resolution radiography of cadaveric kidneys: Unraveling the mystery of Randall's plaque formation. *J. Urol.* **1996**, *156*, 1263–1266. [CrossRef]
58. Kuo, R.L.; Lingeman, J.E.; Evan, A.P.; Paterson, R.F.; Parks, J.H.; Bledsoe, S.B.; Munch, L.C.; Coe, F.L. Urine calcium and volume predict coverage of renal papilla by Randall's plaque. *Kidney Int.* **2003**, *64*, 2150–2154. [CrossRef]
59. Vermooten, V. The Origin and Development in the Renal Papilla of Randall's Calcium Plaques. *J. Urol.* **1942**, *48*, 27–37. [CrossRef]
60. Tournus, M.; Seguin, N.; Perthame, B.; Thomas, S.R.; Edwards, A. A model of calcium transport along the rat nephron. *Am. J. Physiol. Renal,Physiol.* **2013**, *305*, F979–F994. [CrossRef]
61. Granjon, D.; Bonny, O.; Edwards, A. A model of calcium homeostasis in the rat. *Am. J. Physiol. Renal Physiol.* **2016**, *311*, F1047–F1062. [CrossRef]
62. Jungers, D. *Lithiase Urinaire*, 2nd ed.; Lavoisier: Paris, France, 2012; pp. 145–150, ISBN 978-2-257-22597-9.
63. Batlle, D.; Haque, S.K. Genetic causes and mechanisms of distal renal tubular acidosis. *Nephrol. Dial. Transplant.* **2012**, *27*, 3691–3704. [CrossRef]
64. Letavernier, E.; Verrier, C.; Goussard, F.; Perez, J.; Huguet, L.; Haymann, J.-P.; Baud, L.; Bazin, D.; Daudon, M. Calcium and vitamin D have a synergistic role in a rat model of kidney stone disease. *Kidney Int.* **2016**, *90*, 809–817. [CrossRef]
65. Bushinsky, D.A.; Grynpas, M.D.; Nilsson, E.L.; Nakagawa, Y.; Coe, F.L. Stone formation in genetic hypercalciuric rats. *Kidney Int.* **1995**, *48*, 1705–1713. [CrossRef]
66. Russell, R.G.; Hodgkinson, A. The urinary excretion of inorganic pyrophosphate by normal subjects and patients with renal calculus. *Clin. Sci.* **1966**, *31*, 51–62.
67. Letavernier, E.; Daudon, M. Vitamin D, Hypercalciuria and Kidney Stones. *Nutrients* **2018**, *10*, 366. [CrossRef]
68. Bouderlique, E.; Tang, E.; Perez, J.; Coudert, A.; Bazin, D.; Verpont, M.-C.; Duranton, C.; Rubera, I.; Haymann, J.-P.; Leftheriotis, G.; et al. Vitamin D and Calcium Supplementation Accelerates Randall's Plaque Formation in a Murine Model. *Am. J. Pathol.* **2019**, *189*, 2171–2180. [CrossRef]
69. Cheungpasitporn, W.; Thongprayoon, C.; Mao, M.A.; O'Corragain, O.A.; Edmonds, P.J.; Erickson, S.B. The Risk of Coronary Heart Disease in Patients with Kidney Stones: A Systematic Review and Meta-analysis. *N. Am. J. Med. Sci.* **2014**, *6*, 580–585. [CrossRef]
70. Reiner, A.P.; Kahn, A.; Eisner, B.H.; Pletcher, M.J.; Sadetsky, N.; Williams, O.D.; Polak, J.F.; Jacobs, D.R.; Stoller, M.L. Kidney stones and subclinical atherosclerosis in young adults: Coronary Artery Risk Development in Young Adults (CARDIA) study. *J. Urol.* **2011**, *185*. [CrossRef]
71. Fabris, A.; Ferraro, P.M.; Comellato, G.; Caletti, C.; Fantin, F.; Zaza, G.; Zamboni, M.; Lupo, A.; Gambaro, G. The relationship between calcium kidney stones, arterial stiffness and bone density: Unraveling the stone-bone-vessel liaison. *J. Nephrol.* **2015**, *28*, 549–555. [CrossRef]
72. Shavit, L.; Girfoglio, D.; Vijay, V.; Goldsmith, D.; Ferraro, P.M.; Moochhala, S.H.; Unwin, R. Vascular Calcification and Bone Mineral Density in Recurrent Kidney Stone Formers. *Clin. J. Am. Soc. Nephrol.* **2015**, *10*, 278–285. [CrossRef]
73. Schibler, D.; Russell, R.G.; Fleisch, H. Inhibition by pyrophosphate and polyphosphate of aortic calcification induced by vitamin D3 in rats. *Clin. Sci.* **1968**, *35*, 363–372.
74. Villa-Bellosta, R.; O'Neill, W.C. Pyrophosphate deficiency in vascular calcification. *Kidney Int.* **2018**, *93*, 1293–1297. [CrossRef]
75. Lomashvili, K.A.; Garg, P.; Narisawa, S.; Millan, J.L.; O'Neill, W.C. Upregulation of alkaline phosphatase and pyrophosphate hydrolysis: Potential mechanism for uremic vascular calcification. *Kidney Int.* **2008**, *73*, 1024–1030. [CrossRef]
76. Lau, W.L.; Liu, S.; Vaziri, N.D. Chronic kidney disease results in deficiency of ABCC6, the novel inhibitor of vascular calcification. *Am. J. Nephrol.* **2014**, *40*, 51–55. [CrossRef]

16

# Acute Kidney Injury in Patients Undergoing Total Hip Arthroplasty

**Charat Thongprayoon [1], Wisit Kaewput [2], Natanong Thamcharoen [3], Tarun Bathini [4], Kanramon Watthanasuntorn [5], Sohail Abdul Salim [6], Patompong Ungprasert [7], Ploypin Lertjitbanjong [5], Narothama Reddy Aeddula [8], Aldo Torres-Ortiz [6], Michael A. Mao [1] and Wisit Cheungpasitporn [6,*]**

1 Division of Nephrology and Hypertension, Mayo Clinic, Rochester, MN 55905, USA; charat.thongprayoon@gmail.com (C.T.); mao.michael@mayo.edu (M.A.M.)
2 Department of Military and Community Medicine, Phramongkutklao College of Medicine, Bangkok 10400, Thailand; wisitnephro@gmail.com
3 Division of Nephrology, Beth Israel Deaconess Medical Center, Harvard Medical School, Boston, MA 02215, USA; natthamcharoen@gmail.com
4 Department of Internal Medicine, University of Arizona, Tucson, AZ 85721, USA; tarunjacobb@gmail.com
5 Department of Internal Medicine, Bassett Medical Center, Cooperstown, NY 13326, USA; kanramon@gmail.com (K.W.); ploypinlert@gmail.com (P.L.)
6 Division of Nephrology, Department of Medicine, University of Mississippi Medical Center, Jackson, MS 39216, USA; sohail3553@gmail.com (S.A.S.); Aldo_t86@hotmail.com (A.T.-O.)
7 Clinical Epidemiology Unit, Department of Research and Development, Faculty of Medicine, Siriraj Hospital, Mahidol University, Bangkok 10700, Thailand; p.ungprasert@gmail.com
8 Division of Nephrology, Department of Medicine, Deaconess Health System, Evansville, IN 47747, USA; dr.anreddy@gmail.com
* Correspondence: wcheungpasitporn@gmail.com

**Abstract:** Background: The number of total hip arthroplasties (THA) performed across the world is growing rapidly. We performed this meta-analysis to evaluate the incidence of acute kidney injury (AKI) in patients undergoing THA. Methods: A literature search was performed using MEDLINE, EMBASE and Cochrane Database from inception until July 2018 to identify studies assessing the incidence of AKI (using standard AKI definitions of RIFLE, AKIN, and KDIGO classifications) in patients undergoing THA. We applied a random-effects model to estimate the incidence of AKI. The protocol for this meta-analysis is registered with PROSPERO (no. CRD42018101928). Results: Seventeen cohort studies with a total of 24,158 patients undergoing THA were enrolled. Overall, the pooled estimated incidence rates of AKI and severe AKI requiring dialysis following THA were 6.3% (95% CI: 3.8%–10.2%) and 0.5% (95% CI: 0.1%–2.3%). Subgroup analysis based on the countries by continent was performed and demonstrated the pooled estimated incidence of AKI following THA of 9.2% (95% CI: 5.6%–14.8%) in Asia, 8.1% (95% CI: 4.9%–13.2%) in Australia, 7.4% (95% CI: 3.2%–16.3%) in Europe, and 2.8% (95% CI: 1.2%–17.0%) in North America. Meta-regression of all included studies showed significant negative correlation between incidence of AKI following THA and study year (slope = −0.37, $p$ <0.001). There was no publication bias as assessed by the funnel plot and Egger's regression asymmetry test with $p$ = 0.13 for the incidence of AKI in patients undergoing THA. Conclusion: The overall estimated incidence rates of AKI and severe AKI requiring dialysis in patients undergoing THA are 6.3% and 0.5%, respectively. There has been potential improvement in AKI incidence for patients undergoing THA over time.

**Keywords:** acute kidney injury; acute renal failure; hip arthroplasty; hip Surgery; postoperative acute kidney injury; incidence; epidemiology; systematic reviews; meta-analysis

## 1. Introduction

Acute kidney injury (AKI) is a complex clinical syndrome, characterized by an abrupt decrease in glomerular filtration, associated with various etiologies and pathophysiological pathways [1–6]. Globally, AKI is a common condition, affecting 13.3 million patients a year [3,4]. This complex syndrome is associated with significant morbidity, considerable mortality resulting in 1.7 million deaths a year, and increased hospital costs and subsequent burden on national health care budgets across the world [7,8].

Total hip arthroplasty (THA) is one of the most consistently successful and cost-effective orthopedic procedures performed today. It is indicated in patients with severe hip pain from a variety of conditions and ultimately provides significant improved pain relief, functionality and quality of life [9–15]. The total number of THA performed across the world is growing rapidly with close to 522,800 surgeries in the United States alone in 2014, making it the fourth most common operative procedure [16,17].

Previous studies have demonstrated different incidence of AKI following total joint arthroplasties using standard AKI criteria ranging from 0.5% to 22% based on types of joint arthroplasties [5,18–40]. The clinical and economic landscape of joint replacement surgeries including both general orthopedic and more specifically THA is rapidly changing, thus making it imperative for clinicians and administrators to understand the various risk factors and post-operative complications in order to better provide excellence in clinical and financial outcomes. However, despite progress in perioperative medicine, the incidence, incidence trend, and risk factors for AKI in patients following THA remain unclear [18–40]. In addition, complication rates such as reoperation and readmission among patients undergoing THA remain high [18–33]. Thus, we performed this systematic review to summarize the incidence and associated risk factors for AKI in patients undergoing THA.

## 2. Methods

### 2.1. Search Strategy and Literature Review

The protocol for this meta-analysis is registered with PROSPERO (International Prospective Register of Systematic Reviews; no. CRD42018101928). A systematic literature search of EMBASE (1988 to July 2018), MEDLINE (1946 to July 2018), and the Cochrane Database of Systematic Reviews (database inception to July 2018) was performed to evaluate the incidence of AKI in patients undergoing THA. The systematic literature review was undertaken independently by two investigators (C.T. and W.C) using the search strategy that combined the terms of "acute kidney injury" or "renal failure" and "hip arthroplasty" or "hip surgery" which is provided in Online Supplementary Data 1. No language limitation was applied. A manual search for conceivably relevant studies using references of the included articles was also performed. This study was conducted by the Preferred Reporting Items for Systematic Reviews and Meta-Analysis (PRISMA) statement [41] and the Strengthening the Reporting of Observational Studies in Epidemiology (STROBE) [42].

### 2.2. Selection Criteria

Eligible studies must be clinical trials or observational studies (cohort, case-control, or cross-sectional studies) that reported incidence of AKI in patients undergoing THA. Included studies must provide the data to estimate incidence of AKI with 95% confidence intervals (CI). Retrieved articles were individually reviewed for eligibility by the two investigators (C.T. and W.C.). Discrepancies were addressed and solved by mutual consensus. Inclusion was not limited by the size of the study.

*2.3. Data Abstraction*

A structured data collecting form was used to obtain the following information from each study: title, name of the first author, year of the study, publication year, country where the study was conducted, definition of THA, AKI definition, incidence of AKI, and risk factors for AKI.

*2.4. Statistical Analysis*

Analyses were performed utilizing the Comprehensive Meta-Analysis 3.3 software (Biostat Inc, Englewood, NJ, USA). Adjusted point estimates from each study were consolidated by the generic inverse variance approach of DerSimonian and Laird, which designated the weight of each study based on its variance [43]. Given the possibility of between-study variance, we used a random-effect model rather than a fixed-effect model. Cochran's $Q$ test and $I^2$ statistic were applied to determine the between-study heterogeneity. A value of $I^2$ of 0% to 25% represents insignificant heterogeneity, 26% to 50% low heterogeneity, 51% to 75% moderate heterogeneity and 76%–100% high heterogeneity [44]. The presence of publication bias was assessed by the Egger test [45].

**3. Results**

A total of 410 potentially eligible articles were identified using our search strategy. After the exclusion of 162 articles based on title and abstract for clearly not fulfilling inclusion criteria on the basis of type of article, study design, population or outcome of interest, and 209 due to being duplicates, 39 articles were left for full-length review. 11 of them were excluded from the full-length review as they did not report the outcome of interest while 5 articles were excluded because they were not observational studies. Six studies [9–14] were subsequently excluded because they did not use standard AKI definitions of Risk, Injury, Failure, Loss of kidney function, and End-stage kidney disease (RIFLE), Acute Kidney Injury Network (AKIN), and Kidney Disease: Improving Global Outcomes (KDIGO) classifications. Thus, 17 cohort studies [18–33,37] comprising 24,158 patients undergoing THA were included into the meta-analysis of associated AKI incidence. The literature retrieval, review, and selection process are demonstrated in Figure 1. The characteristics of the included studies are presented in Table 1.

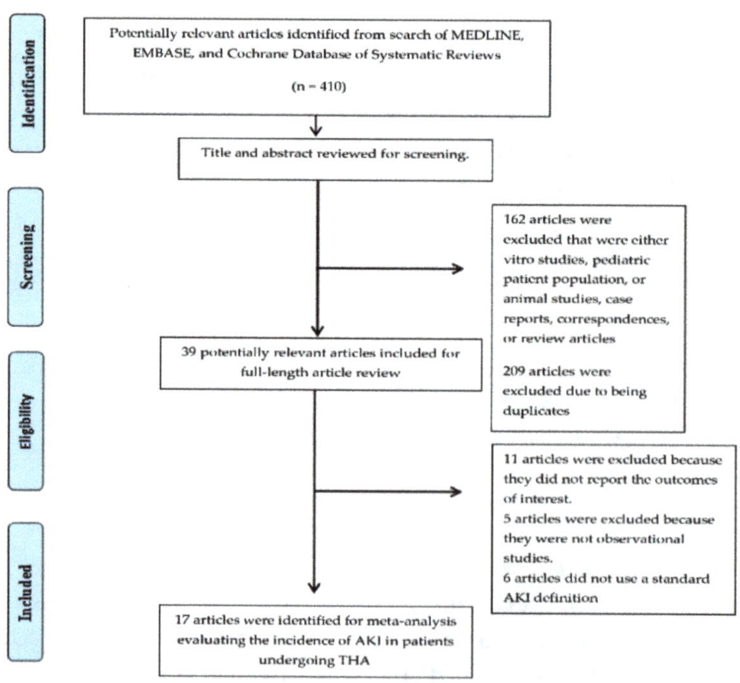


**Figure 1.** Outline of our search methodology.

**Table 1.** Main characteristic of studies included in meta-analysis of AKI incidence in patients undergoing THA [18–33].

| Study | Year | Country | Study Design | Procedures/Patients | Number of Patients | AKI Definition | Incidence |
|---|---|---|---|---|---|---|---|
| Ulucay et al. [18] | 2012 | Turkey | Cohort | Cemented bipolar hip arthroplasty for femur neck fracture; aged ≥65 years | 163 | Acute kidney injury; AKIN criteria | 25/163 (15.3%) Dialysis 3/163 (1.8%) |
| Choi et al. [1,19] | 2013 | South Korea | Cohort | Total hip replacement for avascular necrosis | 489 | Acute kidney injury; AKIN criteria | 47/489 (9.6%) |
| Challagunda et al. [20] | 2013 | UK | Cohort | Elective hip surgery | 112 | Acute kidney injury; RIFLE criteria | 33/112 (29.5%) |
| Craxford et al. [21] | 2014 | UK | Cohort | Total hip replacement | 200 | Acute kidney injury; RIFLE criteria | 7/200 (3.5%) |
| Li et al. [22] | 2014 | China | Cohort | Total hip replacement | 900 | Acute kidney injury; AKIN criteria | 93/900 (10.3%) |
| Kimmel et al. [23] | 2014 | Australia | Cohort | Primary elective total hip arthroplasty | 173 | Acute kidney injury; RIFLE criteria | 14/173 (8.1%) |
| Hassan et al. [37] | 2015 | Denmark | Cohort | Primary hip replacement | 586 | Acute kidney injury; RIFLE criteria | 81/586 (13.8%) |
| Warth et al. [24] | 2016 | USA | Cohort | Total hip arthroplasty | 488 | Acute kidney injury; AKIN criteria | 22/488 (4.5%) Dialysis 0/488 (0%) |
| Nowicka et al. [25] | 2016 | UK | Cohort | Elective hip arthroplasty | 156 | Acute kidney injury; AKIN criteria | 11/156 (7.1%) Dialysis 0/156 (0%) |
| Choi et al. [2,26] | 2016 | South Korea | Cohort | Total hip replacement | 2467 | Acute kidney injury; AKIN criteria | 119/2467 (4.8%) |
| Johansson et al. [27] | 2016 | Denmark | Cohort | Elective total hip replacement | 136 | Acute kidney injury; KDIGO criteria | 27/136 (19.9%) |
| Perregaard et al. [28] | 2016 | Denmark | Cohort | Primary elective total hip replacement | 3416 | Acute kidney injury; KDIGO criteria | 75/3416 (2.2%) |
| Ferguson et al. [29] | 2017 | UK | Cohort | Primary hip arthroplasty | 187 | Acute kidney injury; KDIGO criteria | 20/187 (10.7%) Dialysis 0/187 (0%) |
| Jiang et al. [30] | 2017 | USA | Cohort | Total hip arthroplasty | 411 | Acute kidney injury; RIFLE criteria | 30/411 (7.3%) |
| Gharaibeh et al. [31] | 2017 | USA | Cohort | Total hip arthroplasty | 10323 | Acute kidney injury; KDIGO criteria | 114/10323 (1.1%) |
| Weinstein et al. [32] | 2018 | USA | Cohort | Unilateral total hip arthroplasty with intraoperative controlled hypotension under neuraxial anesthesia | 2431 | Acute kidney injury; RIFLE or AKIN criteria | 45/2431 (1.9%) |
| Tucker et al. [33] | 2018 | UK | Cohort | Primary hip arthroplasty | 1420 | Acute kidney injury; AKIN criteria | 19/1420 (1.3%) |

Abbreviations: AKI, acute kidney injury; AKIN, Acute Kidney Injury Network;KDIGO, Kidney Disease Improving Global Outcomes; RIFLE, Risk, Injury, Failure, Loss of kidney function, and End-stage kidney disease; THA, total hip arthroplasties; UK, United Kingdom; USA, United States of America.

### 3.1. Incidence of AKI in Patients Undergoing THA

Overall, the pooled estimated incidence rates of AKI and severe AKI requiring dialysis following THA were 6.3% (95% CI: 3.8%–10.2%, $I^2$ = 97%, Figure 2A) and 0.5% (95% CI: 0.1%–2.3%, $I^2$ = 42%, Figure 2B), respectively. Subgroup analysis based on AKI definitions was performed and showed the pooled estimated incidence rates of AKI of 5.5% (95% CI: 1.3%–21.0%, $I^2$ = 98%) by RIFLE criteria, 8.4% (95% CI: 5.2%–13.3%, $I^2$ = 95%) by AKIN criteria, and 4.2% (95% CI: 1.9%–9.0%, $I^2$ = 96%) by KDIGO criteria, respectively. We conducted a sensitivity analysis by excluding with patients undergoing THA for hip fractures. The pooled estimated incidence rates of AKI following THA for non-fracture indications was 5.6% (95% CI: 3.3%–9.3%, $I^2$ = 97%). The pooled estimated incidence rates of AKI following THA among patients with fractures was 14.2% (95% CI: 11.8%–16.9%, $I^2$ = 0%).

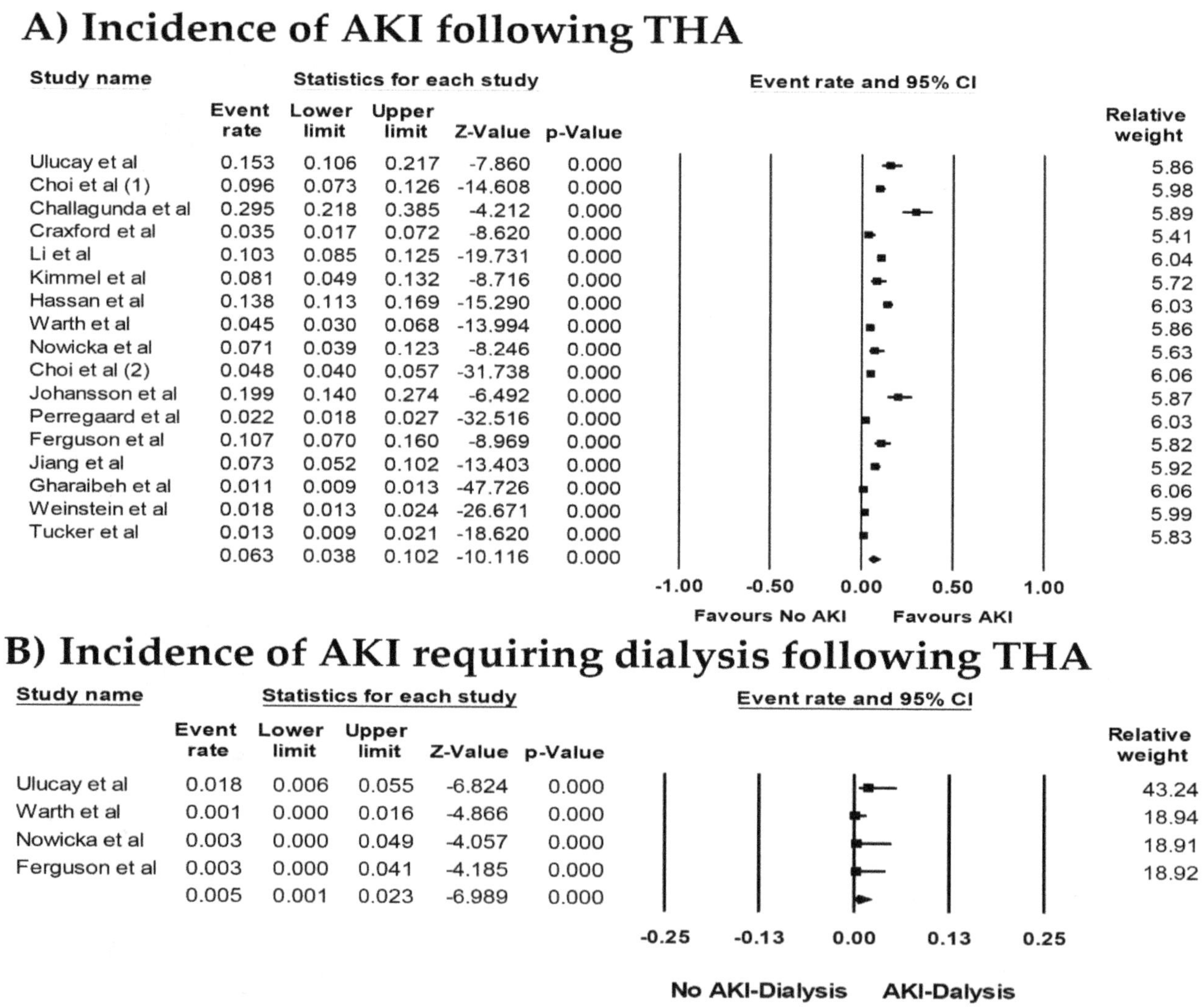


**Figure 2.** Forest plots of the included studies [18–33] assessing (**A**) incidence rates of AKI and (**B**) incidence rates of AKI requiring dialysis following THA. A diamond data marker represents the overall rate from each included study (square data marker) and 95% confidence interval (CI).

Subgroup analysis based on the countries by continent was performed and demonstrated pooled estimated incidence of AKI following THA of 9.2% (95% CI: 5.6%–14.8%) in Asia, 8.1% (95% CI: 4.9%–13.2%) in Australia, 7.4% (95% CI: 3.2%–16.3%) in Europe, and 2.8% (95% CI: 1.2%–17.0%) in North America.

Meta-regression of all included studies showed significant negative correlation between incidence of AKI following THA and the study year (slope = $-0.37$, $p$ <0.001), as shown in Figure 3.

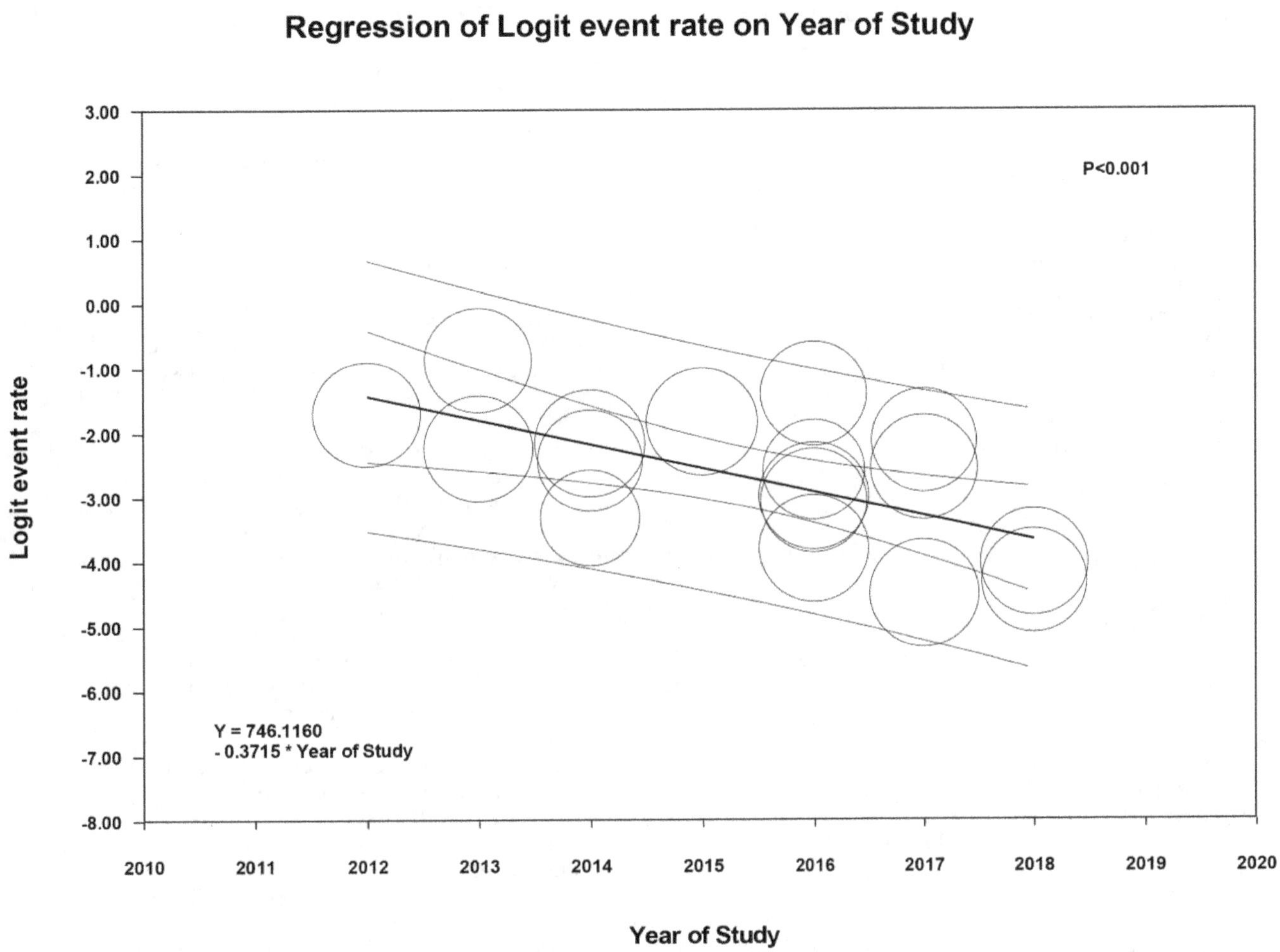


**Figure 3.** Meta-regression analyses showed significant negative correlation between incidence of AKI following THA and the study year (slope = −0.37, $p$ <0.001). The solid black line represents the weighted regression line based on variance-weighted least squares. The inner and outer lines show the 95% confidence interval and prediction interval around the regression line. The circles indicate log event rates in each study.

### *3.2. Risk Factors for AKI in Patients Undergoing THA*

Reported risk factors for AKI in patients undergoing THA are demonstrated in Table 2 [18–20,22–24,26,27,29–33,46–62]. Older age [23,24,26,29,31,55,60], higher body mass index (BMI) [19,22–24,26,30,31,46–49,56,57,59], reduced baseline estimated glomerular filtration rate (eGFR)/chronic kidney disease (CKD) [31,54,55,57,60], diabetes mellitus (DM) [24,26,31,34,47,55,57], nonsteroidal anti-inflammatory drug (NSAID) [23,32,53] use, and perioperative blood transfusion [23,47,53,55] were consistently identified as important risk factors for AKI in patients undergoing THA.

**Table 2.** Reported Risk Factors for AKI in patients undergoing THA [18–20,22–24,26,27,29–33,46–62].

| Study | Risk Factors for AKI |
|---|---|
| Jafari et al. [46] | Elevated BMI, elevated baseline creatinine, history of COPD, liver disease, CHF, hypertension, underlying heart disease |
| Weingarten et al. [47] | Elevated BMI, DM, the number of baseline antihypertensive medications, cerebral or peripheral vascular disease, the use of general anesthesia, perioperative blood transfusion |
| Ulucay et al. [18] | Lower baseline eGFR |
| Choi et al. [1,19] | Transplantation, increased weight |
| Li et al. [22] | Transplantation, increased weight |
| Challagundla et al. [20] | Male, ACEI/ARB |
| Nielson et al. [48] | Preoperative ACEI/ARB, BMI, CAD, intra-operative hypotension |
| Kimmel et al. [23] | Older age, increased BMI, lower baseline eGFR, NSAID use, ACEI/ARB use, blood transfusion |
| Ward et al. [49] | Increased BMI |
| Marty et al. [50] | Postoperative resistive index |
| Courtney et al. [51] | Dual antibiotics prophylaxis (cefazolin + vancomycin vs. cefazolin), ASA classification, preoperative kidney disease |
| Opperer et al. [52] | Perioperative fluid resuscitation with 6% HES or 5% albumin |
| Aeng et al. [53] | Gentamicin in premanufactured bone cement, intraoperative blood transfusion, postoperative NSAID use |
| Warth et al. [24] | Older age, elevated BMI, DM, smoking |
| Tan et al. [54] | CKD |
| Nadkarni et al. [55] | Older age, male sex, black race, CKD, CHF, chronic liver disease, hypertension, DM, atrial fibrillation, HCV infection, postoperative sepsis, acute MI, blood transfusion, urban hospital, small hospital size |
| Meller et al. [56] | Morbid obesity |
| Choi et al. [2,26] | Postoperative anemia, older age, male sex, BMI <22 or ≥25, DM, beta-blocker, ARB use |
| Ferguson et al. [29] | Older age, the use of ≥1 L of postoperative fluid |
| Johansson et al. [27] | Gentamicin, female sex |
| Geller et al. [57] | Higher BMI, lower baseline hemoglobin, history of comorbid condition (DM, CKD, CVD, hypertension) |
| Jiang et al. [30] | Perioperative ACEI/ARB use, vancomycin use, increased BMI |
| Zainudheen et al. [58] | Use of renin-angiotensin antagonists |
| Jamsa et al. [59] | Lower preoperative eGFR, ASA classification, BMI, duration of operation |
| Ghareibeh et al. [31] | Entire cohort: older age, male, CKD, heart failure, diabetes, hypertension<br>Nested case control: elevated BMI, heart failure, DM, hypertension, lower GFR, transfusion |
| Yadav et al. [60] | Older age, surgery for periprosthetic joint infection, CKD, total number of surgeries |
| Weinstein et al. [32] | Lower baseline GFR, lower baseline hemoglobin, previous NSAID use |
| Tucker et al. [33] | Gentamicin use |
| Klement et al. [61] | Co-occurrence of a mental illness and a substance abuse disorder |
| Abar et al. [62] | Elevated preoperative creatinine, larger postoperative drop in hemoglobin, and higher ASA classification |
| Hassan et al. [37] | Older age, hypertension, general anesthesia, high ASA score, low baseline systolic and diastolic blood pressure, hip fracture |
| Dubrovskaya et al. [34] | Hospital stay >1 day prior to surgery, knee or hip surgery, DM |
| Bailey et al. [38] | Prophylactic use of flucloxacillin and gentamicin versus cefuroxime alone |

Abbreviations: ACEI/ARB, angiotensin-converting enzyme inhibitor/angiotensin II receptor blockers; AKI, acute kidney injury; ASA, American Society of Anesthesiologists; BMI, body mass index; CAD, coronary artery disease; CHF, congestive heart failure; CKD, chronic kidney disease; COPD, chronic obstructive pulmonary disease; CVD, cardiovascular disease; DM, diabetes mellitus; eGFR, estimated glomerular filtration rate; HCV, hepatitis C virus; NSAID, nonsteroidal anti-inflammatory drug; THA, total hip arthroplasties.

### 3.3. *Evaluation for Publication Bias*

Funnel plot (Supplementary Figure S1) and Egger's regression asymmetry test were performed to evaluate for publication bias in analysis evaluating incidence of AKI in patients undergoing THA. There was no significant publication bias in meta-analysis assessing incidence of AKI in patients undergoing THA, $p = 0.20$.

## 4. Discussion

In this systematic review and meta-analysis, we found that patients who underwent THA had incidences of AKI (using a standard AKI definition) and AKI requiring dialysis of 6.3% and 0.5%, respectively. In addition, our findings showed a statistically significant negative correlation between incidence of AKI following THA and the study year, representing potential improvement in the AKI incidence for patients undergoing THA over time.

Similar to other types of perioperative AKI, the pathogenesis of THA-related AKI is multifactorial including intraoperative hypotension, perioperative anemia and blood transfusion, antibiotic-related AKI, and nephrotoxic agents such as NSAID use [18–20,22–24,26,27,29–33,46–62]. Our study demonstrated an overall low incidence of AKI following THA of 6.3%, and comparatively much lower than AKI incidence following other types of major surgeries such as coronary artery bypass grafting (AKI incidence approximately 20%) [63,64], vascular surgery (AKI incidence approximately 25%) [35,65], or heart valve replacement surgery (AKI incidence approximately 35% to 47%) [66]. In addition, the majority of AKI following THA is mild in severity [18–33] and only 0.5% of patients undergoing THA developed severe AKI requiring dialysis, as demonstrated by our meta-analysis. Despite the low incidence of AKI among patients undergoing THA, those who develop AKI following THA still carry significant increased mortality and worse outcomes including prolonged hospital stay [39,46,67,68] and hospital readmissions after THA [69,70]. In addition, it is now evident that even mild AKI is still associated with poor long-term outcomes including development of cardiovascular diseases and CKD [71,72]. Thus, perioperative medicine remains critically important in patients undergoing THA in order to prevent perioperative AKI [73].

Our study also showed a potential improvement in the AKI incidence following THA over time. This is likely explained by advances in perioperative medicine care [73]. As described earlier in this systematic review, the pathogenesis of AKI in patients undergoing THA is multifactorial. Risk factors for AKI following THA are summarized in Table 2. Since older age, higher BMI, CKD, DM were consistently identified as important risk factors for AKI in patients undergoing THA [18–20,22–24,26,27,29–33,46–62], clinicians and nephrologists should pay close attention to particular populations of patients. Limitation of nephrotoxic agents such as NSAIDs and a judicious use of perioperative blood transfusion should be considered [23,47,53,55] for preventive measures to reduce AKI following THA. In patients undergoing THA, recent studies have demonstrated significant avoidance of NSAID use in those possessing higher AKI risk, such as patients with CKD and congestive heart failure (CHF) [29,31]. In addition, in recent years, the use of hydroxyethyl starch (HES) solutions, unnecessary blood transfusions, chloride-rich intravenous fluids, and aminoglycosides have been discouraged [29,52,73]. Furthermore, although the use of angiotensin-converting enzyme inhibitors/angiotensin receptor blockers (ACEI/ARB) and perioperative AKI risk remains controversial [2,74,75], ACEIs/ARBs have been commonly discontinued before THA to prevent intraoperative hypotension [29]. Future studies are required to assess if discontinuation of ACEIs/ARBs before THA may affect the incidence of THA-associated AKI, and whether it should be included in AKI preventative strategies and care optimization among patients undergoing THA [37,40].

Several limitations in our meta-analysis are worth mentioning. First, there are statistical heterogeneities in our study. Possible sources for heterogeneities were the differences in patient characteristics between the individual studies. Studies involving large sample size observed lower AKI incidence compared to those with small sample size. Studies outside USA observed higher AKI incidence following THA, suggesting potential differences in operative surgery, antibiotic and blood transfusion, and perioperative care. Subgroup analysis based on the countries by continent demonstrated significantly different AKI incidences in each continent. Furthermore, the meta-regression analysis that demonstrated a significant negative correlation of post-THA AKI incidence with time adds the contribution of study year as a source of heterogeneity in our study. Second, there was limited data on the AKI incidence following THA from countries in South America and Africa. Third, there is a lack of data from the included studies on novel AKI biomarkers and

AKI diagnosis based on urine output criteria. Lastly, this is a systematic review and meta-analysis of cohort studies and the data from population based studies were limited. Thus, future population based studies evaluating the incidence of AKI following THA are required.

In summary, there is an overall low incidence of AKI of 6.3% among patients undergoing THA. There has also been potential improvement in AKI incidence for patients undergoing THA over time.

**Author Contributions:** Conceptualization, C.T., W.K., N.T., W.C.; Data curation, C.T., W.K., W.C.; Formal analysis, C.T., W.C.; Funding acquisition, C.T. and K.W.; Investigation, C.T., W.K., W.C.; Methodology, C.T., W.K., N.T., W.C.; Project administration, K.W., P.L., S.A.S., P.U., A.T.-O., N.R.A.; Resources, K.W.; Software, K.W.; Supervision, M.A.M. and W.C.; Validation, C.T. and W.C.; Writing—original draft, C.T.; Writing—review & editing, C.T., W.K., N.T., T.B., K.W., P.L., S.A.S., P.U., N.R.A., A.T.-O., M.A.M., W.C.

**Acknowledgments:** None. All authors had access to the data and played essential roles in writing of the manuscript.

## References

1. Thongprayoon, C.; Cheungpasitporn, W.; Harrison, A.M.; Kittanamongkolchai, W.; Ungprasert, P.; Srivali, N.; Akhoundi, A.; Kashani, K.B. The comparison of the commonly used surrogates for baseline renal function in acute kidney injury diagnosis and staging. *BMC Nephrol.* **2016**, *17*, 6. [CrossRef] [PubMed]
2. Cheungpasitporn, W.; Thongprayoon, C.; Srivali, N.; O'corragain, O.A.; Edmonds, P.J.; Ungprasert, P.; Kittanamongkolchai, W.; Erickson, S.B. Preoperative renin-angiotensin system inhibitors use linked to reduced acute kidney injury: A systematic review and meta-analysis. *Nephrol. Dial. Transplant.* **2015**, *30*, 978–988. [CrossRef] [PubMed]
3. Hoste, E.A.; Kellum, J.A.; Selby, N.M.; Zarbock, A.; Palevsky, P.M.; Bagshaw, S.M.; Goldstein, S.L.; Cerdá, J.; Chawla, L.S. Global epidemiology and outcomes of acute kidney injury. *Nat. Rev. Nephrol.* **2018**, *14*, 607–625. [CrossRef] [PubMed]
4. Gameiro, J.; Agapito Fonseca, J.; Jorge, S.; Lopes, J.A. Acute Kidney Injury Definition and Diagnosis: A Narrative Review. *J. Clin. Med.* **2018**, *7*, 307. [CrossRef]
5. Sehgal, V.; Bajwa, S.J.; Sehgal, R.; Eagan, J.; Reddy, P.; Lesko, S.M. Predictors of acute kidney injury in geriatric patients undergoing total knee replacement surgery. *Int. J. Endocrinol. Metab.* **2014**, *12*, e16713. [CrossRef] [PubMed]
6. Kim, H.J.; Koh, W.U.; Kim, S.G.; Park, H.S.; Song, J.G.; Ro, Y.J.; Yang, H.S. Early postoperative albumin level following total knee arthroplasty is associated with acute kidney injury: A retrospective analysis of 1309 consecutive patients based on kidney disease improving global outcomes criteria. *Medicine* **2016**, *95*, e4489. [CrossRef] [PubMed]
7. Mehta, R.L.; Burdmann, E.A.; Cerdá, J.; Feehally, J.; Finkelstein, F.; García-García, G.; Godin, M.; Jha, V.; Lameire, N.H.; Levin, N.W.; et al. Recognition and management of acute kidney injury in the International Society of Nephrology 0by25 Global Snapshot: A multinational cross-sectional study. *Lancet* **2016**, *387*, 2017–2025. [CrossRef]
8. Mehta, R.L.; Cerdá, J.; Burdmann, E.A.; Tonelli, M.; García-García, G.; Jha, V.; Susantitaphong, P.; Rocco, M.; Vanholder, R.; Sever, M.S.; et al. International Society of Nephrology's 0by25 initiative for acute kidney injury (zero preventable deaths by 2025): A human rights case for nephrology. *Lancet* **2015**, *385*, 2616–2643. [CrossRef]
9. Coventry, M.B.; Beckenbaugh, R.D.; Nolan, D.R.; Ilstrup, D.M. 2012 total hip arthroplasties. A study of postoperative course and early complications. *J. Bone Joint Surg. Am.* **1974**, *56*, 273–284. [CrossRef]
10. Sharrock, N.E.; Beksac, B.; Flynn, E.; Go, G.; Della Valle, A.G. Hypotensive epidural anaesthesia in patients with preoperative renal dysfunction undergoing total hip replacement. *Br. J. Anaesth.* **2006**, *96*, 207–212. [CrossRef]
11. Jameson, S.S.; Khan, S.K.; Baker, P.; James, P.; Gray, A.; Reed, M.R.; Deehan, D.J. A national analysis of complications following hemiarthroplasty for hip fracture in older patients. *QJM* **2012**, *105*, 455–460. [CrossRef] [PubMed]

12. Horstmann, W.G.; Swierstra, M.J.; Ohanis, D.; Castelein, R.M.; Kollen, B.J.; Verheyen, C.C. Reduction of blood loss with the use of a new combined intra-operative and post-operative autologous blood transfusion system compared with no drainage in primary total hip replacement. *Bone Joint J.* **2013**, *95-B*, 616–622. [CrossRef] [PubMed]
13. Regenbogen, S.E.; Cain-Nielsen, A.H.; Norton, E.C.; Chen, L.M.; Birkmeyer, J.D.; Skinner, J.S. Costs and Consequences of Early Hospital Discharge After Major Inpatient Surgery in Older Adults. *JAMA Surg.* **2017**, *152*, e170123. [CrossRef] [PubMed]
14. Frenkel Rutenberg, T.; Daglan, E.; Heller, S.; Velkes, S. A comparison of treatment setting for elderly patients with hip fracture, is the geriatric ward superior to conventional orthopedic hospitalization? *Injury* **2017**, *48*, 1584–1588. [CrossRef] [PubMed]
15. Pulido, L.; Parvizi, J.; Macgibeny, M.; Sharkey, P.F.; Purtill, J.J.; Rothman, R.H.; Hozack, W.J. In hospital complications after total joint arthroplasty. *J. Arthroplast.* **2008**, *23* (Suppl. 1), 139–145. [CrossRef] [PubMed]
16. McDermott, K.W.; Freeman, W.J.; Elixhauser, A. Overview of Operating Room Procedures During Inpatient Stays in U.S. Hospitals, 2014: Statistical Brief #233. 2006. Available online: https://www.hcup-us.ahrq.gov/reports/statbriefs/sb233-Operating-Room-Procedures-United-States-2014.pdf (accessed on 9 January 2019).
17. Abdel, M.P.; Watts, C.D.; Houdek, M.T.; Lewallen, D.G.; Berry, D.J. Epidemiology of periprosthetic fracture of the femur in 32 644 primary total hip arthroplasties: A 40-year experience. *Bone Joint J.* **2016**, *98-B*, 461–467. [CrossRef] [PubMed]
18. Ulucay, C.; Eren, Z.; Kaspar, E.C.; Ozler, T.; Yuksel, K.; Kantarci, G.; Altintas, F. Risk factors for acute kidney injury after hip fracture surgery in the elderly individuals. *Geriatr. Orthop. Surg. Rehabil.* **2012**, *3*, 150–156. [CrossRef] [PubMed]
19. Choi, Y.J.; Lee, E.H.; Hahm, K.D.; Kwon, K.; Ro, Y.J. Transplantation is a risk factor for acute kidney injury in patients undergoing total hip replacement arthroplasty for avascular necrosis: An observational study. *Transplant. Proc.* **2013**, *45*, 2220–2225. [CrossRef]
20. Challagundla, S.R.; Knox, D.; Hawkins, A.; Hamilton, D.; WVFlynn, R.; Robertson, S.; Isles, C. Renal impairment after high-dose flucloxacillin and single-dose gentamicin prophylaxis in patients undergoing elective hip and knee replacement. *Nephrol. Dial. Transplant.* **2013**, *28*, 612–619. [CrossRef]
21. Craxford, S.; Bayley, E.; Needoff, M. Antibiotic-associated complications following lower limb arthroplasty: A comparison of two prophylactic regimes. *Eur. J. Orthop. Surg. Traumatol.* **2014**, *24*, 539–543. [CrossRef]
22. Li, X.; Guo, D.; Shi, G.; Li, R.; Li, X.; Shen, R.; Wang, H.; Li, Y.; Yuan, F.; Han, G. Role of total hip replacement arthroplasty between transplantation and acute kidney injury. *Ren. Fail.* **2014**, *36*, 899–903. [CrossRef]
23. Kimmel, L.A.; Wilson, S.; Janardan, J.D.; Liew, S.M.; Walker, R.G. Incidence of acute kidney injury following total joint arthroplasty: A retrospective review by RIFLE criteria. *Clin. Kidney J.* **2014**, *7*, 546–551. [CrossRef]
24. Warth, L.C.; Noiseux, N.O.; Hogue, M.H.; Klaassen, A.L.; Liu, S.S.; Callaghan, J.J. Risk of Acute Kidney Injury After Primary and Revision Total Hip Arthroplasty and Total Knee Arthroplasty Using a Multimodal Approach to Perioperative Pain Control Including Ketorolac and Celecoxib. *J. Arthroplast.* **2016**, *31*, 253–255. [CrossRef] [PubMed]
25. Nowicka, A.; Selvaraj, T. Incidence of acute kidney injury after elective lower limb arthroplasty. *J. Clin. Anesth.* **2016**, *34*, 520–523. [CrossRef] [PubMed]
26. Choi, Y.J.; Kim, S.O.; Sim, J.H.; Hahm, K.D. Postoperative Anemia Is Associated with Acute Kidney Injury in Patients Undergoing Total Hip Replacement Arthroplasty: A Retrospective Study. *Anesth. Analg.* **2016**, *122*, 1923–1928. [CrossRef] [PubMed]
27. Johansson, S.; Christensen, O.M.; Thorsmark, A.H. A retrospective study of acute kidney injury in hip arthroplasty patients receiving gentamicin and dicloxacillin. *Acta Orthop.* **2016**, *87*, 589–591. [CrossRef] [PubMed]
28. Perregaard, H.; Damholt, M.B.; Solgaard, S.; Petersen, M.B. Renal function after elective total hip replacement. *Acta Orthop.* **2016**, *87*, 235–238. [CrossRef]
29. Ferguson, K.B.; Winter, A.; Russo, L.; Khan, A.; Hair, M.; MacGregor, M.S.; Holt, G. Acute kidney injury following primary hip and knee arthroplasty surgery. *Ann. R. Coll. Surg. Engl.* **2017**, *99*, 307–312. [CrossRef] [PubMed]
30. Jiang, E.X.; Gogineni, H.C.; Mayerson, J.L.; Glassman, A.H.; Magnussen, R.A.; Scharschmidt, T.J. Acute Kidney Disease After Total Hip and Knee Arthroplasty: Incidence and Associated Factors. *J. Arthroplast.* **2017**, *32*, 2381–2385. [CrossRef]

31. Gharaibeh, K.A.; Hamadah, A.M.; Sierra, R.J.; Leung, N.; Kremers, W.K.; El-Zoghby, Z.M. The Rate of Acute Kidney Injury After Total Hip Arthroplasty Is Low but Increases Significantly in Patients with Specific Comorbidities. *J. Bone Joint Surg. Am.* **2017**, *99*, 1819–1826.
32. Weinstein, S.M.; YaDeau, J.T.; Memtsoudis, S.G. Lack of Association Between Levels and Length of Intraoperative Controlled Hypotension and Acute Kidney Injury in Total Hip Arthroplasty Patients Receiving Neuraxial Anesthesia. *Reg. Anesth. Pain Med.* **2018**, *43*, 725–731. [CrossRef] [PubMed]
33. Tucker, A.; Hegarty, P.; Magill, P.J.; Blaney, J.; Armstrong, L.V.; McCaffrey, J.E.; Beverland, D.E. Acute Kidney Injury After Prophylactic Cefuroxime and Gentamicin in Patients Undergoing Primary Hip and Knee Arthroplasty-A Propensity Score-Matched Study. *J. Arthroplast.* **2018**, *33*, 3009–3015. [CrossRef] [PubMed]
34. Dubrovskaya, Y.; Tejada, R.; Bosco, I.I.I.J.; Stachel, A.; Chen, D.; Feng, M.; Rosenberg, A.; Phillips, M. Single high dose gentamicin for perioperative prophylaxis in orthopedic surgery: Evaluation of nephrotoxicity. *SAGE Open Med.* **2015**, *3*. [CrossRef] [PubMed]
35. Bell, S.; Davey, P.; Nathwani, D.; Marwick, C.; Vadiveloo, T.; Sneddon, J.; Patton, A.; Bennie, M.; Fleming, S.; Donnan, P.T. Risk of AKI with gentamicin as surgical prophylaxis. *J. Am. Soc. Nephrol.* **2014**, *25*, 2625–2632. [CrossRef] [PubMed]
36. Ross, A.D.; Boscainos, P.J.; Malhas, A.; Wigderowitz, C. Peri-operative renal morbidity secondary to gentamicin and flucloxacillin chemoprophylaxis for hip and knee arthroplasty. *Scott. Med. J.* **2013**, *58*, 209–212. [CrossRef] [PubMed]
37. Hassan, B.K.; Sahlstrom, A.; Dessau, R.B. Risk factors for renal dysfunction after total hip joint replacement; a retrospective cohort study. *J. Orthop. Surg. Res.* **2015**, *10*, 158. [CrossRef] [PubMed]
38. Bailey, O.; Torkington, M.S.; Anthony, I.; Wells, J.; Blyth, M.; Jones, B. Antibiotic-related acute kidney injury in patients undergoing elective joint replacement. *Bone Joint J.* **2014**, *96-B*, 395–398. [CrossRef]
39. Bennet, S.J.; Berry, O.M.; Goddard, J.; Keating, J.F. Acute renal dysfunction following hip fracture. *Injury* **2010**, *41*, 335–338. [CrossRef]
40. Bjerregaard, L.S.; Jorgensen, C.C.; Kehlet, H. Serious renal and urological complications in fast-track primary total hip and knee arthroplasty; a detailed observational cohort study. *Minerva Anestesiol.* **2016**, *82*, 757–776.
41. Moher, D.; Liberati, A.; Tetzlaff, J.; Altman, D.G. Preferred reporting items for systematic reviews and meta-analyses: The PRISMA statement. *PLoS Med.* **2009**, *6*, e1000097. [CrossRef]
42. Von Elm, E.; Altman, D.G.; Egger, M.; Pocock, S.J.; Gotzsche, P.C.; Vandenbroucke, J.P. The Strengthening the Reporting of Observational Studies in Epidemiology (STROBE) statement: Guidelines for reporting observational studies. *PLoS Med.* **2007**, *4*, e296. [CrossRef] [PubMed]
43. DerSimonian, R.; Laird, N. Meta-analysis in clinical trials. *Control. Clin. Trials* **1986**, *7*, 177–188. [CrossRef]
44. Higgins, J.P.; Thompson, S.G.; Deeks, J.J.; Altman, D.G. Measuring inconsistency in meta-analyses. *BMJ* **2003**, *327*, 557–560. [CrossRef] [PubMed]
45. Easterbrook, P.J.; Berlin, J.A.; Gopalan, R.; Matthews, D.R. Publication bias in clinical research. *Lancet* **1991**, *337*, 867–872. [CrossRef]
46. Jafari, S.M.; Huang, R.; Joshi, A.; Parvizi, J.; Hozack, W.J. Renal impairment following total joint arthroplasty: Who is at risk? *J. Arthroplast.* **2010**, *25*, 49–53. [CrossRef] [PubMed]
47. Weingarten, T.N.; Gurrieri, C.; Jarett, P.D.; Brown, D.R.; Berntson, N.J.; Calaro, R.D., Jr.; Kor, D.J.; Berry, D.J.; Garovic, V.D.; Nicholson, W.T.; et al. Acute kidney injury following total joint arthroplasty: Retrospective analysis. *Can. J. Anaesth.* **2012**, *59*, 1111–1118. [CrossRef] [PubMed]
48. Nielson, E.; Hennrikus, E.; Lehman, E.; Mets, B. Angiotensin axis blockade, hypotension, and acute kidney injury in elective major orthopedic surgery. *J. Hosp. Med.* **2014**, *9*, 283–288. [CrossRef]
49. Ward, D.T.; Metz, L.N.; Horst, P.K.; Kim, H.T.; Kuo, A.C. Complications of Morbid Obesity in Total Joint Arthroplasty: Risk Stratification Based on BMI. *J. Arthroplast.* **2015**, *30*, 42–46. [CrossRef]
50. Marty, P.; Szatjnic, S.; Ferre, F.; Conil, J.M.; Mayeur, N.; Fourcade, O.; Silva, S.; Minville, V. Doppler renal resistive index for early detection of acute kidney injury after major orthopaedic surgery: A prospective observational study. *Eur. J. Anaesthesiol.* **2015**, *32*, 37–43. [CrossRef]
51. Courtney, P.M.; Melnic, C.M.; Zimmer, Z.; Anari, J.; Lee, G.C. Addition of Vancomycin to Cefazolin Prophylaxis Is Associated With Acute Kidney Injury After Primary Joint Arthroplasty. *Clin. Orthop. Relat. Res.* **2015**, *473*, 2197–2203. [CrossRef]

52. Opperer, M.; Poeran, J.; Rasul, R.; Mazumdar, M.; Memtsoudis, S.G. Use of perioperative hydroxyethyl starch 6% and albumin 5% in elective joint arthroplasty and association with adverse outcomes: A retrospective population based analysis. *BMJ* **2015**, *350*, h1567. [CrossRef] [PubMed]
53. Aeng, E.S.; Shalansky, K.F.; Lau, T.T.; Zalunardo, N.; Li, G.; Bowie, W.R.; Duncan, C.P. Acute Kidney Injury With Tobramycin-Impregnated Bone Cement Spacers in Prosthetic Joint Infections. *Ann. Pharmacother.* **2015**, *49*, 1207–1213. [CrossRef] [PubMed]
54. Tan, T.L.; Kheir, M.M.; Tan, D.D.; Filippone, E.J.; Tischler, E.H.; Chen, A.F. Chronic Kidney Disease Linearly Predicts Outcomes After Elective Total Joint Arthroplasty. *J. Arthroplast.* **2016**, *31*, 175–179. [CrossRef]
55. Nadkarni, G.N.; Patel, A.A.; Ahuja, Y.; Annapureddy, N.; Agarwal, S.K.; Simoes, P.K.; Konstantinidis, I.; Kamat, S.; Archdeacon, M.; Thakar, C.V. Incidence, Risk Factors, and Outcome Trends of Acute Kidney Injury in Elective Total Hip and Knee Arthroplasty. *Am. J. Orthop.* **2016**, *45*, E12–E19. [PubMed]
56. Meller, M.M.; Toossi, N.; Gonzalez, M.H.; Son, M.S.; Lau, E.C.; Johanson, N. Surgical Risks and Costs of Care are Greater in Patients Who Are Super Obese and Undergoing THA. *Clin. Orthop. Relat. Res.* **2016**, *474*, 2472–2481. [CrossRef]
57. Geller, J.A.; Cunn, G.; Herschmiller, T.; Murtaugh, T.; Chen, A. Acute Kidney Injury After First-Stage Joint Revision for Infection: Risk Factors and the Impact of Antibiotic Dosing. *J. Arthroplast.* **2017**, *32*, 3120–3125. [CrossRef]
58. Zainudheen, A.; Scott, I.A.; Caney, X. Association of renin angiotensin antagonists with adverse perioperative events in patients undergoing elective orthopaedic surgery: A case-control study. *Intern. Med. J.* **2017**, *47*, 999–1005. [CrossRef]
59. Jamsa, P.; Jamsen, E.; Lyytikainen, L.P.; Kalliovalkama, J.; Eskelinen, A.; Oksala, N. Risk factors associated with acute kidney injury in a cohort of 20,575 arthroplasty patients. *Acta Orthop.* **2017**, *88*, 370–376. [CrossRef]
60. Yadav, A.; Alijanipour, P.; Ackerman, C.T.; Karanth, S.; Hozack, W.J.; Filippone, E.J. Acute Kidney Injury Following Failed Total Hip and Knee Arthroplasty. *J. Arthroplast.* **2018**, *33*, 3297–3303. [CrossRef]
61. Klement, M.R.; Nickel, B.T.; Bala, A.; Penrose, C.T.; Green, C.L.; Wellman, S.S.; Bolognesi, M.P.; Seyler, T.M. Dual Diagnosis and Total Hip Arthroplasty. *Orthopedics* **2018**, *41*, e321–e327. [CrossRef]
62. Abar, O.; Toossi, N.; Johanson, N. Cost and determinants of acute kidney injury after elective primary total joint arthroplasty. *Arthroplast. Today.* **2018**, *4*, 335–339. [CrossRef] [PubMed]
63. Cheungpasitporn, W.; Thongprayoon, C.; Kittanamongkolchai, W.; Srivali, N.; O'Corragain, O.A.; Edmonds, P.J.; Ratanapo, S.; Spanuchart, I.; Erickson, S.B. Comparison of renal outcomes in off-pump versus on-pump coronary artery bypass grafting: A systematic review and meta-analysis of randomized controlled trials. *Nephrology* **2015**, *20*, 727–735. [CrossRef] [PubMed]
64. Sakhuja, A.; Kashani, K.; Schold, J.; Cheungpasitporn, W.; Soltesz, E.; Demirjian, S. Hospital procedure volume does not predict acute kidney injury after coronary artery bypass grafting-a nationwide study. *Clin. Kidney J.* **2017**, *10*, 769–775. [CrossRef] [PubMed]
65. Cheungpasitporn, W.; Thongprayoon, C.; Kashani, K. Transcatheter Aortic Valve Replacement: A Kidney's Perspective. *J. Ren. Inj. Prev.* **2016**, *5*, 1–7. [CrossRef] [PubMed]
66. Thongprayoon, C.; Cheungpasitporn, W.; Lin, J.; Mao, M.A.; Qian, Q. Acute kidney injury in octogenarians after heart valve replacement surgery: A study of two periods over the last decade. *Clin. Kidney J.* **2017**, *10*, 648–654. [CrossRef] [PubMed]
67. Napier, R.J.; Spence, D.; Diamond, O.; O'Brien, S.; Walsh, T.; Beverland, D.E. Modifiable factors delaying early discharge following primary joint arthroplasty. *Eur. J. Orthop. Surg. Traumatol.* **2013**, *23*, 665–669. [CrossRef] [PubMed]
68. Panteli, M.; Habeeb, S.; McRoberts, J.; Porteous, M.J. Enhanced care for primary hip arthroplasty: Factors affecting length of hospital stay. *Eur. J. Orthop. Surg. Traumatol.* **2014**, *24*, 353–358. [CrossRef] [PubMed]
69. Schairer, W.W.; Vail, T.P.; Bozic, K.J. What are the rates and causes of hospital readmission after total knee arthroplasty? *Clin. Orthop. Relat. Res.* **2014**, *472*, 181–187. [CrossRef] [PubMed]
70. Pugely, A.J.; Callaghan, J.J.; Martin, C.T.; Cram, P.; Gao, Y. Incidence of and risk factors for 30-day readmission following elective primary total joint arthroplasty: Analysis from the ACS-NSQIP. *J. Arthroplast.* **2013**, *28*, 1499–1504. [CrossRef]

71. Coca, S.G.; Yusuf, B.; Shlipak, M.G.; Garg, A.X.; Parikh, C.R. Long-term risk of mortality and other adverse outcomes after acute kidney injury: A systematic review and meta-analysis. *Am. J. Kidney Dis.* **2009**, *53*, 961–973. [CrossRef]
72. Murugan, R.; Kellum, J.A. Acute kidney injury: what's the prognosis? *Nat. Rev. Nephrol.* **2011**, *7*, 209–217. [CrossRef] [PubMed]
73. Goren, O.; Matot, I. Perioperative acute kidney injury. *Br. J. Anaesth.* **2015**, *115* (Suppl. 2), ii3–ii14. [CrossRef] [PubMed]
74. Xu, N.; Long, Q.; He, T.; Liu, X.; Dai, H.; Lu, Y.; Wen, J.; Wu, Q.; Yuan, H. Association between preoperative renin-angiotensin system inhibitor use and postoperative acute kidney injury risk in patients with hypertension. *Clin. Nephrol.* **2018**, *89*, 403–414. [CrossRef] [PubMed]
75. Tagawa, M.; Ogata, A.; Hamano, T. Pre- and/or Intra-Operative Prescription of Diuretics, but Not Renin-Angiotensin-System Inhibitors, Is Significantly Associated with Acute Kidney Injury after Non-Cardiac Surgery: A Retrospective Cohort Study. *PLoS ONE* **2015**, *10*, e0132507. [CrossRef] [PubMed]

17

# Why Have Detection, Understanding and Management of Kidney Hypoxic Injury Lagged behind Those for the Heart?

**Zaid Abassi [1,2,*], Seymour Rosen [3], Simon Lamothe [3] and Samuel N. Heyman [4]**

1 Department of Physiology, Ruth & Bruce Rappaport Faculty of Medicine, Technion-IIT, Haifa 31096, Israel
2 Department of Laboratory Medicine, Rambam Health Care Campus, Haifa 31096, Israel
3 Department of Pathology, Beth Israel Deaconess Medical Center and Harvard Medical School, Boston, MA 02215, USA; srosen@bidmc.harvard.edu (S.R.); slamoth1@bidmc.harvard.edu (S.L.)
4 Department of Medicine, Hadassah Hebrew University Hospital, Mt. Scopus, Jerusalem 91240, Israel; heyman@cc.huji.ac.il
* Correspondence: abassi@tx.technion.ac.il

**Abstract:** The outcome of patients with acute myocardial infarction (AMI) has dramatically improved over recent decades, thanks to early detection and prompt interventions to restore coronary blood flow. In contrast, the prognosis of patients with hypoxic acute kidney injury (AKI) remained unchanged over the years. Delayed diagnosis of AKI is a major reason for this discrepancy, reflecting the lack of symptoms and diagnostic tools indicating at real time altered renal microcirculation, oxygenation, functional derangement and tissue injury. New tools addressing these deficiencies, such as biomarkers of tissue damage are yet far less distinctive than myocardial biomarkers and advanced functional renal imaging technologies are non-available in the clinical practice. Moreover, our understanding of pathogenic mechanisms likely suffers from conceptual errors, generated by the extensive use of the wrong animal model, namely warm ischemia and reperfusion. This model parallels mechanistically type I AMI, which properly represents the rare conditions leading to renal infarcts, whereas common scenarios leading to hypoxic AKI parallel physiologically type II AMI, with tissue hypoxic damage generated by altered oxygen supply/demand equilibrium. Better understanding the pathogenesis of hypoxic AKI and its management requires a more extensive use of models of type II-rather than type I hypoxic AKI.

**Keywords:** acute kidney injury; myocardial infarction; ischemia; biomarkers; management; diversity outcome

---

## 1. Introduction

Despite the high incidence of acute kidney injury (AKI) and its association with an alarming increase in morbidity and mortality, the therapeutic approaches for AKI are still disappointing and rely mainly on supportive measures [1,2]. This deficiency stems from the poor understanding of the pathogenesis of AKI and due to the delayed detection of AKI, as this syndrome is often asymptomatic during its early stages. Concerning the latter, the diagnosis of AKI is challenging since it mainly relies on serum creatinine (Scr), which suffers from major limitations as reliable biomarker for measurement of kidney function [3]. Specifically, in the setting of AKI, the time relationship between changes in SCr and concomitant changes in GFR does not allow accurate estimation regarding timing and reversibility of renal injury and the severity of kidney dysfunction, thus delaying diagnosis and intervention [3].

As opposed to the lack of breakthroughs in the diagnosis and management of AKI, great leaps took place in the setup of acute myocardial infarction (AMI). Mortality following AMI declined dramatically over the last 40 years and post-MI morbidity and mortality improved substantially, thanks to the early detection of evolving myocardial hypoxic injury and the achievement of myocardial salvage by the prompt restoration of coronary blood flow, first with early thrombolysis, and later with immediate or delayed coronary interventions and surgery. Currently, early mortality among patients treated for acute ST-elevation MI (STEMI) is about 4%, some 80% lower than a few decades ago, underscoring the importance of early detection of AMI and of prompt intervention to restore regional blood flow.

Renal parenchymal hypoxia plays a pivotal role in various conditions leading to AKI, and a major clinical challenge is its early detection and the differentiation between hypoxic injury and other factors leading to AKI.

The aim of this review is to compare the clinical tools available for the timely detection of incipient or evolving acute hypoxic organ damage in the heart and kidney and to analyze the causes leading to the lack of advances in the diagnosis and management of hypoxic AKI, as compared with the outstanding clinical achievements in ischemic myocardial injury. This review will encompass the physiologic complexity of acute hypoxic kidney dysfunction, as compared with the heart, and as summarized in Table 1 putting side-by-side clinical features and available techniques detecting real-time organ injury. We shall further underscore what we believe are basic misconceptions regarding hypoxic AKI that have for decades diverted interventional efforts in the attempt to prevent or amend AKI in the wrong direction.

**Table 1.** Types of acute kidney injury (AKI) and acute myocardial infarction (AMI)-similarities and differences.

| | Type I Ischemic AKI | Type II Hypoxic AKI | Type I AMI | Type II AMI |
|---|---|---|---|---|
| **Pathophysiology** | Ischemia and reperfusion | Altered oxygen supply/demand balance | Ischemia and reperfusion | Altered oxygen supply/demand balance |
| **Tissue blood supply** | ceases | Maintained or reduced | ceases | Maintained or reduced |
| **Workload and oxygen consumption** | ceases | continued/enhanced | Rapidly declines | enhanced |
| **Clinical scenario** | Rare Renal infarct | Common Hypotension, CKD, diabetes, NSAIDs, iodinated contrast media, osmotic dieresis etc. | AMI Due to ruptured plaque | Increased workload in the presence of coronary stenosis (hypotension, anemia, tachycardia etc.) |
| **Symptoms** | Flank pain, hematuria | None related to AKI | Chest pain and accompanying complaints | Chest pain and accompanying complaints |
| **Immediate evidence of functional impairment** | None if unilateral/segmental | None | Occasionally evidence of impaired circulation and heart failure | Occasionally evidence of impaired circulation and heart failure |
| **Rapid functional diagnostic tools** | None | None | Echocardiography (ECG) | Echocardiography (ECG) |
| **Specific biomarkers** | Available and sensitive, limited specificity † | Available, limited specificity and sensitivity † | Highly specific and sensitive in detecting injury | Highly specific and sensitive in detecting injury |

† Specificity is limited especially in the presence of pre-existing renal disease and in aged patients. Tubular segment-type-specificity of the various biomarkers require panel assays. CKD: Chronic kidney diseases; NSAIDs: Non-steroidal anti-inflammatory drugs.

## 2. Comparing the Pathogenesis of Renal and Cardiac Hypoxic Injury

Myocardial ischemia is caused by interrupted blood supply, either as an acute coronary occlusion (caused by a ruptured plaque within an atheromatous plaque), or as a chronic narrowing of the coronary lumen, mostly due to an atheromatous plaque. The former clinical scenario leads to what is called Type I AMI, reflecting organ ischemia (i.e., anoxia due to total cessation of regional blood flow), whereas chronic narrowing of the coronary lumen leads to a transient and usually reversible regional hypoxia with an anginal syndrome (typically characterized by reversible pain), appearing whenever oxygen demand surpasses the restricted oxygen supply, for instance during exercise or tachycardia, and resolving as oxygen demand declines. If severe and protracted enough, myocardial hypoxia related to anginal syndrome may evolve into frank tissue injury, termed Type II MI [4]. The myocardium is characterized by an oxygenation gradient, with $pO_2$ declining from the sub-pericardial to the innermost sub-endocardial regions, especially in regions with coronary stenosis, whenever oxygen demand/supply balance is altered: for instance when diastolic intraventricular pressure increases, undermining sub-endocardial myocardial blood flow and oxygen supply [5–7]. Consequently, a trans-myocardial gradient of hypoxia-induced response appears, such as enhanced expression of hypoxia-inducible factors (HIF) specifically in subendocardial regions [8], or ultimate myocardial injury, first manifested at the innermost portions of the myocardium and spreads outwards as hypoxia persists or intensifies. Intermediate degrees of sub-lethal hypoxia may invoke functional impairment, with altered myocyte contraction and relaxation, myocardial hibernation and apoptosis, whereas prolonged ischemia invokes tissue necrosis and a local inflammatory response [9,10]. Adaptive responses to chronic hypoxia such as the development of collateral microcirculation, as happens in patients with multi-vessel disease, often mitigate the outcome of acute vessel occlusion, leading to subtler tissue damage, in the form of limited subendothelial necrosis (often presented as non-Q wave myocardial infarction). By contrast, acute coronary occlusion due to ruptured plaque without prior chronic hypoxia, as occurs in young smokers with a single vessel disease, is usually manifested as STEMI, with en-block trans-mural myocardial infarction that spreads from the sub-endocardial myocardium outwards along time as ischemia persists. Rapid restoration of regional blood flow by thrombolysis, endovascular interventions (transluminal angioplasty and stenting) or with bypass operations provide myocardial salvage and may restrict the spread of necrosis. Cellular mechanisms of injury are beyond the scope of this short review but the outcome of ischemia and subsequent reperfusion in these settings are the consequence of energy store depletion and access formation of free-radicals, leading to the impairment of vital cellular functions and irreversible structural damage.

As compared with the heart, the kidney presents with only a few uncommon clinical conditions that physiologically mimic Type I AMI with extensive ischemia and reperfusion injury. Acute main- or segmental renal arterial occlusion, for instance due to arterial emboli, is one example. Functional impairment may be subtle in these instances, reflecting enhanced filtration in remnant nephrons, unless an embolus affects a single functioning kidney, or in the presence of a-priori renal failure without functional reserve [11]. Acute global renal ischemia with AKI may develop also in kidneys harvested for transplantation or during cross-clamping of the aorta or cardiopulmonary bypass operations, where the organ is subjected to cold ischemia-reperfusion injury. Acute global warm renal ischemia with AKI may also very rarely develop due to profound and protracted shock in post-partum settings [12], or as shown in Figure 1, following prolonged pulseless cardiorespiratory resuscitation with the use of huge amounts of catecholamines [13].

However, most cases of hypoxic AKI encountered in the clinical practice are not associated with total or near-total cessation of renal blood flow, and is believed to represent a Type II organ injury pattern, reflecting imbalanced regional renal oxygen supply and consumption, especially in regions which are a-priori physiologically hypoxic. As with the heart, the renal parenchymal oxygenation profile is also non-homogenous, with a cortico-medullary oxygen gradient and an inner medullary $pO_2$ as low as 20 mmHg under normal physiologic conditions [14]. Physiological medullary hypoxia reflects very limited blood supply (some 10% of total renal blood flow, delivered by vasa recta), medullary oxygen shunts across descending and ascending vasa recta, and intense regional tubular transport and oxygen consumption. Medullary physiologic hypoxia is the price paid for the construction of the countercurrent urine concentrating apparatus and the very low regional blood flow required for the generation of medullary hyperosmolality. Complex mechanisms are designed to maintain safe oxygen levels in the medulla by the regulation and matching of regional blood flow and oxygen consumption for tubular transport. Prostaglandins, nitric oxide and adenosine are key regulators of these mechanisms [15]. Additional physiologic factors that affect distal tubular transport activity and oxygen consumption are glomerular filtration rate (GFR) and the extent of proximal tubular reabsorption. Enhanced GFR and diminished proximal tubular transport increase distal tubular transport workload, while reduced GFR and enhanced proximal tubular reabsorption reduce oxygen consumption by distal tubular segments and may paradoxically improve medullary oxygenation [16]. Renal oxygenation profile may diversely be affected in the cortex and medulla. For instance, controlled moderate hypotension (with reduced cortical oxygenation but maintained vasa recta blood flow) may result in declined cortical oxygenation, while medullary $pO_2$ paradoxically increases as tubular transport workload diminishes. By contrast, medullary oxygenation eventually declines when mean blood pressure falls below 60–65 mmHg, as vasa recta blood flow and medullary oxygen delivery eventually decline [17]. The term "renal angina syndrome" has been proposed to describe the situation of the renal medulla, which functions on the verge of hypoxia, comparable to the myocardial anginal syndrome. Pre-renal failure exists in this setup, when mean blood pressure is kept above 60–65 mmHg, without structural damage or tubular functional defects. As medullary hypoxia intensifies with a further decline of blood pressure, tubular injury and dysfunction develops, with an activation of tubulo-glomerular feedback mechanisms that reduce GFR. Indeed, this condition of transformation from pre-renal failure to hypoxic AKI has been termed "acute renal success", with renal parenchymal injury remaining limited and often undetected in biopsies (Figure 2) thanks to reduced GFR, as long as medullary blood supply is not critically diminished [15].

As opposed to the rare scenarios leading to total cessation of blood flow with ischemic injury, there is a host of clinical conditions leading to renal parenchymal hypoxia and to the propensity to develop hypoxic AKI due to imbalanced regional oxygen supply and consumption. Chronic kidney disease leads to renal hypoxia through rarefication of microvasculature, interstitial fibrosis and increased workload imposed on remnant nephrons [18,19]. The diabetic kidney is also hypoxic, reflecting both altered medullary flow, combined with enhanced tubular transport and oxygen requirements [20,21]. As detailed above, all conditions leading to reduced renal perfusion may affect the renal parenchymal oxygenation profile. Administration of hypertonic saline [22], mannitol [23] or SGLT2 inhibitors [24,25] increase distal solute delivery and may intensify transport workload and medullary hypoxia. Inhibition of prostaglandins synthesis with non-steroidal anti-inflammatory agents or altered nitric oxide production invokes profound medullary hypoxia by both the selective reduction of vasa recta blood flow and augmentation of sodium transport in medullary thick ascending limbs (mTALs) [26]. Likewise, iodinated contrast agents cause intense medullary hypoxia by reducing vasa recta flow and enhancing tubular transport [27]. Other nephrotoxins may induce hypoxic injury by the reduction of regional blood flow alone (cyclosporine, heme-containing molecules) or in association with enhancement of tubular transport (amphotericin) [26]. Near-drowning in seawater is an archetype of renal oxygenation imbalance, due to both reduced renal oxygen supply (because of systemic hypoxemia, intense sympathetic activity and perhaps a transient hypotension) and enhanced oxygen consumption (with large amounts of absorbed hypertonic saline profoundly enhancing solute delivery for re-uptake in the distal nephron) [28]. Worth noting is that we often induce predictable iatrogenic type II hypoxic AKI in justified clinical settings such as coronary interventions using iodinated contrast media in very high-risk patients with cardiogenic shock. Yet, understanding this disorder might reduce it by measures aimed to maintain renal oxygen balance, as outlined in Future Challenges.

Unlike the homogenous myocardium, renal morphology is highly complex and tubular segments and other parenchymal components differ in their ability to cope with hypoxic stress. The proximal tubule is highly susceptible to hypoxic injury since it cannot tolerate prolonged anaerobic glycolysis. By contrast, mTALs are capable to endure prolonged hypoxia as long as transport activity stops, but rapidly develop hypoxic damage in proportion to oxygen consumption for ion transport [29,30]. Transport activity also intensifies hypoxic injury to S3 segments [31], while collecting ducts are highly resistant to hypoxia and are able to express large amounts of HIF in response to intensified ambient hypoxia [32]. In the outer medulla, seemingly tubular segments compete with each other on sparse oxygen availability, and excess tubular transport in on segment intensify damage in others [33]. A further complicating factor is the often complex and multifactorial nature of renal parenchymal injury and dysfunction, with renal hypoxic injury act in concert with direct tubular toxicity (as with amphothericin, or in hemo/myoglobinuric renal failure), or with altered renal hemodynamics (for instance in sepsis) [26]. It is, therefore, often impossible to assess the independent impact of hypoxia on AKI in these settings.

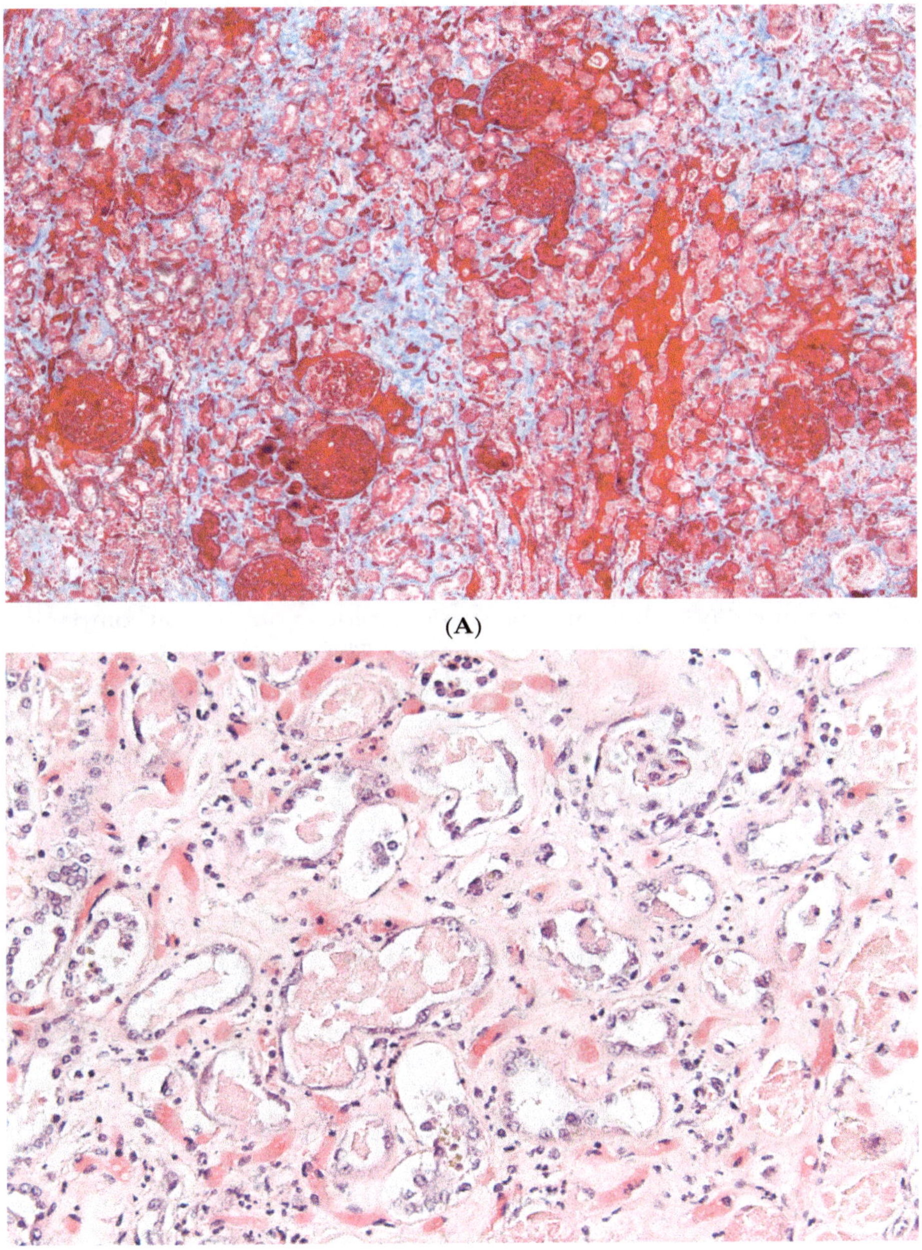

(A)

(B)

**Figure 1.** Renal cortical morphology of type I ischemic AKI. Resuscitation was initiated in a 71 years old patient with AMI who remained pulseless for an hour before the restoration of effective cardiac rhythm. The patient's blood pressure was only briefly maintained by intravenous pressors, but he subsequently developed intractable cardiogenic shock and anuria, dying 5 days after the initial incident. Autopsy findings resemble renal morphology following prolonged WIR in rodents: In (**A**) changes of ischemic hemorrhagic necrosis are shown, superimposed on renal parenchymal tissue with fibrotic changes. Proximal tubules are illustrated in high-power photograph (**B**). The tubular epithelium is flattened and shows extensive regenerative changes and formation of casts. Scattered polymorphonuclear infiltration is also noted. (Masson's trichrome and H&E, original magnifications ×40 and ×200, respectively).

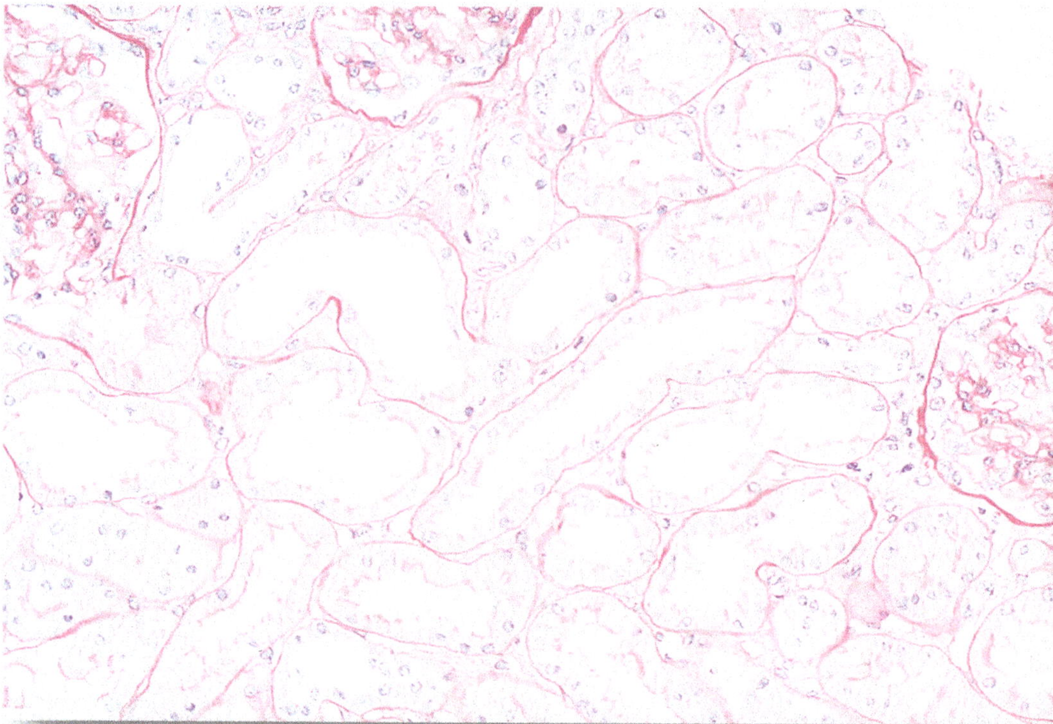

**Figure 2.** Renal cortical morphology of type II hypoxic acute kidney injury (AKI). A 18 year old male who presented with a one-day history of nausea and copious vomiting, accompanied by low-back and lower abdominal pain for which he took ibuprofen. The previous day he had consumed a fifth of Jack Daniels, smoked marijuana and played drums all night. Initial creatinine upon admission was 6.0 mg/dL with laboratory evidence of mild rhabdomyolysis (creatine kinase 2025u, normal 90–250u). Anuric AKI developed, requiring a single hemodialysis. Biopsy, obtained at peak creatinine of 14.7 mg/dL on 7th day shows maintained cortical parenchyma. (Periodic Acid-Schiff (PAS), original magnification ×200).

In conclusion, renal ischemia, i.e., total cessation of renal blood flow is a rare form of hypoxic AKI that resembles Type I AMI, with tissue ischemia and reperfusion injury. By contrast, in most cases, renal parenchymal- and particularly medullary hypoxic injury may develop whenever oxygen supply/demand balance is disrupted, resembling pathophysiologically Type II AMI in patients with fixed stenotic coronary arteries [4]. We propose using the terminology of type I and type II hypoxic AKI, for these two different conditions, respectively.

### 3. Conceptual Errors in the Understanding of Hypoxic AKI

For decades, renal warm ischemia-reperfusion has been adopted by nephrologists as the representative of hypoxic AKI. Extensive research and large budgets have been invested in studying rodent models of ischemia generated by arterial cross-clamping of the renal artery for 30 and up to 60 min in mice and rats, respectively, followed by reperfusion. These models of ischemia and reperfusion (type I hypoxic AKI) parallel animal models of Type I AMI. Morphologic characteristics of tissue injury in these AKI models are ischemic time-dependent extensive proximal tubular injury predominantly in the outer stripe of the outer medulla, accompanied by congestion and substantial inflammation [34], with renal functional impairment grossly proportional to the extent of injury. Medullary thick limb injury in these models does not occur since tubular transport ceases upon cross-clamping, and is low during reperfusion, likely because of reduced GFR and downstream solute delivery [35]. Renal morphology in these models resembles en-bloc necrosis and inflammation, noted in the uncommon clinical cases of global renal ischemia, as shown in Figure 1.

As outlined above, this injury mechanism with global organ ischemia does not physiologically mimic type II hypoxic AKI, where near-complete cessation of renal blood flow does not occur. Over the years models of hypoxic AKI were constructed, both in isolated perfused kidneys and in intact animals in vivo, based on medullary oxygen imbalance, where renal oxygen supply and tubular transport persist throughout the induction of injury [36,37]. Tubular hypoxic stress and injury in these models is principally noted in mTALs and to a lesser extent in S3 segments in the outer medulla, ranging from stabilization of HIF signals, through apoptosis or reversible phases of cell injury (nuclear pyknosis, mitochondrial swelling) to frank necrosis with cell membrane disruption. Injury gradient is evident, most prominent in the inner layers of the outer medulla and in the interbundle zone, most remote from vasa recta and oxygen supply [32,38,39]. In these models tissue injury may be focal, without prominent inflammation, and with functional impairment (reduced GFR) often out-of-proportion to the very limited focal tubular injury. We believe that such models are physiologically relevant to type II hypoxic AKI, with limited tubular injury as in Figure 2. Using the warm ischemia-reperfusion AKI models for years has been a formidable obstacle in the development of clinically relevant therapeutic strategies, treating animals with an artificial disease that is irrelevant to the human scenario [36,40].

## 4. Clinical Presentation of Hypoxic Cardiac vs. Renal Injury

Myocardial ischemia is most often manifested immediately with chest pain and accompanying complains, such as radiating pain, nausea and vomiting, cold perspiration, shortness of breath and doom feeling. Angina pectoris is initiated or aggravated by physical activity and enhanced myocardial oxygen demand. Yet, some patients, especially elderly and diabetic individuals might undergo painless myocardial ischemia or hypoxia due to altered sensorium.

As opposed to protean overt symptoms in most cases of myocardial injury, clinical symptoms in the clinical settings of hypoxic AKI are most often absent, likely since tissue injury in subtle and focal, and out of proportion to the extent of functional impairment. Rare exceptions are type I hypoxic injury due to acute total or segmental renal infarction that may be manifested as flank pain mimicking renal colic. Gradual renal artery stenosis may be revealed among patients during the evaluation of secondary hypertension, and symptoms of severe hypertension or pulmonary congestion may develop in the case of renal arterial occlusion of a single functioning kidney or in the rare cases of bilateral renal ischemia.

## 5. Detection and Assessment of Myocardial Hypoxic Injury

A large and easily accessible arsenal of diagnostic tools is available in the clinical practice for the immediate detection of myocardial hypoxia. Myocardial ischemia can be detected in real time as it evolves by typical electrocardiographic changes and by altered regional wall motion, easily sensed by echocardiography, which also helps ruling out major differential diagnoses. Dynamics in these parameters can be assessed in type II ischemia during enhanced workload and oxygen consumption, with exercise test or its equivalents. Myocardial perfusion can be identified by radiolabled scans and by MRI, and tissue injury can be validated by the detection of released myocardial constituents, such as troponin isoforms, myoglobin and others. The extent of myocardial necrosis grossly correlates with the rise in these biomarkers of cardiac muscle injury. With all these technologies myocardial hypoxia or ischemia is usually easily detected and intravascular lesions can be located and managed by non-invasive and invasive coronary imaging and interventions.

Altogether, cardiologists possess reliable and readily available diagnostic tools that provide immediate assessment of cardiac function and indices of tissue injury, studies that can be performed repeatedly with grossly clear-cut threshold definitions of myocyte injury.

## 6. Detection of Hypoxic Renal Injury

Delayed involvement of nephrologists is an important obstacle in achieving real-time identification, appropriate management and improved outcome of AKI. Furthermore, comparable tools for the prompt and timely diagnosis of AKI in general and specifically of hypoxic renal injury are unfortunately lacking. The parameters used by AKIN or RIFLE criteria for grading of AKI stages [41,42], namely the rates of urine output and rise in plasma creatinine, are non-specific and non-immediate upon injury. The clinical scenario and the presence of orthostatic hypotension may suggest pre-renal failure, and renal Doppler-ultrasound can rule out post-renal causes and assess renal vascular resistance, and may identify features of chronic renal disease. Urinalysis and microscopy may help detecting glomerulopathies and might identify typical features of acute tubular necrosis or crystal nephropathy. Analysis of urine osmolality, sodium and creatinine, and their corresponding plasma values further may help differing pre-renal failure from tubular injury. Yet, often results are within a very wide gray zone with low specificity, and these parameters are markedly affected by the use of fluids and diuretics and in the presence of pre-existing renal disease. Enhancement imaging with iodine-containing- or gadolinium-based contrast agents is associated with the risk of further renal injury or nephrogenic systemic fibrosis, respectively.

Novel technologies currently under development provide non-enhanced imaging of renal morphology, function, microcirculation and oxygenation [43]. Additional promising diagnostic tools are biomarkers of renal tissue injury [44]. The potential use of these two advanced tools in the early detection of AKI in general and in are briefly discussed below.

### 7. Biomarkers of Acute Kidney Injury

The great development in molecular biology during recent decades has led to a major advance in the search for novel biomarkers for early detection of AKI [45], as evident by the discovery of several key biomarkers of myocardial injury with various specificity and sensitivity, including neutrophil gelatinase-associated lipocalin (NGAL), kidney injury molecule-1 (KIM-1), liver-type fatty acid-binding protein (L-FABP), netrin-1 and IL18 [45–48]. NGAL is one of the most prominently up-regulated genes in the kidney after AKI, particularly in distal nephron segments and damaged renal tubule [45,46]. This biomarker is increased in urine and plasma early after renal ischemia in mouse and rat models [49], and following cardiopulmonary bypass, radiocontrast administration, sepsis, and kidney transplantation, specifically in patients who subsequently developed AKI [50]. Meta-analysis of data from 19 studies, which included more than 2500 patients, revealed that rises in serum or urine NGAL levels are diagnostic for AKI [51]. As opposed to NGAL, KIM-1 is a biomarker for proximal tubular injury, and is a hallmark of toxic and ischemic proximal tubular injury [46,47]. Double labeling immunohistochemistry in various experimental and human renal diseases revealed that KIM-1-positive tubules are associated with macrophages and areas with increased expression of $\alpha$-smooth muscle actin ($\alpha$-SMA), a marker of myofibroblast transformation [46,52,53]. Interleukin 18 (IL-18), a pro-inflammatory cytokine belonging to the IL-1 superfamily has been reported to mediate experimental ischemic proximal tubular injury and its accompanied pro-inflammatory responses [54]. IL-18 is produced by phagocytes attracted to injured proximal tubules, activated by caspase 1, and excreted into the urine upon renal ischemic injury [54]. Although IL-18 was found to be a helpful biomarker for early detection of AKI, it is less sensitive than NGAL [55,56]. Most recently additional two cycle arrest biomarkers were added to the growing list of AKI biomarkers, namely, insulin-like growth factor-binding protein 7 (IGFBP7) and tissue inhibitor of metalloproteinases-2 (TIMP-2), with the potential to provide new mechanistic insights into the pathogenesis of AKI on one hand and the ability for early detection of this clinical setting, on the other [48,57].

Despite the expectations from these novel biomarkers to be sensitive, practical, and accurate in predicting AKI, the results were not unambiguous. Indeed, some of these biomarkers show unequivocal ability to predict AKI in certain settings as mentioned above. However, many of them suffer from drawbacks mainly due to broad range of its predictive accuracy. Moreover, the circulatory concentration profile of most biomarkers is adversely affected by the fluid balance and diuretic therapy. Though this concern regarding urinary biomarkers could be overcome by correcting their excretion to urinary creatinine, in certain clinical settings the creatinine kinetics is dramatically altered as the case in critical ill patients where most of the AKI cases are witnessed. Additional concern is the fact the most of the tested biomarkers are present in the circulation and their excretion in the urine does not necessarily reflect renal origin/damage. For instance, NGAL is expressed by several cell types, including endothelial cells, smooth muscle cells and macrophages in atherosclerotic plaques, where it assumedly plays a role in the pathogenesis of atherosclerosis, endothelial dysfunction, inflammatory processes and extracellular matrix remodeling [58]. Moreover, since the urinary origin of the various biomarkers are cell-specific, and AKI could be due various aetiologies, i.e., ischemia, nephrotoxicity, inflammation and renal outflow obstruction, with differential involvement of cell types, it is unlikely that a single biomarker would predict AKI reliably, the mechanisms underlying AKI or the identity of the damaged renal cells: proximal, distal, collecting duct epithelial cells, or interstitial cells [48]. Support for the use of combined biomarkers to improve their predictability value came from a study in adult patients who underwent CPB surgery, where using urinary biomarkers KIM-1, NAG, and NGAL predicted AKI 3 h from the operation by 0.65 for KIM-1; 0.63 for NAG; and 0.65 for NGAL [59]. When two biomarker was applied, the sensitivity of AKI prediction 3 h from surgery was enhanced to 0.78 [60], and escalated even to a higher specificity (0.94) when four biomarkers were used [59]. Finally, the specificity and sensitivity of most of these biomarkers are deleteriously affected by confounding factors as the presence background diseases such as CKD, cancer, heart failure, atherosclerosis or inflammation, which may cause false positive diagnosis [45]. This may explain the high specificity and sensitivity of the initial results where the reliability of theses biomarkers were tested in children who underwent CPB or radiocontrast administration [45,46], as compared with the lower accuracy when the studies were repeated in adult patients (usually with background diseases) who underwent similar clinical procedures [48].

In sum, the AKI biomarkers field is evolving. Despite their advantage as noninvasive and reasonable specificity for renal injury, more comprehensive studies are still requested to determine their clinical application.

## 8. Renal Functional Imaging

Although determination of vital organs function and dysfunction still largely relies on biochemical analysis of blood/serum and/or urine, imaging of these organs is evolving rapidly and holds great promise for improving detection of structural, functional and even molecular changes in these tissues [61]. The kidney is of special interest yet challenging, as it has unique anatomic and ultrastructural features. Specifically, the multi functions of the kidney require different types of epithelial cells, regional blood flow and oxygen consumption along the nephron and the cortical and medullary tissues. Therefore, development of functional imaging is crucial for diagnosis of physiological and pathophysiological alterations in the kidney.

Historically, renal perfusion and oxygenation under various conditions was determined either invasively via laser-Doppler flowmeter and oxygen microelectrodes [17,23,33] or indirectly via measurement of urinary $pO_2$ [22]. Subsequently, imaging of renal perfusion and GFR were developed, with arterial spin labeling (ASL), an MRI methodology applied to determine total RBF [62]. ASL uses magnetically tagged water with a radiofrequency pulse. Briefly, a control image is obtained without contrast, followed by a radiofrequency pulse of the blood before it enters the kidney. The labeled image is then subtracted from the baseline image, generating a map of the signal difference created by the perfused blood [63]. Although initially ASL was not considered sensitive, upgrading imaging acquisition techniques improved its performance, where it can currently discriminate between medulla and cortex according to meta-analysis of 53 studies [64]. For instance, ASL allows detecting early renal damage following cardiopulmonary bypass procedures, where the incidence of AKI may reach up to one third of patients [50,65]. As cardiopulmonary bypass-induced AKI was associated with renal hypoperfusion and vasoconstriction, ASL was sensitive enough to detect reduced RBF and GFR [49]. This methodology was found to be valid in kidney-transplanted patients with delayed graft function [66]. Similarly, ASL exhibited high sensitivity in detecting impaired regional blood perfusion along kidney injury and histological changes in correlation with the severity of the renal insult in experimental models of AKI induced by ischemic/reperfusion for 35–45 min [67]. Moreover, ASL detected long term outcome of renal remodeling and hypo perfusion/remodeling or full recovery a few weeks after the AKI induction [61,67].

In the last two decades, blood oxygen level-dependent (BOLD) MRI and related technologies provided the most striking advance in non-invasive measurement of intra renal oxygenation profile in humans and in experimental animals [61,68]. Bold MRI uses the different properties of oxygenated and non-oxygenated hemoglobin, where the latter is magnetic, to determine tissue oxygen levels [61]. Several studies have shown that R2* relaxation rate is inversely correlated with tissue $pO_2$ and can be mapped throughout BOLD MRI of the kidneys [69–71]. Specifically, using BOLD MRI revealed that administration of furosemide to normal subjects significantly decreased outer medullary R2* [72], indicating improved oxygenation, in agreement with findings with oxygen microelectrodes [23]. Yet it did not cause such reduction in patients with CKD and among hypertensive subjects, although basal R2* was comparable in the three studied groups [72]. Despite the increasing popularity of this convenient method, there are several confounding factors that may adversely affect its reliability, such as fluid balance, salt intake, smoking, and pulmonary function [69]. Respiratory gating is also required to overcome kidney motion-related artifacts. Dynamic contrast-enhanced (DCE) MRI is an additional imaging approach aimed at measuring GFR and renal blood flow, using gadolinium-based contrast agents [73,74]. For this purpose, serial images of the kidney are obtained as the contrast is filtered and used to calculate GFR. The DCE MRI method was found to be superior to other MRI techniques that use radionuclides for the measurements of GFR [75]. Finally, hemodynamic response imaging (HRI), a non-enhanced functional MRI method, provides insights regarding renal perfusion and vascular reactivity in response to alternating hypercapnia and hyperoxia [76,77].

Sodium MRI provides an additional unique capability of the assessment of outer medullary function. In healthy state and especially in pre-renal impairment, this gradient reflects the efficient concentrating mechanism generated in part by avid sodium transport across mTALs. Disruption of the normal cortico-medullary sodium gradient that appears within a few hours following the disruption of medullary oxygenation balance is a very early indicator of medullary hypoxic injury, when morphologic indices of tubular damage are still very focal and perhaps reversible, and plasma creatinine hardly rises [78]. This finding likely goes together with increased fractional sodium excretion and the transformation from highly concentrated urine to isosthenuria [79]. Thus, renal sodium MRI might provide the equivalent of the detection of compromised myocardium with segmental wall-motion disturbances by stress-echocardiography.

These wonderful non-invasive tools alone or in combination provide tremendous insight about real-time changes in renal structure, hemodynamics, glomerular filtration, oxygenation and function. Unfortunately, while they may serve as advanced experimental probes, their clinical use is limited, as they are not available in most institutes. Furthermore, most patients requiring diagnostic evaluation of AKI are in critical care settings, connected to monitoring and life-maintaining equipment that preclude bedside usage of MRI. A more feasible and promising technology for the early real-time detection of evolving medullary hypoxia and for assessing the risk of hypoxic AKI is a continuous determination of urinary $pO_2$ at the catheter tip, as recently shown in the settings of cardiac surgery [80].

Imaging that enables the detection of injured tissues is another exciting plausible technology to be studied [81]. Focal tubular apoptosis and necrosis were traced by a specific small molecule in evolving hypoxic and septic models of AKI [82]. Radiolabeling of this molecule enables detection by PET, and has been used to spot apoptotic malignant cells in response to chemotherapy or the development of neuronal damage. However, the renal clearance of this compound currently precludes its use in the assessment of tissue damage in AKI. In that respect, recently introduced advanced Doppler ultrasound technologies provide fine assessment of the renal microcirculation at the bedside [83] and may be clinically more applicable.

## 9. Future Challenges

Current technologies enable the precise mapping of hypoxic regions (such as BOLD MRI in vivo, or immunostaining for HIF isoforms or for pimonidazole adducts in kidney samples) and the detection of renal parenchymal injury in animal models with biomarkers. To better appreciate the pathophysiology and the impact of interventions, such endpoints should be included in experimental settings in whole animal studies, in parallel with precise morphology, since looking only at parameters of glomerular filtration, or even of tubular function may not suffice. For instance, the use of loop diuretics in clinical trials for the prevention of hypoxic AKI induced by radiocontrast agents has been abandoned as plasma creatinine increased [84]. Likely, the rise in creatinine reflected insufficient volume replacement and pre-renal failure [85], while in fact medullary oxygenation and tubular viability have been improved [38,86]. In later clinical trials in high-risk patients, large fluid replacements combined with furosemide attenuated the risk of radiocontrast-induced nephropathy [87]. Most importantly, the correlation of urine biomarker levels with the extent and distribution of tubular injury has not been studied in depth. As mentioned above, some urine biomarkers, such as KIM-1 are generated by proximal tubular segments while others, such as NGAL originate from distal segments. Precise quantitation of injury at specified nephron segments at various locations within the renal parenchyma, as well as the extent of chronic fibrotic changes and the renal distribution of hypoxia (with pimonidazole) and hypoxia-response (HIF detection) can be achieved in perfusion-fixed thin section preparations in experimental models of AKI [88,89]. It is about time to try and correlate the extent of tubular injury at different segments with their corresponding cell-specific biomarkers in order to validate the sensitivity and specificity of these biomarkers in animal models of acute- and acute on chronic AKI. Such studies may improve our understanding of human AKI and may direct us in the generation of appropriate panels of biomarkers to appropriate for varied clinical conditions, for instance biomarkers for proximal tubular injury for suspected aminoglycoside nephrotoxicity, or a panel of distal tubular biomarkers following near drowning, or in AKI following the administration of SGLT2 antagonists.

Most non-invasive functional imaging techniques are not applicable for patients in critical care settings, and their use is restricted to animal studies and to human studies under ambulatory settings. Further development is needed of technologies that will enable bedside mapping of renal oxygenation profile and of real-time renal functional parameters.

## 10. Conclusions

The detection, prevention and successful treatment of hypoxic AKI have only moderately been advanced over recent decades, as compared to the substantial achievements in the diagnosis and management of ischemic heart disease. Disorders of renal parenchymal oxygenation are much more compound than those of the heart muscle. Furthermore, nephrology lags far behind cardiology in the diagnosis and management of hypoxic injury because of the lack of clinical symptoms and overt early physiologic signs, and the absence of diagnostic tools that provide immediate and highly specific results during the evolution of kidney injury. Changes in urine volume and the pattern of the rise in creatinine are non-specific and often retarded crude indices of renal dysfunction. Novel biomarkers provide new tools for the early detection of renal parenchymal injury, yet, the heterogeneity of damage patterns affecting different tubular segments in various toxic and hypoxic insults may differently affect some segment-specific biomarkers. There is no available human data regarding the correlation of biomarker levels and tissue injury extent and pattern, and such data should be evaluated in animal studies. The specificity and sensitivity of biomarkers in the detection of acute-on-chronic renal injury need improvement. Functional imaging is a fantastic experimental tool, but its availability and potential use in the clinical practice are currently limited.

The pathogenesis of AKI is often complex, with direct nephrotoxicity, hypoxia, altered microcirculation and other factors playing in concert. Differentiation between the causative factors is therefore principally based on clinical judgment and the assessment of the individual contribution of hypoxia may be based only on hypoxia mapping by functional imaging or by the determination of urine $pO_2$.

Differing between type I and type II organ injury pattern should be based principally on the clinical scenario, both for the heart and kidney. Yet, this distinction, easily confirmed by angiography in AMI, might not be possible to establish unequivocally for AKI.

Finally, nephrologists lag behind cardiologists regarding hypoxic AKI also because of conceptual errors. Research projects have failed to distinguish between conditions with protracted renal warm ischemia and reperfusion, and those with maintained renal blood flow and transport activity but imbalanced oxygen supply and expenditure. We propose to differently address these conditions as type I and type II hypoxic AKI, terms physiologically parallel to type I and type II AMI. Whereas type I AKI is infrequent and rarely presents with renal functional impairment, most research studies use type I ischemic AKI animal models, which bear little relevance to the far more frequent conditions leading to type II hypoxic AKI. Better understanding and advances in the management of hypoxic AKI will require more studies using animal models of type II-, rather than type I renal parenchymal hypoxic injury.

**Author Contributions:** Conceptualization, Z.A., S.R., S.L. and S.N.H.; methodology, Z.A., S.R., S.L. and S.N.H.; software, Z.A., S.R., S.L. and S.N.H.; validation, Z.A., S.R., S.L. and S.N.H.; formal analysis, Z.A., S.R., S.L. and S.N.H.; investigation, Z.A., S.R., S.L. and S.N.H.; resources, Z.A., S.R., S.L. and S.N.H.; data curation, Z.A., S.R., S.L. and S.N.H.; writing-original draft preparation Z.A., S.R., S.L. and S.N.H.; writing-review and editing, Z.A., S.R., S.L. and S.N.H.; visualization, Z.A., S.R., S.L. and S.N.H.; project administration, S.R. and S.N.H.

## References

1. Bonventre, J.V.; Yang, L. Cellular pathophysiology of ischemic acute kidney injury. *J. Clin. Investig.* **2011**, *121*, 4210–4221. [CrossRef] [PubMed]
2. Schrier, R.W.; Wang, W.; Poole, B.; Mitra, A. Acute renal failure: definitions, diagnosis, pathogenesis, and therapy. *J. Clin. Investig.* **2004**, *114*, 5–14. [CrossRef] [PubMed]
3. Moran, S.M.; Myers, B.D. Course of acute renal failure studied by a model of creatinine kinetics. *Kidney Int.* **1985**, *27*, 928–937. [CrossRef] [PubMed]
4. Smilowitz, N.R.; Naoulou, B.; Sedlis, S.P. Diagnosis and Management of Type II Myocardial Infarction: Increased Demand for a Limited Supply of Evidence. *Curr. Atheroscler. Rep.* **2015**, *17*, 478. [CrossRef] [PubMed]
5. Bache, R.J.; Dai, X.Z. Myocardial oxygen consumption during exercise in the presence of left ventricular hypertrophy secondary to supravalvular aortic stenosis. *J. Am. Coll. Cardiol.* **1990**, *15*, 1157–1164. [CrossRef]
6. Watanabe, H.; Ohtsuka, S.; Kakihana, M.; Sugishita, Y. Decreased aortic compliance aggravates subendocardial ischaemia in dogs with stenosed coronary artery. *Cardiovasc. Res.* **1992**, *26*, 1212–1218. [CrossRef] [PubMed]
7. Nagao, N.; Yamasaki, Y.; Kawanami, S.; Kamitani, T.; Sagiyama, K.; Higo, T.; Ide, T.; Takemura, A.; Ishizaki, U.; Fukushima, K.; et al. Quantification of myocardial oxygenation in heart failure using blood-oxygen-level-dependent T2* magnetic resonance imaging: Comparison with cardiopulmonary exercise test. *Magn. Reson. Imaging* **2017**, *39*, 138–143. [CrossRef] [PubMed]
8. May, D.; Gilon, D.; Djonov, V.; Itin, A.; Lazarus, A.; Gordon, O.; Rosenberger, C.; Keshet, E. Transgenic system for conditional induction and rescue of chronic myocardial hibernation provides insights into genomic programs of hibernation. *Proc. Natl. Acad. Sci. USA* **2008**, *105*, 282–287. [CrossRef] [PubMed]
9. Frangogiannis, N.G.; Smith, C.W.; Entman, M.L. The inflammatory response in myocardial infarction. *Cardiovasc. Res.* **2002**, *53*, 31–47. [CrossRef]
10. Buja, L.M. Myocardial ischemia and reperfusion injury. *Cardiovasc. Pathol.* **2005**, *14*, 170–175. [CrossRef] [PubMed]
11. Hazanov, N.; Somin, M.; Attali, M.; Beilinson, N.; Thaler, M.; Mouallem, M.; Maor, Y.; Zaks, N.; Malnick, S. Acute renal embolism: Forty-four cases of renal infarction in patients with atrial fibrillation. *Medicine (Baltimore)* **2004**, *83*, 292–299. [CrossRef] [PubMed]

12. Matlin, R.A.; Gary, N.E. Acute cortical necrosis. Case report and review of the literature. *Am. J. Med.* **1974**, *56*, 110–118. [CrossRef]
13. Rosen, S.; Stillman, I.E. Acute Tubular Necrosis Is a Syndrome of Physiologic and Pathologic Dissociation. *J. Am. Soc. Nephrol.* **2008**, *19*, 871–875. [CrossRef] [PubMed]
14. Brezis, M.; Rosen, S. Hypoxia of the Renal Medulla-Its Implications for Disease. *N. Engl. J. Med.* **1995**, *332*, 647–655. [CrossRef] [PubMed]
15. Heyman, S.N.; Evans, R.G.; Rosen, S.; Rosenberger, C. Cellular adaptive changes in AKI: mitigating renal hypoxic injury. *Nephrol. Dial. Transplant.* **2012**, *27*, 1721–1728. [CrossRef] [PubMed]
16. Stillman, I.E.; Brezis, M.; Heyman, S.N.; Epstein, F.H.; Spokes, K.; Rosen, S. Effects of salt depletion on the kidney: changes in medullary oxygenation and thick ascending limb size. *J. Am. Soc. Nephrol.* **1994**, *4*, 1538–1545. [PubMed]
17. Brezis, M.; Heyman, S.N.; Epstein, F.H. Determinants of intrarenal oxygenation. II. Hemodynamic effects. *Am. J. Physiol.* **1994**, *267*, F1063–F1068. [CrossRef] [PubMed]
18. Nangaku, N.; Rosenberger, C.; Heyman, S.N.; Eckardt, K.U. Regulation of hypoxia-inducible factor in kidney disease. *Clin. Exp. Pharmacol. Physiol.* **2013**, *40*, 148–157. [CrossRef] [PubMed]
19. Heyman, S.N.; Khamaisi, M.; Rosen, S.; Rosenberger, C. Renal parenchymal hypoxia, hypoxia response and the progression of chronic kidney disease. *Am. J. Nephrol.* **2008**, *28*, 998–1006. [CrossRef] [PubMed]
20. Franzén, S.; Palm, F. Endothelin type A receptor inhibition normalises intrarenal hypoxia in rats used as a model of type 1 diabetes by improving oxygen delivery. *Diabetologia* **2015**, *58*, 2435–2442. [CrossRef] [PubMed]
21. Heyman, S.N.; Rosenberger, C.; Rosen, S.; Khamaisi, M. Why is diabetes mellitus a risk factor for contrast-induced nephropathy? *BioMed Res. Int.* **2013**, *2013*, 123589. [CrossRef] [PubMed]
22. Washington, J.A., 2nd; Holland, J.M. Urine oxygen tension: effects of osmotic and saline diuresis and of ethacrynic acid. *Am. J. Physiol.* **1966**, *210*, 243–250. [CrossRef] [PubMed]
23. Brezis, M.; Agmon, Y.; Epstein, F.H. Determinants of intrarenal oxygenation. I. Effects of diuretics. *Am. J. Physiol.* **1994**, *267*, F1063–F1068. [CrossRef] [PubMed]
24. O'Neill, J.; Fasching, A.; Pihl, L.; Patinha, D.; Franzén, S.; Palm, F. Acute SGLT inhibition normalizes $O_2$ tension in the renal cortex but causes hypoxia in the renal medulla in anaesthetized control and diabetic rats. *Am. J. Physiol. Renal Physiol.* **2015**, *309*, F227–F234. [CrossRef] [PubMed]
25. Szalat, A.; Perlman, A.; Muszkat, M.; Khamaisi, M.; Abassi, Z.; Heyman, S.N. Can SGLT2 Inhibitors Cause Acute Renal Failure? Plausible Role for Altered Glomerular Hemodynamics and Medullary Hypoxia. *Drug Saf.* **2018**, *41*, 239–252. [CrossRef] [PubMed]
26. Rosenberger, C.; Rosen, S.; Heyman, S.N. Renal parenchymal oxygenation and hypoxia adaptation in acute kidney injury. *Clin. Exp. Pharmacol. Physiol.* **2006**, *33*, 980–988. [CrossRef] [PubMed]
27. Heyman, S.N.; Rosen, S.; Rosenberger, C. Renal parenchymal hypoxia, hypoxia adaptation, and the pathogenesis of radiocontrast nephropathy. *Clin. J. Am. Soc. Nephrol.* **2008**, *3*, 288–296. [CrossRef] [PubMed]
28. Heyman, S.N.; Gorelik, Y.; Zorbavel, D.; Rosenberger, C.; Abassi, Z.; Rosen, S. Near drowning: New perspectives for human hypoxic AKI. *Nephrol Dial. Transplant.* **2019**. [CrossRef] [PubMed]
29. Brezis, M.; Shanley, P.; Silva, P.; Spokes, K.; Lear, S.; Epstein, F.H.; Rosen, S. Disparate mechanisms for hypoxic cell injury in different nephron segments. Studies in the isolated perfused rat kidney. *J. Clin. Investig.* **1985**, *76*, 1796–1806. [CrossRef] [PubMed]
30. Brezis, M.; Rosen, S.; Silva, P.; Epstein, F.H. Transport activity modifies thick ascending limb damage in the isolated perfused kidney. *Kidney Int.* **1984**, *25*, 65–72. [CrossRef] [PubMed]
31. Shanley, P.F.; Brezis, M.; Spokes, K.; Silva, P.; Epstein, F.H.; Rosen, S. Transport-dependent cell injury in the S3 segment of the proximal tubule. *Kidney Int.* **1986**, *29*, 1033–1037. [CrossRef] [PubMed]
32. Rosenberger, C.; Rosen, S.; Shina, A.; Bernhardt, W.; Wiesener, M.S.; Frei, U.; Eckardt, K.U.; Heyman, S.N. Hypoxia-inducible factors and tubular cell survival in isolated perfused kidneys. *Kidney Int.* **2006**, *70*, 60–70. [CrossRef] [PubMed]
33. Heyman, S.N.; Rosen, S.; Epstein, F.H.; Spokes, K.; Brezis, M.L. Loop diuretics reduce hypoxic damage to proximal tubules of the isolated perfused rat kidney. *Kidney Int.* **1994**, *45*, 981–985. [CrossRef] [PubMed]
34. Shanley, P.F.; Rosen, M.D.; Brezis, M.; Silva, P.; Epstein, F.H.; Rosen, S. Topography of focal proximal tubular necrosis after ischemia with reflow in the rat kidney. *Am. J. Pathol.* **1985**, *122*, 462–468.

35. Heyman, S.N. Proximal tubular injury attenuates outer medullary hypoxic damage: studies in perfused rat kidneys. *Exp. Nephrol.* **2001**, *10*, 259–266. [CrossRef] [PubMed]
36. Heyman, S.N.; Rosen, S.; Rosenberger, C. Critical assessment of experimental models of acute renal failure. *Crit. Care Nephrol.* **2009**, *169*, 237–250.
37. Heyman, S.N.; Rosen, S.; Rosenberger, C. Animal models of renal dysfunction: acute kidney injury. *Expert Opin. Drug Discov.* **2009**, *4*, 629–641. [CrossRef] [PubMed]
38. Heyman, S.N.; Brezis, M.; Epstein, F.H.; Spokes, K.; Silva, P.; Rosen, S. Early renal medullary hypoxic injury from radiocontrast and indomethacin. *Kidney Int.* **1991**, *40*, 632–642. [CrossRef] [PubMed]
39. Heyman, S.N.; Brezis, M.; Reubinoff, C.A.; Greenfeld, Z.; Lechene, G.; Epstein, F.H.; Rosen, S. Acute renal failure with selective medullary injury in the rat. *J. Clin. Investig.* **1988**, *82*, 401–412. [CrossRef] [PubMed]
40. Heyman, S.N.; Rosenberger, C.; Rosen, S. Experimental ischemia-reperfusion: Biases and mythsthe proximal vs. distal hypoxic tubular injury debate revisited. *Kidney Int.* **2010**, *77*, 9–16. [CrossRef] [PubMed]
41. Bellomo, R.; Ronco, C.; Kellum, J.A.; Mehta, R.L.; Palevsky, P.; Acute Dialysis Quality Initiative Workgroup. Acute renal failure-definition, outcome measures, animal models, fluid therapy and information technology needs: the Second International Consensus Conference of the Acute Dialysis Quality Initiative (ADQI) Group. *Crit. Care* **2004**, *8*, R204–R212. [PubMed]
42. Bagga, A.; Bakkaloglu, A.; Devarajan, P.; Mehta, R.L.; Kellum, J.A.; Shah, S.V.; Molitoris, B.A.; Ronco, C.; Warnock, D.G.; Joannidis, M.; et al. Improving outcomes from acute kidney injury: Report of an initiative. *Pediatr. Nephrol.* **2007**, *22*, 1655–1658. [CrossRef] [PubMed]
43. Ronco, C. Acute kidney injury: from clinical to molecular diagnosis. *Crit. Care* **2016**, *20*, 201–204. [CrossRef] [PubMed]
44. Cox, E.F.; Buchanan, C.E.; Bradley, C.R.; Prestwich, B.; Mahmoud, H.; Taal, M.; Selby, N.M.; Francis, S.T. Multiparametric renal magnetic resonance imaging: Validation, interventions, and alterations in chronic kidney disease. *Front. Physiol.* **2017**, *8*, 696. [CrossRef] [PubMed]
45. Devarajan, P. Review: Neutrophil gelatinase-associated lipocalin: A troponin-like biomarker for human acute kidney injury. *Nephrology (Carlton)* **2010**, *15*, 419–428. [CrossRef] [PubMed]
46. Vaidya, V.S.; Ferguson, M.A.; Bonventre, J.V. Biomarkers of acute kidney injury: early diagnosis, pathogenesis, and recovery. *Annu. Rev. Pharmacol. Toxicol.* **2008**, *48*, 463–493. [CrossRef] [PubMed]
47. Vanmassenhove, J.; Vanholder, R.; Nagler, E.; Van Biesen, W. Urinary and serum biomarkers for the diagnosis of acute kidney injury: An in-depth review of the literature. *Nephrol. Dial. Transplant.* **2013**, *28*, 254–273. [CrossRef] [PubMed]
48. Beker, B.M.; Corleto, M.G.; Fieiras, C.; Musso, C.G. Novel acute kidney injury biomarkers: Their characteristics, utility and concerns. *Int. Urol. Nephrol.* **2018**, *50*, 705–713. [CrossRef] [PubMed]
49. Mishra, J.; Qing, M.A.; Prada, A.; Mitsnefes, M.; Zahedi, K.; Yang, J.; Barasch, J.; Devarajan, P. Identification of neutrophil gelatinase-associated lipocalin as a novel early urinary biomarker for ischemic renal injury. *J. Am. Soc. Nephrol.* **2003**, *14*, 2534–2543. [CrossRef] [PubMed]
50. Mishra, J.; Dent, C.; Tarabishi, R.; Mitsnefes, M.M.; Ma, Q.; Kelly, C.; Ruff, S.M.; Zahedi, K.; Shao, M.; Bean, J.; et al. Neutrophil gelatinase-associated lipocalin (NGAL) as a biomarker for acute renal injury after cardiac surgery. *Lancet* **2005**, *365*, 1231–1238. [CrossRef]
51. Haase, M.; Bellomo, R.; Devarajan, P.; Schlattmann, P.; Haase-Fielitz, A.; Bagshaw, S.M.; Bogle, R.; Changchun, C.; Constantin, J.M.; Cruz, D.; et al. Accuracy of Neutrophil Gelatinase-Associated Lipocalin (NGAL) in Diagnosis and Prognosis in Acute Kidney Injury: A Systematic Review and Meta-analysis. *Am. J. Kidney Dis.* **2009**, *54*, 1012–1024. [CrossRef] [PubMed]
52. Ichimura, T.; Asseldonk, E.J.; Humphreys, B.D.; Gunaratnam, L.; Duffield, J.S.; Bonventre, J.V. Kidney injury molecule-1 is a phosphatidylserine receptor that confers a phagocytic phenotype on epithelial cells. *J. Clin. Investig.* **2008**, *118*, 1657–1668. [CrossRef] [PubMed]
53. Ichimura, T.; Bonventre, J.V.; Bailly, V.; Wei, H.; Hession, C.A.; Cate, R.L.; Sanicola, M. Kidney injury molecule-1 (KIM-1), a putative epithelial cell adhesion molecule containing a novel immunoglobulin domain, is up-regulated in renal cells after injury. *J. Biol. Chem.* **1998**, *273*, 4135–4142. [CrossRef] [PubMed]
54. Melnikov, V.Y.; Ecder, T.; Fantuzzi, G.; Siegmund, B.; Lucia, M.S.; Dinarello, C.A.; Schrier, R.W.; Edelstein, C.L. Impaired IL-18 processing protects caspase-1-deficient mice from ischemic acute renal failure. *J. Clin. Investig.* **2001**, *107*, 1145–1152. [CrossRef] [PubMed]

55. Gan, J.; Zhou, X. Comparison of urine neutrophil gelatinase-associated lipocalin and interleukin-18 in prediction of acute kidney injury in adults. *Medicine (Baltimore)* **2018**, *97*, e12570. [CrossRef] [PubMed]
56. Liu, Y.; Guo, W.; Zhang, J.; Xu, C.; Yu, S.; Mao, Z.; Wu, J.; Ye, C.; Mei, C.; Dai, B. Urinary interleukin 18 for detection of acute kidney injury: A meta-analysis. *Am. J. Kidney Dis.* **2013**, *62*, 1058–1067. [CrossRef] [PubMed]
57. Jia, H.M.; Huang, L.F.; Zheng, Y.; Li, W.X. Diagnostic value of urinary tissue inhibitor of metalloproteinase-2 and insulin-like growth factor binding protein 7 for acute kidney injury: A meta-analysis. *Crit. Care* **2017**, *21*, 77. [CrossRef] [PubMed]
58. Hemdahl, A.L.; Gabrielsen, A.; Zhu, C.; Eriksson, P.; Hedin, U.; Kastrup, J.; Thorén, P.; Hansson, G.K. Expression of neutrophil gelatinase-associated lipocalin in atherosclerosis and myocardial infarction. *Arterioscler. Thromb. Vasc. Biol.* **2006**, *26*, 136–142. [CrossRef] [PubMed]
59. Elmedany, S.M.; Naga, S.S.; Elsharkawy, R.; Mahrous, R.S.; Elnaggar, A.I. Novel urinary biomarkers and the early detection of acute kidney injury after open cardiac surgeries. *J. Crit. Care* **2017**, *40*, 171–177. [CrossRef] [PubMed]
60. Ghatanatti, R.; Teli, A.; Tirkey, S.S.; Bhattacharya, S.; Sengupta, G.; Mondal, A. Role of renal biomarkers as predictors of acute kidney injury in cardiac surgery. *Asian Cardiovasc. Thorac. Ann.* **2014**, *22*, 234–241. [CrossRef] [PubMed]
61. Buddenkotte, J.; Steinhoff, M. Recent advances in understanding and managing. *F1000 Res.* **2018**, *7*, 1–10. [CrossRef] [PubMed]
62. Petcharunpaisan, S. Arterial spin labeling in neuroimaging. *World J. Radiol.* **2010**, *2*, 384–398. [CrossRef] [PubMed]
63. Nery, F.; Gordon, I.; Thomas, D. Non-Invasive Renal Perfusion Imaging Using Arterial Spin Labeling MRI: Challenges and Opportunities. *Diagnostics (Basel)* **2018**, *8*, 2. [CrossRef] [PubMed]
64. Odudu, A.; Nery, F.; Harteveld, A.A.; Evans, R.G.; Pendse, D.; Buchanan, C.E.; Francis, S.T.; Fernández-Seara, M.A. Arterial spin labelling MRI to measure renal perfusion: a systematic review and statement paper. *Nephrol. Dial. Transplant.* **2018**, *33*, ii15–ii21. [CrossRef] [PubMed]
65. O'Neal, J.B.; Shaw, A.D.; Billings, F.T. Acute kidney injury following cardiac surgery: Current understanding and future directions. *Crit. Care* **2016**, *20*, 187. [CrossRef] [PubMed]
66. Hueper, K.; Gueler, F.; Bräsen, J.H.; Gutberlet, M.; Jang, M.S.; Lehner, F.; Richter, N.; Hanke, N.; Peperhove, M.; Martirosian, P.; et al. Functional MRI detects perfusion impairment in renal allografts with delayed graft function. *Am. J. Physiol. Ren. Physiol.* **2015**, *308*, F1444–F1451. [CrossRef] [PubMed]
67. Hueper, K.; Gutberlet, M.; Rong, S.; Hartung, D.; Mengel, M.; Lu, X.; Haller, H.; Wacker, F.; Meier, M.; Gueler, F. Acute Kidney Injury: Arterial Spin Labeling to Monitor Renal Perfusion Impairment in Mice-Comparison with Histopathologic Results and Renal Function. *Radiology* **2014**, *270*, 117–124. [CrossRef] [PubMed]
68. Prasad, P.V.; Priatna, A.; Spokes, K.; Epstein, F.H. Changes in intrarenal oxygenation as evaluated by BOLD MRI in a rat kidney model for radiocontrast nephropathy. *J. Magn. Reson. Imaging* **2001**, *13*, 744–747. [CrossRef] [PubMed]
69. Pruijm, M.; Mendichovszky, I.A.; Liss, P.; Van der Niepen, P.; Textor, S.C.; Lerman, L.O.; Krediet, C.T.P.; Caroli, A.; Burnier, M.; Prasad, P.V. Renal blood oxygenation level-dependent magnetic resonance imaging to measure renal tissue oxygenation: a statement paper and systematic review. *Nephrol. Dial. Transplant.* **2018**, *33*, ii22–ii28. [CrossRef] [PubMed]
70. Prasad, P.V.; Edelman, R.R.; Epstein, F.H. Noninvasive evaluation of intrarenal oxygenation with BOLD MRI. *Circulation* **1996**, *94*, 3271–3275. [CrossRef] [PubMed]
71. Prasad, P.V.; Chen, Q.; Goldfarb, J.W.; Epstein, F.H.; Edelman, R.R. Breath-hold R2 mapping with a multiple gradient-recalled echo sequence: Application to the evaluation of intrarenal oxygenation. *J. Magn. Reson. Imaging* **1997**, *7*, 1163–1165. [CrossRef] [PubMed]
72. Textor, S.C.; Glockner, J.F.; Lerman, L.O.; Misra, S.; McKusick, M.A.; Riederer, S.J.; Grande, J.P.; Gomez, S.I.; Romero, J.C. The Use of Magnetic Resonance to Evaluate Tissue Oxygenation in Renal Artery Stenosis. *J. Am. Soc. Nephrol.* **2008**, *19*, 780–788. [CrossRef] [PubMed]
73. Zhang, J.L.; Morrell, G.; Rusinek, H.; Sigmund, E.E.; Chandarana, H.; Lerman, L.O.; Prasad, P.V.; Niles, D.; Artz, N.; Fain, S.; et al. New magnetic resonance imaging methods in nephrology. *Kidney Int.* **2014**, *85*, 768–778. [CrossRef] [PubMed]

74. Bokacheva, L.; Rusinek, H.; Chen, Q.; Oesingmann, N.; Prince, C.; Kaur, M.; Kramer, E.; Lee, V.S. Quantitative determination of Gd-DTPA concentration in T1-weighted MR renography studies. *Magn. Reson. Med.* **2007**, *57*, 1012–1018. [CrossRef] [PubMed]
75. Bokacheva, L.; Rusinek, H.; Zhang, J.L.; Chen, Q.; Lee, V.S. Estimates of glomerular filtration rate from MR renography and tracer kinetic models. *J. Magn. Reson. Imaging* **2009**, *29*, 371–382. [CrossRef] [PubMed]
76. Milman, Z.; Heyman, S.N.; Corchia, N.; Edrei, Y.; Axelrod, J.H.; Rosenberger, C.; Tsarfati, G.; Abramovitch, R. Hemodynamic response magnetic resonance imaging: Application for renal hemodynamic characterization. *Nephrol. Dial. Transplant.* **2013**, *28*, 1150–1156. [CrossRef] [PubMed]
77. Milman, Z.; Axelrod, J.H.; Heyman, S.N.; Nachmansson, N.; Abramovitch, R. Assessment with unenhanced MRI techniques of renal morphology and hemodynamic changes during acute kidney injury and chronic kidney disease in mice. *Am. J. Nephrol.* **2014**, *39*, 268–278. [CrossRef] [PubMed]
78. Maril, N.; Margalit, R.; Rosen, S.; Heyman, S.N.; Degani, H. Detection of evolving acute tubular necrosis with renal 23Na MRI: Studies in rats. *Kidney Int.* **2006**, *69*, 765–768. [CrossRef] [PubMed]
79. Kleeman, C.R.; Maxwell, M.H.; Witlin, S. Functional isosthenuria; an isolated reversible renal tubular defect. *AMA Arch. Intern. Med.* **1958**, *101*, 1023–1028. [CrossRef] [PubMed]
80. Zhu, M.Z.L.; Martin, A.; Cochrane, A.D.; Smith, J.A.; Thrift, A.G.; Harrop, G.K.; Ngo, J.P.; Evans, R.G. Urinary hypoxia: an intraoperative marker of risk of cardiac surgery-associated acute kidney injury. *Nephrol Dial Transplant.* **2018**, *33*, 2191–2201. [CrossRef] [PubMed]
81. Reshef, A.; Shirvan, A.; Akselrod-Ballin, A.; Wall, A.; Ziv, I. Small-Molecule Biomarkers for Clinical PET Imaging of Apoptosis. *J. Nucl. Med.* **2010**, *51*, 837–840. [CrossRef] [PubMed]
82. Damianovich, M.; Ziv, I.; Heyman, S.N.; Rosen, S.; Shina, A.; Kidron, D.; Aloya, T.; Grimberg, H.; Levin, G.; Reshef, A.; et al. *ApoSense*: A novel technology for functional molecular imaging of cell death in models of acute renal tubular necrosis. *Eur. J. Nucl. Med. Mol. Imaging* **2006**, *33*, 281–291. [CrossRef] [PubMed]
83. Correas, J.M.; Anglicheau, D.; Joly, D.; Gennisson, J.L.; Tanter, M.; Hélénon, O. Ultrasound-based imaging methods of the kidney-recent developments. *Kidney Int.* **2016**, *90*, 1199–1210. [CrossRef] [PubMed]
84. Solomon, R.; Werner, C.; Mann, D.; D'Elia, J.; Silva, P. Effects of Saline, Mannitol, and Furosemide on Acute Decreases in Renal Function Induced by Radiocontrast Agents. *N. Engl. J. Med.* **1994**, *331*, 1416–1420. [CrossRef] [PubMed]
85. Weinstein, J.M.; Heyman, S.; Brezis, M. Potential deleterious effect of furosemide in radiocontrast nephropathy. *Nephron* **1992**, *62*, 413–415. [CrossRef] [PubMed]
86. Heyman, S.N.; Brezis, M.; Greenfeld, Z.; Rosen, S. Protective Role of Furosemide and Saline in Radiocontrast-Induced Acute Renal Failure in the Rat. *Am. J. Kidney Dis.* **1989**, *14*, 377–385. [CrossRef]
87. Briguori, C.; Visconti, G.; Focaccio, A.; Airoldi, F.; Valgimigli, M.; Sangiorgi, G.M.; Golia, B.; Ricciardelli, B.; Condorelli, G. Renal Insufficiency After Contrast Media Administration Trial II (REMEDIAL II). *Circulation* **2011**, *124*, 1260–1269. [CrossRef] [PubMed]
88. Goldfarb, M.; Rosenberger, C.; Abassi, Z.; Shina, A.; Zilbersat, F.; Eckardt, K.U.; Rosen, S.; Heyman, S.N. Acute-on-chronic renal failure in the rat: Functional compensation and hypoxia tolerance. *Am. J. Nephrol.* **2006**, *26*, 22–33. [CrossRef] [PubMed]
89. Rosenberger, C.; Heyman, S.N.; Rosen, S.; Shina, A.; Goldfarb, M.; Griethe, W.; Frei, U.; Reinke, P.; Bachmann, S.; Eckardt, K.U. Up-regulation of HIF in experimental acute renal failure: Evidence for a protective transcriptional response to hypoxia. *Kidney Int.* **2005**, *67*, 531–542. [CrossRef] [PubMed]

# Permissions

All chapters in this book were first published by MDPI; hereby published with permission under the Creative Commons Attribution License or equivalent. Every chapter published in this book has been scrutinized by our experts. Their significance has been extensively debated. The topics covered herein carry significant findings which will fuel the growth of the discipline. They may even be implemented as practical applications or may be referred to as a beginning point for another development.

The contributors of this book come from diverse backgrounds, making this book a truly international effort. This book will bring forth new frontiers with its revolutionizing research information and detailed analysis of the nascent developments around the world.

We would like to thank all the contributing authors for lending their expertise to make the book truly unique. They have played a crucial role in the development of this book. Without their invaluable contributions this book wouldn't have been possible. They have made vital efforts to compile up to date information on the varied aspects of this subject to make this book a valuable addition to the collection of many professionals and students.

This book was conceptualized with the vision of imparting up-to-date information and advanced data in this field. To ensure the same, a matchless editorial board was set up. Every individual on the board went through rigorous rounds of assessment to prove their worth. After which they invested a large part of their time researching and compiling the most relevant data for our readers.

The editorial board has been involved in producing this book since its inception. They have spent rigorous hours researching and exploring the diverse topics which have resulted in the successful publishing of this book. They have passed on their knowledge of decades through this book. To expedite this challenging task, the publisher supported the team at every step. A small team of assistant editors was also appointed to further simplify the editing procedure and attain best results for the readers.

Apart from the editorial board, the designing team has also invested a significant amount of their time in understanding the subject and creating the most relevant covers. They scrutinized every image to scout for the most suitable representation of the subject and create an appropriate cover for the book.

The publishing team has been an ardent support to the editorial, designing and production team. Their endless efforts to recruit the best for this project, has resulted in the accomplishment of this book. They are a veteran in the field of academics and their pool of knowledge is as vast as their experience in printing. Their expertise and guidance has proved useful at every step. Their uncompromising quality standards have made this book an exceptional effort. Their encouragement from time to time has been an inspiration for everyone.

The publisher and the editorial board hope that this book will prove to be a valuable piece of knowledge for researchers, students, practitioners and scholars across the globe.

# List of Contributors

**Caterina Savriè**
Faculty of Medicine, Surgery and Prevention, University of Ferrara, via Ludovico Ariosto 35, 44121 Ferrara, Italy

**Alfredo De Giorgi, Emanuele Di Simone, Benedetta Boari, Alda Storari and Massimo Gallerani**
Azienda Ospedaliero-Universitaria 'S. Anna', Via Aldo Moro 8, 44123 Cona, Ferrara, Italy

**Fabio Fabbian, Rosaria Cappadona and Roberto Manfredini**
Faculty of Medicine, Surgery and Prevention, University of Ferrara, via Ludovico Ariosto 35, 44121 Ferrara, Italy
Azienda Ospedaliero-Universitaria 'S. Anna', Via Aldo Moro 8, 44123 Cona, Ferrara, Italy

**Ha-Jung Kim, Hee-Sun Park, Yon-Ji Go, Won Uk Koh, Hyungtae Kim, Jun-Gol Song and Young-Jin Ro**
Department of Anesthesiology and Pain Medicine, Asan Medical Center, University of Ulsan, College of Medicine, Seoul 05505, Korea

**Domenico De Rasmo and Anna Ferretta**
Institute of Biomembranes, Bioenergetics and Molecular Biotechnology (IBIOM), National Research Council (CNR), 70124 Bari, Italy

**Anna Signorile and Silvia Russo**
Department of Basic Medical Sciences, Neurosciences and Sense Organs, University of Bari "Aldo Moro", 70124 Bari, Italy

**Ester De Leo, Roberto Raso and Francesco Bellomo**
Renal Diseases Research Unit, Genetics and Rare Diseases Research Division, Bambino Gesù Children's Hospital—IRCCS, 00146 Rome, Italy

**Francesco Emma**
Division of Nephrology, Department of Pediatric Subspecialties, Bambino Gesù Children's Hospital—IRCCS, 00165 Rome, Italy

**Vin-Cent Wu**
Division of Nephrology, National Taiwan University Hospital, No. 7 Chung-Shan South Road, Zhong-Zheng District, Taipei 100, Taiwan
Department of Internal Medicine, National Taiwan University Hospital, Taipei 100, Taiwan
NSARF, National Taiwan University Study Group on Acute Renal Failure, Taiwan

**Elena V. Polishchuk and Roman Polishchuk**
Telethon Institute of Genetics and Medicine, 80078 Pozzuoli, Italy

**Shih-Chieh Jeff Chueh**
Glickman Urological and Kidney Institute, Cleveland Clinic Lerner College of Medicine, Cleveland Clinic, Cleveland, 9500 Euclid Ave., Cleveland, OH 44195, USA

**Jui-Ting Chang**
Division of Nephrology, Department of Internal Medicine, Shin Kong Memorial Wu Ho-Su Hospital, Taipei 111, Taiwan

**Bang-Gee Hsu**
Division of Nephrology, Hualien Tzu Chi Hospital, Buddhist Tzu Chi Medical Foundation; and School of Medicine, Tzu Chi University, Hualien 970, Taiwan

**Marlies Ostermann**
Department of Critical Care and Nephrology, King's College London, Guy's and St Thomas Hospital, London SE1 7EH, UK

**Tzong-Shinn Chu**
Division of Nephrology, National Taiwan University Hospital, No. 7 Chung-Shan South Road, Zhong-Zheng District, Taipei 100, Taiwan
NSARF group (National Taiwan University Hospital Study Group of ARF), Zhong-Zheng District, Taipei 100, Taiwan
CAKS group (Taiwan Consortium for Acute Kidney Injury and Renal Diseases), Guishan District, Taoyuan City 333, Taiwan

**Che-Hsiung Wu**
Division of Nephrology, Taipei Tzu Chi Hospital, Buddhist Tzu Chi Medical Foundation, New Taipei City 231, Taiwan
School of Medicine, Tzu Chi University, Hualien 970, Taiwan

**Huang-Ming Chang and Hao-Chien Wang**
Department of Internal Medicine, National Taiwan University Hospital, Taipei 100, Taiwan

**Cheng-Yi Wang**
Department of Internal Medicine, College of Medicine, Fu Jen Catholic University, New Taipei City 242, Taiwan

**Likwang Chen**
Institute of Population Health Sciences, National Health Research Institutes, Zhunan 350, Taiwan

**Liang-Wen Chen, Chien-Heng Lai and Shuenn-Wen Kuo**
Department of Surgery, National Taiwan University Hospital, National Taiwan University, Taipei 100, Taiwan

**Ying-Ying Chen**
Division of Nephrology, Department of Internal Medicine, MacKay Memorial Hospital, No. 92, Sec. 2, Zhongshan North Road, Taipei 10449, Taiwan
Graduate Institute of Clinical Medicine, College of Medicine, National Taiwan University, No.7. Chung San South Road, Taipei 10002, Taiwan

**Kwan-Dun Wu**
Division of Nephrology, Department of Internal Medicine, National Taiwan University Hospital, No.7. Chung San South Road, Taipei 10002, Taiwan

**Wei-Chieh Huang**
Division of Cardiology, Department of Internal Medicine, Taipei Veterans General Hospital, No.201, Sec. 2, Shipai Road, Taipei 11217, Taiwan

**Yu-Chang Yeh**
Department of Anesthesiology, National Taiwan University Hospital, No.7. Chung San South Road, Taipei 10002, Taiwan

**Mai-Szu Wu**
Division of Nephrology, Department of Internal Medicine, Taipei Medical University-Shuang Ho Hospital, No.291, Zhongzheng Road, Zhonghe District, New Taipei City 23561, Taiwan

**Chiu-Ching Huang**
Division of Nephrology, Department of Internal Medicine, China Medical University Hospital, No. 2, Yude Road, North District, Taichung 40447, Taiwan

**Ji-Tseng Fang**
Chang Gung University College of Medicine, Taoyuan, Taiwan; Kidney Research Center, Department of Nephrology, Chang Gung Memorial Hospital, 5. Fu-Hsing Street, Kuei Shan Hsiang, Taoyuan City 333, Taiwan

**Wei-Chih Kan**
Division of Nephrology, Department of Internal medicine, Chi Mei Medical Center, Yongkang District, Tainan City 710, Taiwan
Department of Biological Science and Technology, Chung Hwa University of Medical Technology, Rende District, Tainan City 717, Taiwan

**Chih-Jen Wu**
Division of Nephrology, Department of Internal Medicine, MacKay Memorial Hospital, No. 92, Sec. 2, Zhongshan North Road, Taipei 10449, Taiwan
Department of Medicine, Mackay Medical College, No.46, Sec. 3, Zhongzheng Road, Sanzhi District, New Taipei City 252, Taiwan
Graduate Institute of Medical Sciences and Department of Pharmacology, School of Medicine, College of Medicine, Taipei Medical University, 250 Wuxing St., Taipei 11031, Taiwan
Department of Medical Research, China Medical University Hospital, China Medical University, No.91, Hsueh-Shih Road, Taichung 40402, Taiwan
Mackay Junior College of Medicine, Nursing and Management, No.92, Shengjing Road, Taipei 11260, Taiwan

**Maurizio Bruschi and Giovanni Candiano**
Laboratory of Molecular Nephrology, IRCCS Istituto Giannina Gaslini, 16147 Genova, Italy

**Simona Granata, Antonia Fabris, Giovanni Gambaro and Gianluigi Zaza**
Renal Unit, Department of Medicine, University/Hospital of Verona, Piazzale A. Stefani 1, 37126 Verona, Italy

**Andrea Petretto**
Laboratory of Mass Spectrometry—Core Facilities, IRCCS Istituto Giannina Gaslini, 16147 Genova, Italy

**Gian Marco Ghiggeri**
Division of Nephrology, Dialysis and Transplantation, IRCCS Istituto Giannina Gaslini, 16147 Genova, Italy

**Chih-Chung Shiao**
Division of Nephrology, Department of Internal Medicine, Saint Mary's Hospital Luodong, Loudong 265, Yilan, Taiwan
Saint Mary's Junior College of Medicine, Nursing and Management, Sanxing Township, Yilan County 266, Taiwan

**Jian-Jhong Wang**
Division of Nephrology, Department of Internal Medicine, Chi Mei Medical Center, Liouying, Tainan City 736, Taiwan

**Yu-Feng Lin**
Graduate Institute of Clinical Medicine, National Taiwan University College of Medicine, Taipei 106, Taiwan
Division of Nephrology, Department of Internal Medicine, National Taiwan University Hospital, Taipei 100, Taiwan
Division of Hospital Medicine, Department of Internal Medicine, National Taiwan University Hospital, Taipei 100, Taiwan

**Eric Chueh**
Case Western Reserve University, No. 10900 Euclid Ave., Cleveland, OH 44106, USA

**Ya-Ting Huang**
Department of Nursing, Saint Mary's Hospital Luodong, Loudong 265, Yilan, Taiwan

**Wen-Po Chiang, Li-Jung Tseng and Chih-Hsien Wang**
Department of Surgery, National Taiwan University Hospital, Taipei 100, Taiwan

**Hyung-Chul Lee and Leerang Lim**
Department of Anesthesiology and Pain Medicine, Seoul National University Hospital, Seoul 03080, Korea

**Won Ho Kim, Ho-Geol Ryu and Chul-Woo Jung**
Department of Anesthesiology and Pain Medicine, Seoul National University Hospital, Seoul 03080, Korea
Department of Anesthesiology and Pain Medicine, Seoul National University College of Medicine, Seoul 03080, Korea

**Ho-Jin Lee, Jinyoung Bae, Yongsuk Kwon, Hwan Suk Jang, Seokha Yoo, Jin-Tae Kim and Won Ho Kim**
Department of Anesthesiology and Pain Medicine, Seoul National University Hospital, Seoul National University College of Medicine, Seoul 03080, Korea

**Chang Wook Jeong**
Department of Urology, Seoul National University Hospital, Seoul National University College of Medicine, Seoul 03080, Korea

**Eleftherios Papadakis, Alexandra Papaioannou and Helen Askitopoulou**
Departments of Anaesthesiology, University Hospital of Heraklion, 71110 Crete, Greece

**Diamantina Marouli**
Departments of Anaesthesiology, University Hospital of Heraklion, 71110 Crete, Greece
Intensive Care, University Hospital of Heraklion, 71110 Crete, Greece

**Dimitris Georgopoulos**
Intensive Care, University Hospital of Heraklion, 71110 Crete, Greece

**Kostas Stylianou, Nikolaos Kroustalakis and Eugene Daphnis**
Nephrology, University Hospital of Heraklion, 71110 Crete, Greece

**Stavroula Kolyvaki**
Clinical Biochemistry, University Hospital of Heraklion, 71110 Crete, Greece

**Georgios Papadopoulos and Christos Ioannou**
Vascular Surgery, University Hospital of Heraklion, 71110 Crete, Greece

**Michele Rossini**
Department of Emergency and Organ Transplantation, Renal Unit, University of Bari, 70124 Bari, Italy

**Francesco Paolo Schena**
Department of Emergency and Organ Transplantation, Renal Unit, University of Bari, 70124 Bari, Italy
Schena Foundation, European Center for the Study of Renal Diseases, 70010 Valenzano, Italy

**Pasquale Esposito**
Department of Internal Medicine, Division of Nephrology, Dialysis and Transplantation, University of Genoa and IRCCS Ospedale Policlinico San Martino, 16132 Genova, Italy

**Victor Ortiz-Soriano, Katherine Donaldson, Mark Rudy and Javier A. Neyra**
Division of Nephrology, Bone and Mineral Metabolism, Department of Internal Medicine, University of Kentucky Medical Center, Lexington, KY 40506, USA

**Dan Cleland and Gaixin Du**
Center for Health Services Research, University of Kentucky, Lexington, KY 40506, USA

**Joshua Lambert and Ye Li**
Department of Statistics, University of Kentucky, Lexington, KY 40506, USA

**Alice Thornton and Laura C. Fanucchi**
Division of Infectious Diseases, Department of Internal Medicine, University of Kentucky Medical Center, Lexington, KY 40506, USA

**Moises A. Huaman**
Division of Infectious Diseases, Department of Internal Medicine, University of Kentucky Medical Center, Lexington, KY 40506, USA
Division of Infectious Diseases, Department of Internal Medicine, University of Cincinnati, Cincinnati, OH 45221, USA

**Christina Fitzner, Tatjana Levkovich, Michael Sobotta, Jil Vieten, Gernot Marx and Christian Stoppe**
Department of Intensive Care Medicine, RWTH Aachen University Hospital, 52074 Aachen, Germany

**Luisa Averdunk**
Department of Intensive Care Medicine, RWTH Aachen University Hospital, 52074 Aachen, Germany
Institute of Human Genetics, Medical Faculty, Heinrich Heine University, 40225 Düsseldorf, Germany

**David E. Leaf**
Division of Renal Medicine, Brigham and Women's Hospital, Boston, MA 02115, USA
Department of Medicine, Harvard Medical School, Boston, MA 02115, USA

**Akinobu Ochi and Gilbert Moeckel**
Department of Nephropathology, Yale University School of Medicine, New Haven, CT 06510, USA

**Emmanuel Letavernier, Elise Bouderlique, Jeremy Zaworski and Michel Daudon**
UMR S 1155 and Physiology Unit, AP-HP, Hôpital Tenon, Sorbonne Université and INSERM, F-75020 Paris, France

**Ludovic Martin**
PXE Consultation Center, MAGEC Reference Center for Rare Skin Diseases, Angers University Hospital, MITOVASC Institute, UMR CNRS 6015 INSERM U1083 Angers University, 49000 Angers, France

**Charat Thongprayoon and Michael A. Mao**
Division of Nephrology and Hypertension, Mayo Clinic, Rochester, MN 55905, USA

**Wisit Kaewput**
Department of Military and Community Medicine, Phramongkutklao College of Medicine, Bangkok 10400, Thailand

**Natanong Thamcharoen**
Division of Nephrology, Beth Israel Deaconess Medical Center, Harvard Medical School, Boston, MA 02215, USA

**Tarun Bathini**
Department of Internal Medicine, University of Arizona, Tucson, AZ 85721, USA

**Kanramon Watthanasuntorn and Ploypin Lertjitbanjong**
Department of Internal Medicine, Bassett Medical Center, Cooperstown, NY 13326, USA

**Sohail Abdul Salim, Wisit Cheungpasitporn and Aldo Torres-Ortiz**
Division of Nephrology, Department of Medicine, University of Mississippi Medical Center, Jackson, MS 39216, USA

**Narothama Reddy Aeddula**
Division of Nephrology, Department of Medicine, Deaconess Health System, Evansville, IN 47747, USA

**Patompong Ungprasert**
Clinical Epidemiology Unit, Department of Research and Development, Faculty of Medicine, Siriraj Hospital, Mahidol University, Bangkok 10700, Thailand

**Zaid Abassi**
Department of Physiology, Ruth & Bruce Rappaport Faculty of Medicine, Technion-IIT, Haifa 31096, Israel
Department of Laboratory Medicine, Rambam Health Care Campus, Haifa 31096, Israel

**Seymour Rosen and Simon Lamothe**
Department of Pathology, Beth Israel Deaconess Medical Center and Harvard Medical School, Boston, MA 02215, USA

**Samuel N. Heyman**
Department of Medicine, Hadassah Hebrew University Hospital, Mt. Scopus, Jerusalem 91240, Israel

# Index

## N



## O



## P



## R



## S



## T



## U



## V

www.ingramcontent.com/pod-product-compliance
Lightning Source LLC
LaVergne TN
LVHW081039210926
848485LV00004B/1061